Introduction to
CARE COORDINATION
and NURSING
MANAGEMENT

Laura J. Fero, PhD, MSN, RN
Assistant Professor
University of North Carolina at Greensboro
School of Nursing
Greensboro, North Carolina

Charlotte A. Herrick, PhD, RN
Professor Emerita
University of North Carolina at Greensboro
School of Nursing
Greensboro, North Carolina

Jie Hu, PhD, RN
Associate Professor
University of North Carolina at Greensboro
School of Nursing
Greensboro, North Carolina

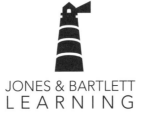

JONES & BARTLETT
LEARNING

World Headquarters

Jones & Bartlett Learning
40 Tall Pine Drive
Sudbury, MA 01776
978-443-5000
info@jblearning.com
www.jblearning.com

Jones & Bartlett Learning
Canada
6339 Ormindale Way
Mississauga, Ontario L5V 1J2
Canada

Jones & Bartlett Learning
International
Barb House, Barb Mews
London W6 7PA
United Kingdom

Jones & Bartlett Learning books and products are available through most bookstores and online booksellers. To contact Jones & Bartlett Learning directly, call 800-832-0034, fax 978-443-8000, or visit our website, www.jblearning.com.

Substantial discounts on bulk quantities of Jones & Bartlett Learning publications are available to corporations, professional associations, and other qualified organizations. For details and specific discount information, contact the special sales department at Jones & Bartlett Learning via the above contact information or send an email to specialsales@jblearning.com.

The authors, editor, and publisher have made every effort to provide accurate information. However, they are not responsible for errors, omissions, or for any outcomes related to the use of the contents of this book and take no responsibility for the use of the products and procedures described. Treatments and side effects described in this book may not be applicable to all people; likewise, some people may require a dose or experience a side effect that is not described herein. Drugs and medical devices are discussed that may have limited availability controlled by the Food and Drug Administration (FDA) for use only in a research study or clinical trial. Research, clinical practice, and government regulations often change the accepted standard in this field. When consideration is being given to use of any drug in the clinical setting, the health care provider or reader is responsible for determining FDA status of the drug, reading the package insert, and reviewing prescribing information for the most up-to-date recommendations on dose, precautions, and contraindications, and determining the appropriate usage for the product. This is especially important in the case of drugs that are new or seldom used.

Production Credits

Publisher: Kevin Sullivan
Acquisitions Editor: Amy Sibley
Associate Editor: Patricia Donnelly
Editorial Assistant: Rachel Shuster
Associate Production Editor: Katie Spiegel
Marketing Manager: Rebecca Wasley
V.P., Manufacturing and Inventory Control: Therese Connell
Composition: Toppan Best-set Premedia Limited
Cover Design: Scott Moden
Cover Image: © Georgy Shafeev/ShutterStock, Inc.
Printing and Binding: Malloy, Inc.
Cover Printing: Malloy, Inc.

Library of Congress Cataloging-in-Publication Data
Fero, Laura J.
   Introduction to care coordination and nursing management / Laura J. Fero, Charlotte A. Herrick, Jie Hu.
       p. ; cm.
   Includes bibliographical references and index.
   ISBN 978–0-7637–7160–7 (pbk.)
   1. Nursing care plans.   2. Hospitals–Care management services.   I. Herrick, Charlotte A. (Charlotte Anne), 1933–   II. Hu, Jie, Ph. D.   III. Title.
   [DNLM: 1. Nursing Care.   2. Case Management.   3. Models, Nursing. WY 100 F367i 2011]
   RT49.F47 2011
   610.73—dc22

                                                                        2010017553
6048

Printed in the United States of America
14 13 12 11 10   10 9 8 7 6 5 4 3 2 1

Dedication

The authors of this book dedicate it to patients with complex health issues, who are either chronically or acutely ill and who need a care coordinator (case manager) to facilitate and integrate care across the health continuum. We also dedicate this book to the nurses, social workers, and other healthcare professionals who function as collaborators, to the care coordinators, and to the patient advocates, who ensure that patients and families are knowledgeable about their therapeutic options and can exercise their right to self-determination.

Contents

1   Introduction to Nursing Case Management   1

2   Cultural Competence   43

3   Managed Care: Examining Today's Healthcare System   67

As nursing case management has evolved as a healthcare discipline; as health care has become more complex and fragmented; and as outcomes-oriented care has become more important, a new role for nurses has gained prominence in hospitals and community health centers. The development of this role—that of the nurse case manager—actually preceded the inclusion of educational content about this role in schools of nursing. Many of the case managers now working in various healthcare settings were previously clinical nurse specialists. Other case managers are nurses who received their education through associate's degree in nursing (ADN) or bachelor of science in nursing (BSN) programs.

Few nurses have received any education geared specifically toward nursing case management and, until the last few years, many students knew nothing about the role. On the first day of class, when I asked students what they thought a nurse case manager did, they answered, "Case managers walk around in white lab coats looking at charts." But they really did not know anything about the role. When I first started attending the Case Management Society of America (CMSA) meetings, there were fewer than 10 people in attendance. Ten years later, I have seen as many as 70 attendees at the same meetings. Clearly, nursing case management is a rapidly growing professional role.

Our purpose in developing a course in case management/care coordination was to expose future nurse administrators to the benefits of a case management nursing service. On numerous occasions during fiscally tight periods, case management services have been deleted. However, through experience and education, nurse managers and administrators have found that when case management services are cut out of the budget, lengths of stay for patients tend to increase, and medical and nursing services become fragmented or resources are duplicated. Ultimately, these trends cost the hospital, the healthcare agency, or the third-party payers more money than was saved by eliminating the case management function. Coordinated transitions from one level of care to the next are smoother when the transition is planned and coordinated by a nurse case manager, as the quality of care is maintained throughout this process.

The nurse case managers/care coordinators who are our students' preceptors have often recruited those nursing students to their case management services once they have graduated. We do not claim to prepare students specifically for the role of case manager/care coordinator or for the certification exam, however. Instead, our goal is to ensure the ongoing viability of case management programs in healthcare agencies through the supportive endeavors of nursing administrators/managers.

There was long (and in some cases still is) a paucity of information in schools of nursing that is focused on case management. At the time when we developed our course, for example, few textbooks on case management were available for use as resources. As the profession has grown to include disease management, we have required students to buy two textbooks and recommended others that focus on both case management/care coordination and disease management. To supplement the material in those books, we developed learning modules to address the topics to which students were exposed in their clinical settings. After receiving feedback from the students about the learning modules for a period of 2 years, we wrote this text based on the learning modules and taking into consideration the students' comments. It is our hope that students and faculty, as well as working nurse case managers, will find this textbook useful. It describes the traditional and developing roles in nursing case management, both "within the walls" and beyond them.

Chapters 1 through 4 of this book address the historical development of nursing case management/care coordination, the cultural issues involved with coordinating care for a culturally diverse population, and the development of the various case management roles during the advent of managed care. Chapters 5 and 6 then address the skills necessary to carry out the roles and the various models that have been developed to guide the roles across the healthcare continuum. Chapters 7 through 9 address the case manager in private practice either as a consultant or an entrepreneur, as well as the avenues through which to market these services. Developments in case management such as faith community nursing (congregational nursing), telehealth case management, and disease management are discussed in Chapters 10 through 12. Chapter 13 addresses outcomes management, which is an important aspect of case management/care coordination in today's evolving healthcare marketplace.

We consider the final two chapters (Chapters 14 and 15) to be "umbrella chapters," in the sense that the topics covered here affect all aspects of medicine, including nursing and case management. These chapters include the ethical and legal issues that govern decision making in health care.

Acknowledgments

From the editors of this book:

- To all of the contributors of the various book chapters, thank you for making this book a valuable one for current and future students of nursing case management and care coordination.
- To the members of the Piedmont Triad chapter of the Case Management Society of America and the local chapter of the American Case Management Association, for their continuing support of a course in nursing case management at the University of North Carolina at Greensboro, School of Nursing. Since the inception of this course, these organizations have provided lecturers and preceptors whose contributions have enriched the educational experiences of countless students. Thanks to their generosity, the students have received a broad overview of nursing case management/care coordination, "within the walls" care including hospital case management, psychiatric mental health nursing case management, and "beyond the walls" care including topics such as home health, hospice, geriatric care, employee health care, and faith community nursing (congregational nursing).

Laura J. Fero:

- To my family, who has provided me the love, encouragement, and support to continue moving forward in my career.
- To the healthcare organizations for which I had the privilege of working during my career as a case manager, the experience you provided allowed me to expand my knowledge base and truly understand the very complicated road of healthcare delivery.

Charlotte A. Herrick:

- To Bob Herrick, my husband, who has supported my various endeavors as a nurse, an academician, and an author, and to our children, whom I am proud to say have become successful professionals and parents.

- To Dr. Hazel Brown, who was my partner in developing the course in nursing case management (NCM) during the first year of teaching this course, and who has continued to support the NCM course as part of the master's program in nursing administration.

Jie Hu:

- To the memory of my parents, Hu Jianfei and Li Min.
- To Qi Xue, my husband, and Jiayin Xue, my daughter, for their support.
- To Dr. Charlotte A. Herrick, who has mentored me in teaching nursing case management.

Contributors

Sandra Blaha, MSN
Assistant Director, Faith Community Nursing
Moses Cone Health System
Greensboro, North Carolina

Jacqueline DeBrew, PhD, APRN, BC
Clinical Associate Professor
University of North Carolina at Greensboro
School of Nursing
Greensboro, North Carolina

Laura J. Fero, PhD, MSN, RN
Assistant Professor
University of North Carolina at Greensboro
School of Nursing
Greensboro, North Carolina

Charlotte A. Herrick, PhD, RN
Professor Emerita
University of North Carolina at Greensboro
School of Nursing
Greensboro, North Carolina

Jie Hu, PhD, RN
Associate Professor
University of North Carolina at Greensboro
School of Nursing
Greensboro, North Carolina

Jeanne B. Jenkins, MSN, RN, MBA
Graduate Student
University of North Carolina at Greensboro
School of Nursing
Greensboro, North Carolina

Leila Moore, BSN
Director, Faith Community Nursing
Moses Cone Health System
Greensboro, North Carolina

Introduction to Nursing Case Management

Laura J. Fero
Charlotte A. Herrick

1

■ OUTLINE

Introduction
Definitions of Case Management
Case Management: Its Process and Characteristics
Case Management Organizations: An Alphabet Soup
Managed Care
Case Management as a Process
Historical Perspectives and Current Trends
Maintaining Quality

■ OBJECTIVES

1. Be able to discuss case management in a managed care environment.
2. Have a basic knowledge of case management, including its process and characteristics.
3. Be able to discuss how case management evolved historically as a means for delivering nursing care and other healthcare services.
4. Have a basic knowledge of ways to maintain quality, including education, standards of practice, credentialing, and certification.
5. Be able to describe the benefit of multistate licensing.

DEFINITIONS OF CASE MANAGEMENT

The definition of **case management (CM)** varies depending on the discipline, setting, or model (Table 1-1). Kersbergen (1996) has stated that there is no clear definition of case management and that, in fact, cases are not managed but services are (cited in Herrick, 2008; Herrick & Bartlett, 2004). The lack of a clear definition or generally recognized parameters for CM has resulted in wide variations in models. However, even though definitions may vary along with the various settings and target populations, the definitions have certain identifiable characteristics, which overlap from definition to definition. These characteristics include collaboration, coordination, and the integration of the delivery

TABLE 1-1 Definitions of Case Management

- The **case manager** is the "catalyst" who sifts through possible paths, selects the best plan of care, and then coordinates the expertise and support of other professionals, family members, agencies, and suppliers (Mullahy, 2010, p. 9). Mullahy has called the case manager a "catalyst, problem solver, and educator" (p. 3), stating that the case manager is an "advocate for the patient, an empowering agent for the family, and a facilitator of communication among the patient, family, care providers and payers." She described the nurse case manager as the "sentinel for quality assurance and cost effectiveness" (p. 9).
- The Commission for Case Management Certification (CCMC, 2003) defined **case management (CM)** as a "collaborative process that assesses, plans, implements, coordinates, monitors and evaluates options and services to meet the individual's health care needs using communication and available resources to promote quality cost-effective outcomes" (CCMC, 2003; Mullahy, 2010, p. 11).
- The Case Management Society of America (CMSA) defined **case management** as a "collaborative process of assessment, planning, facilitation and advocacy for options and services to meet an individual's health care needs through communication and available resources to promote quality cost-effective outcomes" (Moreo & Lamb, 2003a, 2003b; cited in Mullahy, 2010, p. 11).
- **Case management** is a healthcare delivery system that places responsibility for planning, delivery, and coordination of services on a person (a **care coordinator** or **case manager**) or an **interdisciplinary CM team,** whose members work with the client and the family. The responsibilities of the **case manager** are to develop an appropriate plan to ensure access to needed services; to monitor the delivery of those services; to advocate for the client to meet his or her healthcare and other needs, such as psychosocial and educational needs; and to evaluate the outcomes (Bower, 1992; cited in Herrick, 2008).
- **Case management** represents a shift from traditional discipline-specific tasks to a more integrated outcomes-oriented approach, which has a holistic perspective, provided by an interdisciplinary partnership. There is no standardized job description for a case manager (Tahan, 1999; cited in Herrick, 2008).

of health care and other services, with the goal of achieving care that is both of high quality and cost-effective.

Communication, cultural competence, and collaboration are essential ingredients to working with the client and family, other healthcare providers, ancillary services, vendors, insurance companies, and employers.

CASE MANAGEMENT: ITS PROCESS AND CHARACTERISTICS

Table 1-2 identifies the characteristics that are found in case management, no matter which discipline, setting, or target population is involved. The disease manager's role characteristics are similar (see Table 1-3), although there are

TABLE 1-2 Characteristics of Case Management/Disease Management

Case management/disease management:
- Is both episode based and longitudinally based.
- Promotes a timely discharge.
- Facilitates the patient's care by ensuring that the patient and family have access to the right resources provided by the right healthcare providers at the right time.
- Is directed toward selected populations (usually those who are at risk for expensive treatments, who are prone to repeated emergency room visits, or who may be admitted to the hospital frequently and repeatedly within a short period of time.
- Is quality- and outcomes-driven.
- Works toward strengthening the cost–quality link for clients and healthcare institutions.
- Emphasizes collaboration among interdisciplinary team members to provide holistic care.
- Enhances the accessibility of services.
- Is proactive—the focus is on preventing problems and issues from developing into cyclical patterns.
- Encourages the development of care maps and critical pathways to monitor and document patient's progress and identify variances, which lead to unexpected outcomes.

Sources: Adapted from Bower, 1992; Cohen & Cesta, 2005; Herrick, 2008.

TABLE 1-3 The Roles of a Case Manager/Disease Manager

The case manager/disease manager:
- Is a **broker** who links patient needs with healthcare resources.
- Is a **communicator/educator,** sharing information with other healthcare professionals to better coordinate care, and providing information to patients and families to empower them for self-care.
- Is a **facilitator** who assists the patient in obtaining access to care and provides for smooth transitions from one level of care to another.
- Is the **coordinator of care,** with the goal to provide continuity across the healthcare continuum from primary care to long-term care.
- Is not necessarily a **direct care provider,** except in mental health (social workers/ therapists) or rural settings where healthcare providers must wear many hats.
- Is the **gatekeeper**—the steward of healthcare resources, who allocates resources cost-effectively to meet the patient's needs.
- Is an **advocate** for the patient and family, ensuring that they receive quality care.
- Is **accountable** for standards, use of resources, and outcomes.

some differences between the case manager and the disease manager. The disease manager usually has a long-term relationship with the patient rather than a time-limited relationship, and the target population of the disease manager typically includes chronically ill patients who are at high risk of readmission to an acute care facility. The focus of NCM is more often on the acute care patient.

Both CM and DM are family-oriented services. While many case managers work in acute care settings, others work in community settings providing worker's compensation services, in hospices, and in community clinics. Other case managers focus on the elderly. A few nurses work in child welfare, acting as a liaison between social work and public health agencies.

The Roles of a Case Manager/Disease Manager

Case managers provide care at four levels:

1. The case manager works with the client and family at the primary level.
2. Managers/leaders/administrators/directors of CM programs have responsibilities for personnel and outcomes management.
3. Consultants for CM systems advise other case managers and/or health-care providers, as well as insurance companies and other institutions.
4. Teachers of CM are found in academic settings or continuing education programs in hospitals and chronic care facilities. They educate future case managers or nursing leader/managers, or they provide continuing education for those already in practice—for example, either nurses, nurse case managers, or other healthcare providers, such as social workers.

The case manager's patients are front and center and are the focus of care. Patient and family-centered care builds on the patient's and the family's strengths and helps the patient and family to use their current resources to empower them toward self-care.

Continuity of care is another important value that must be coordinated by the case manager/disease manager and/or the CM interdisciplinary team. Interdisciplinary and interagency collaboration improves transitions from one level of care to another so as to maintain the quality of care and provide for continuity. Delivery of high-quality care in a cost-effective manner is the overall goal. Case managers are accountable both for their patients' progress and to the interdisciplinary team. In this model, clinical research has high value as part of evidence-based practice.

The nurse case manager is the patient's and the family's advocate. To fully represent patients and families from all backgrounds, the nurse case manager must continually strive to achieve cultural competence. If this professional is to successfully adapt his or her practice to the continual changes in nursing and medical care, he or she must be flexible and open to new paradigms for delivering services and must continue to stay up-to-date on new technologies.

The Philosophy of Case Management

According to the Case Management Society of America (CMSA), CM serves as a means for achieving the patient's wellness and autonomy through advocacy, communication, and education. The nurse case manager identifies needed services and resources. The case manager facilitates access to various services and coordinates these services to avoid fragmentation and duplication. The case manager helps to identify the appropriate providers and coordinates the care across the continuum of care, while ensuring that available resources are being used in a timely and cost-effective manner so as to provide the optimal value for both the client and the reimbursement sources. CM services are best offered in a climate that allows direct communication between the case manager, the client, and appropriate service personnel, thereby optimizing the outcomes for all parties.

CM is not a profession in itself, but rather an area of practice within a specific profession, most often social work or nursing (CCMC, 2003; CMSA, 2003). Table 1-4 lists the goals that CMSA has identified for the organization that represents nurses, social workers, and other professional healthcare providers.

TABLE 1-4 The Goals of Case Management, According to the Case Management Society of America (CMSA)

The goals of CM are to:
- Coordinate and integrate healthcare delivery for consistency and continuity of care to provide a seamless system of care.
- Maximize care in the appropriate setting or the least restrictive alternative (LRA).
- Facilitate access to services in a timely manner.
- Ensure quality of care, while containing costs by decreasing the length of stay (LOS).
- Be an effective steward and manage healthcare resources so as to optimize their use, which will help to maintain institutional financial stability.
- Empower patients and families for self-care, including improved compliance with medical regimens.
- Enhance the patient's and family's quality of life.
- Focus on prevention.
- Maintain or improve patient/family and provider satisfaction.
- Reduce variances that impede the patient's progress.
- Improve outcomes, such as LOS, costs, and quality, and reduce hospital recidivism.

Source: CMSA, 2003.

Other Characteristics of Case Management

Case management is *population based*. The focus is generally on a specific group of people or people who are in a specific setting, such as a hospital, a community mental health center, or a hospice, and who may have a similar disorder or have similar characteristics. For example, target populations may include the elderly, mentally ill and mentally retarded persons, children and adults with disabilities or chronic diseases, and children or families who are at risk for abuse.

Treatment settings may vary from inpatient/acute care to outpatient, community-based care; primary care clinics; and tertiary care treatment centers including rehabilitation facilities. These settings may focus on serving populations found in urban health centers, serving the poor or persons in rural home care settings, or serving farmers and their families. It should be noted that the *case manager.*

- Is the only healthcare professional who is fully involved with all stakeholders.
- Is the only professional to successfully navigate the entire health management sea.
- Is the only professional agent with the win-win potential for patients, providers, and payers because of the ongoing communication with all stakeholders.
- Is the only health professional to address issues of waste, abuse, and fraud, while preserving quality care and maximizing cost-efficiency (CMSA, 2003).

CASE MANAGEMENT ORGANIZATIONS: AN ALPHABET SOUP

More than 20 organizations have developed over time to address case management, disease management, and managed care issues in nursing practice. Many of these organizations have certifying, accreditation, and credentialing responsibilities, culminating in an "alphabet soup" of case management organizations (Lessard, 2007). Only a few of these organizations are listed in Table 1-5.

MANAGED CARE

Managed care (MC) is a system of healthcare delivery aimed at managing the cost and the quality of care as well as access to care (Mullahy, 2010). A managed care health plan is a combination of interdependent systems that

TABLE 1-5 An Alphabet Soup

- The **Case Management Society of America (CMSA)** represents case managers—mostly nurses and social workers—whose focus is on the community, rather than the acute care tertiary care setting. (www.cmsa.org)
- The **Disease Management Association of America (DMAA)** focuses on special populations with specific diseases, usually chronic conditions (Howe, 2005, p. xxiv). It serves as an advocacy group for those who are disease managers to educate the public about the important role that disease management programs play in improving the quality and outcomes for persons with chronic conditions (DMAA, cited in Huber, 2005). Most disease managers are nurses. (www.dmaa. org)
- The **National Social Work Association** serves case managers who are also social workers (BSW or MSW). It is an advocacy group for all social workers, regardless of where they work. Its orientation tends to focus more on the community case manager, but the organization also represents social workers who practice in hospitals and community agencies. (www.nswa.org)
- The **American Case Management Association (ACMA)** focuses more on hospital case management. Its membership consists of both nurses and social workers. Its goals are the achievement of optimal health, access to care, and appropriate utilization of resources, balanced with the patient's right to self-determination. (www.acmaweb.org)
- The **American Association of Managed Care Nurses** describes the nurse case manager as a person who wears many hats (Lessard, 2007). This organization represents case managers who work for the insurance industry or the managed care industry with the goal of assisting the nurse case manager to coordinate services for patients/members so as to provide the best quality of care available at the most reasonable cost to patients/members and their providers. The organization assists the nurse case manager in collaborating with other case managers in the hospital and the community. These nurse case managers usually work for a particular managed care network. (www.aamcn.org)
- The **American Association of Nurse Life Care Planners** is oriented toward catastrophic case management and life care planning for patients with a long-term illness or disability. (www.aanlcp.org)

include the financing and delivery of healthcare services. Managed care and case management are not interchangeable concepts. MC is a delivery system that focuses on cost containment, while CM is a process and is only one component of managed care. Today's CM grew out of the MC movement. MC utilizes the following elements:

- Arrangements with selected providers to furnish a comprehensive set of healthcare services to its members
- Explicit standards for the selection of healthcare providers
- Programs for ongoing quality assurance and utilization review

- Financial incentives for members to use providers and procedures associated with the plan

Managed care is used by several types of payers to improve the delivery of services and to contain costs (Mullahy, 2010).

- **Health maintenance organizations (HMOs)** serve well-defined populations of patients. An employer group usually enrolls its employees (the patients) in the HMO for a set period of time. This approach stands in contrast to the traditional **fee-for-service** arrangement, under which the physician serves an ill-defined population. With the latter approach, the patient seeks the services of the physician on a voluntary basis, rather than being assigned to a provider by the insurance company (i.e., by the HMO).
- **Preferred provider organizations (PPOs)** are a mixture of the traditional fee-for-service indemnity insurance plans and HMOs. PPOs comprise organized networks of hospitals and physicians. Unlike HMOs, however, PPOs do not contract for full responsibility to provide certain services. Instead, they serve as service brokers to insurance companies, employers, the government, third-party intermediaries, and other major buyers; that is, the plan contracts with a group of providers to furnish services at reduced fees (Mullahy, 2010).
- **Indemnity plans** reimburse for care at a predetermined amount or through a fee-for-service arrangement. Although no restrictions are placed on the choice of a provider, there are limited incentives to achieve cost containment. (Finkelman, 2001, 2006).

Managed care first emerged as a response to the rapid inflation of healthcare costs and employers' demands for a mechanism for cost containment. It continues to evolve today as the demands of society change and as mergers occur. At the moment, the balance of power is shifting from insurance companies to large corporate providers. Table 1-6 outlines some key differences between managed care, case management, and disease management.

There are five key factors for success in the field of case management:

1. Clearly stated eligibility requirements (i.e., inclusion and exclusion criteria used to select patients from the general population)
2. Specially trained nurse case managers and community case managers
3. Organizational support and infrastructure, including information systems
4. Collection and reporting of outcomes for accountability and validation of effectiveness
5. Physician involvement (Kibbe, 2001)

TABLE 1-6 Differences Between Managed Care, Case Management, and Disease Management

Characteristic	Managed Care	Case Management	Disease Management
Focus	■ Financial cost containment ■ Focus on the providers	■ Quality patient care ■ Interdisciplinary ■ Focus on the individual	■ Target population with a specific disease ■ Group focus
Goals	■ Reduce costs ■ Implement standards to ensure quality care ■ Manage resources	■ Maintain the patient in the most cost-effective environment ■ Avoid emergency department visits, hospitalizations, medical errors ■ Improve patient satisfaction with quality of care ■ Attain evidence-based outcomes ■ Provide quality care	■ Maintain the patient in the most cost-effective environment ■ Attain evidence-based outcomes to manage a specific disease ■ Improve patient satisfaction with care ■ Improve the quality of care
Major changes	■ Delivery systems	■ Healthcare provider roles	■ Nursing roles
Continuum of care	■ Across services and providers	■ Coordinated continuum of care delivery systems	■ Continuum of care during the course of a disease
Obligations	■ Tied to the employer ■ Governed by a contract between the MC company and the employer ■ Governed by federal regulations: Medicare and Medicaid	■ Episodic care ■ Long-term care ■ Health promotion ■ Disease prevention ■ Early case finding	■ Continuous long-term care across the life span of the person who has a chronic debilitating disease or a long-term injury

Sources: Cohen & Cesta, 2005; Finkelman, 2001, 2006; Howe, 2005; Huber, 2005; Mullahy, 2010; Tahan, 1999.

CASE MANAGEMENT AS A PROCESS

Table 1-7 outlines the steps in the CM process, focusing on the features and functions of this approach when applied to a capitated (MC) environment.

Like any process, the case management process and the nursing process progress through steps prior to reaching the final stage of examining outcomes and evaluation. Table 1-8 compares the case management process and the nursing process. Notice that the initial step of CM comprises early case finding, screening, and referral; this step is lacking in the nursing process. In the monitoring step, the case manager closely follows the patient's progress to identify variances and examines the quality of care versus the costs to ascertain the appropriate utilization of resources; the nursing process does not have this step either. The rest of the steps in the two processes are similar.

The case management process is intended to deliver the outcomes identified in Table 1-9.

HISTORICAL PERSPECTIVES AND CURRENT TRENDS

Recent Changes in Healthcare Delivery

In recent years, changes in the delivery of health care have occurred rapidly, driven by several key factors. In particular, the following driving forces have contributed to the development of case management as a new and evolving healthcare profession:

- The escalating costs of health care, along with increasing complaints from business leaders, government officials, and consumers about the rising costs of health insurance premiums
- The complexity of the U.S. healthcare system, including duplication of services and fragmentation, necessitating the establishment of a coordinated continuum of care delivery system (i.e., CM)
- Changing demographics—increasing numbers of older adults with chronic diseases and the increasing incidence of chronic diseases, especially HIV and diabetes
- Increasing government budget deficits
- Increasing numbers of uninsured persons, who often use expensive emergency department (ED) services
- Increasing government regulations (such as diagnostically related groups [DRGs])

TABLE 1-7 Steps in the CM Process: Features and Functions of CM in a Capitated Environment

Case finding, screening, and referral	■ Members, who are eligible for all services covered in the healthcare contract ■ Identify patients who need specific services ■ Early case finding
Screening and intake	■ Screen out patients who do not need specific services ■ Screen out patients outside the contract (carve out) ■ Screen in patients who qualify for services
Assessment and needs identification	■ Assess needs and capabilities of the patient ■ Determine the resources available under the capitated contract ■ Assess resources available from other providers in the network ■ Identify problems and interventions
Planning	■ Plan strategies to meet diagnostic, therapeutic, and educational needs ■ Select the guidelines that will be used to monitor care ■ Find the least restrictive level of care ■ Plan efficient use of services ■ Establish expected outcomes ■ Match resources with needs ■ Decide on, facilitate, coordinate, integrate, and expedite needed services
Implementation and coordination	■ Use as few resources as possible ■ Direct the interdisciplinary team ■ Ensure that access to services is timely ■ Promote cost-effective, efficient care ■ Eliminate duplications ■ Coordinate healthcare resources to meet individual and family needs
Monitoring	■ Follow the patient's progress ■ Change the level of care as needed ■ Maintain the patient's and family's satisfaction ■ Analyze variances ■ Monitor the over- and underutilization of resources ■ Oversee the quality of care, according to standards of care
Evaluation	■ Use data collected to evaluate the care according to patient care guidelines, protocols, and standards of care ■ Examine the relationship between access, quality, and cost ■ Collect utilization and outcomes data, and compare all data in relationship to cost, quality, and access
Termination and documentation	■ Prepare for discharge ■ Plan for community resources available to the patient and family ■ Facilitate a smooth transition to the next level of care to ensure continuity of care ■ Educate the patient and family for self-care ■ Document all pertinent data, including the discharge plan
Outcomes evaluation and managed care utilization review	■ Analyze data ■ Monitor both managerial outcomes and clinical outcomes ■ Negotiate and/or confirm MC authorizations

Sources: Adapted from Birmingham, 1996; Cohen & Cesta, 2005; Mullahy, 2010; Tahan, 1999.

TABLE 1-8 Differences Between the Case Management Process and the Nursing Process

Case Management Process	Nursing Process
Case finding, screening, and referral Screening and intake	
Assessment Diagnosis	*Assessment* Diagnosis
Planning	Planning
Implementation Assess resources Facilitating, networking, brokering, and coordinating	*Implementation* Gathering resources Applying nursing care
Monitoring **Follow the patient's progress; change the level of care PRN** Analyze variances Oversee quality versus cost Utilization of resources and services Patient and family satisfaction	
Evaluation Outcomes: patient, quality, costs	*Evaluation* Patient outcomes
Documentation Analyze the outcome data and document cost, quality, LOS, and patient's health status Transition to home or another facility	*Documentation* Review and analyze patient outcomes Describe the discharge plan Document patient and family teaching

Source: Herrick, 2008.

TABLE 1-9 The Identified Outcomes

Patients	Systems	Healthcare Providers
Increased satisfaction with services	Decreased costs	Increased job satisfaction
Improved quality of care	Increased productivity	Increased support as part of a team and decreased burnout
Decreased costs	Decreased turnover of personnel	Decreased on-the-job stress
Improved quality of life	Increased earnings	Improved problem solving More innovative and creative

Source: Herrick, 2008.

Other forces have also promoted the development of MC, CM, and DM. For example, traditional care has been largely replaced by MC entities that include CM and DM as part of their standard practice.

Traditional Care		*MC/CM/DM*
Institutional acute care	➔	Community-based care
Episodic care/acute care	➔	Chronic care across the continuum of care (continuity of care)
Process-oriented care	➔	Outcomes-oriented care
Fee-for-service	➔	Capitation
Technology poor	➔	Technology rich
Quality assurance	➔	Variance analysis
Individual healthcare provider	➔	Collaborative team or primary care provider
Long hospital stays	➔	Decreased length of stay

Source: Herrick, 2008.

The Evolution of Case Management

The goal throughout history has been the coordination of services across the healthcare continuum, while controlling costs. Sources for historical issues and trends include the following: Arbuckle & Herrick, 2006; Ball, 2000; Brown & Magilvy, 2001; Cohen & Cesta, 2005; Furman & Jackson, 2001; "A Grand 2004!," 2004; Handron, Dosser, McCammon, & Powell, 1998; Herrick & Bartlett, 2004; Huber, 2005; Kersbergen, 1996; Lamb & Zazworsky, 2005; Mullahy, 2010; Tahan, 1998, 1999; Zander, 1988a, 1988b; Zander, 2002.

The 1800s

1860s: Case management developed in response to immigrant populations from Europe flooding into U.S. cities, where there was a lack of coordination of health care and human services. New York City, for example, established CM under the auspices of the Henry Street Settlement; Chicago established Hull House for much the same purpose. Case managers were needed to organize, coordinate, manage, and facilitate the delivery of patient care. Nurses and social workers banded together to provide medical and social services to the needy in these areas. Thus case managers have a long history of an interdisciplinary focus; CM services have been implemented by individuals from the public health, social work, nursing, and medicine areas. According to Tahan (1998), CM transcends all healthcare settings across the continuum of care (cited in Herrick, 2008). The model linking patient needs to healthcare resources was developed during the early 1900s by social workers, who acted as brokers between the healthcare system and individual patients. This was the beginning of the traditional social work model—the **broker model**.

1863: Massachusetts established the first board of charities in the United States to coordinate public services, while conserving the public funds being used to care for the sick and the poor.

1877: The first major effort at interagency cooperation and coordination was made by the Charity Organization Societies, which became a dominant force in providing services to the poor, while emphasizing the need to deliver services in a cost-effective, efficient manner.

1890: American Public Health Nursing was founded by Lillian Wald with the goals of encouraging clients to engage in self-help and promoting the ability of patients to make healthy choices. Wald organized CM services to emphasize clients' participation in choosing their healthcare services. The U.S. Public Health Service also established coordinated services, primarily dealing with sanitation and immunizations.

The 1900s

1900s: The U.S. Public Health Service developed an embryonic system of case management, in which the client was the community and services were coordinated to deal with environmental problems.

1901: Mary Richardson published a model of **case coordination** that featured concern for the client as the center of care—a value that persists today. During the same era, Annie Goodrich wrote about the services provided by community health nurses, which included direct nursing care, housekeeping services, social services, and spiritual care to meet the needs of families in a holistic manner. Under this model, the nurse brokered and facilitated the services needed by families.

1909: All states had organized some form of a health department. Lillian Wald convinced Metropolitan Life Insurance Company to provide visiting nurse services to care for its clients during periods of illness in an attempt to forestall paying death benefits. This proved to be a money saver for the insurance company. New York City's Visiting Nurse Association (VNA) still exists today. It represented the first venture between insurance companies and healthcare providers; such partnerships proliferated with the advent of managed care, during the 1980s and 1990s.

1920s: The Community Chest Movement began to garner donations to support human services agencies. Child Guidance Centers were founded and experimented with the concept of multidisciplinary team planning in an effort to provide needed services for children and families and to prevent duplication and fragmentation of services.

Also during the 1920s, Metropolitan Life Insurance Company documented that it had saved $43 million as a result of implementing a nurse case management system.

1935: The Social Security Act allowed for funding to support activities directed toward individualized health care.

1940s: Following World War II, veterans returned home with many health and mental health problems. The Veterans Administration (VA) established the first "one-stop" center for veterans benefits in Los Angeles. From there, the VA developed centers all over the country to provide healthcare services across the healthcare continuum, which included the establishment of CM programs.

1960s: A variety of human services were established as part of the Civil Rights movement and President Johnson's War on Poverty. The Civil Rights movement affected the role of the client by changing it from a passive one to an active one. Deinstitutionalization of the mentally ill was legislated so that large numbers of mentally ill persons were discharged into their communities; CM programs were funded by the federal government for local mental health centers to assist these patients with making the transition back to the community. The term "case management" was coined during this time and paved the way for today's healthcare delivery system, which functions across the healthcare continuum.

1970s: The Department of Health, Education, and Welfare recognized the need to improve the coordination of its programs and proposed the Allied Services Act to facilitate the integration of services across a continuum of care. The 1970s were a legislative era: CM services were developing in long-term care settings, funded by Medicare and Medicaid. The Area Agencies on Aging were established in 1973 to coordinate services for older adults. Legislation was passed on behalf of children and the mentally ill to promote better interagency cooperation across the continuum of care.

1975–1979: Many mentally disabled persons were deinstitutionalized and became dependent on community service agencies for support. Legislation passed included the Developmentally Disabled Assistant and Bill of Rights Acts, which mandated that each client receive services coordinated by a service coordinator or case manager. CM services became the hallmark for mental health services for developmentally disabled and mentally ill persons, with case managers coordinating their housing, social services, and medical and mental health services, as well as facilitating their entry into community support systems, such as rehabilitation or vocational programs.

1980s: Lawmakers continued to pass legislation that provided federal funding of demonstration projects to establish a continuum of care for service delivery. The goals were to improve accountability by coordinating services around the severely mentally ill person. The case manager was responsible for the client as well as the service delivery system. A federal program developed on behalf of children and their families, called the Child and Adolescent Service System Program (CASSP), was established in 1984 to assist state mental health departments to coordinate care for severely emotionally disturbed (SED) children and adolescents, and their families. Interagency projects were funded in an attempt to overcome the problems associated with a fragmented mental health/healthcare delivery system. Interdisciplinary CM programs, under the auspices of CASSP, included assessment, coordination of care, advocacy, and referrals to community resources. Additional services were outlined for the CM team, to include outreach to the home, crisis intervention, teaching child management skills to parents, medication monitoring, outreach to schools, and the establishment of day treatment programs. This so-called **system of care model** "wrapped" services from across the continuum of care around the family. Services included social services, mental health, public health, educational concerns, and juvenile justice coordinated by the CM team. The **wraparound** concept was developed to depict the coordination of professional and community resources around the family, providing a safety net for distressed families.

The Education and Handicapped Act of 1986 was passed to improve services to all infants and toddlers with special needs.

DRGs and the prospective payment system were implemented to reduce costs. Consequently, innovative approaches to healthcare delivery emerged. New England Medical Center in Boston established an acute care CM model; Carondelet–St. Mary's Hospital and Health Center in Tucson developed a continuum-of-care CM model that integrated community care with an acute care CM model, thus spanning inpatient and outpatient services.

1990s: Case management programs were established in hospitals, insurance companies, and communities as a means of facilitating, coordinating, and monitoring both the quality and the costs of health care.

The 2000s: Today and the Future

New models will continue to evolve as the healthcare scene continues to change. Consider the following developments, which suggest the scope of

TABLE 1-10 Predictions

- Increasing numbers of uninsured people
- Concerns about patient safety in hospitals and nursing homes
- Calls for more collaborative interdisciplinary practice
- Increasing costs, including for pharmaceuticals
- Greater emphasis on wellness and complementary and alternative medicine (CAM)
- More technology
- Increasing use of computerized records
- Greater emphasis on quality management
- Politics mixing with healthcare issues (e.g., universal health insurance, healthcare reform)
- Aging of the workforce
- Higher costs for educating healthcare professionals
- Providing time for interdisciplinary collaboration in a cost-conscious healthcare environment
- Ethical questions about extending life, saving premature babies, abortion, in vitro fertilization, stem cell research, long-term care, and Medicare services for baby boomers and others
- An increasing role for the case manager as a patient and family advocate
- More research on roles and functions for the CM certification exam
- More research for evidence-based practice, including the connections between interventions and outcomes
- Formation of a hospitalist–case manager connection, as collaborative partners
- Lack of primary care providers, especially in poor rural areas
- Pay-for-performance (no reimbursements by Medicare and Medicaid for preventable consequences from hospitalization, such as falls, lack of hospital infection control, bed sores, and other hospital errors)
- Use of Recovery Audit Contractors (RAC) program

Sources: Adapted from Ball, 2000; Carver, 2001; CMSA, Piedmont Chapter State Convention, 2006, 2009; "A Grand 2004!," 2004; Joers, 2001; Park, 2006; Terra, 2009; Thurkettle & Noji, 2003.

changes ahead: disease management, telephonic CM, telehealth, and congregational or parish nursing (recently renamed faith community nursing).

Today's and Tomorrow's Issues

Table 1-10 predicts some things to come that may influence the delivery of health care.

The Recovery Audit Contractors (RAC; www.racinfo.com) program was established as part of the Tax Relief and Health Care Act of 2006, to be implemented in all 50 states by 2010. It was piloted in Florida, California, and New York—these states were chosen because they had the largest number of

Medicare claims in 2005. The pilot study was completed in 2008. RAC will audit claims that are unclear and claims for improper payments by the Centers for Medicare and Medicaid (CMS) in an attempt to recoup erroneous payments. An appeals process is available if the medical facility does not agree with the adverse determination. RAC does not have to consider any new information submitted during the appeals process. Under this program, the government can deny claims for incorrect coding, services that are not deemed medically necessary, excessive billing expenses, payments that should have been made by another insurance carrier, and Medicare/Medicaid payments made erroneously to the medical facility.

Terra (2009) has suggested a three-step process for dealing with a RAC review:

1. Identify an error in the form of incorrect coding. Eliminate any further review.
2. Group the medical necessity denial claims by the presenting complaint (e.g., chest pain, congestive heart failure, pneumonia). Doing this would streamline the review process. Terra has suggested this step could be handled by clerical staff.
3. Write a comprehensive response to the denial and make an appeal to the next level in the five-level appeal process. The response should include the following elements:
   a. All identifying information for the claim in question
   b. Criteria related to the disease
   c. Additional information that establishes a justification for inpatient admission
   d. The reason for the admission to an inpatient setting
   e. All necessary RAC

All of the patient's records should be reviewed against the relevant criteria, using InterQual documents and the CMS guidelines, as well as federal, state, and local coverage determinations. Include any additional forms as requested by RAC. InterQual provides evidence-based criteria on how patients progress through the continuum of care (McKesson, 2010).

Complex claims reviews for denials may have a direct impact on CM departments, making case managers' workloads significantly heavier. The CM department should track and systematically review each denial and appeal.

Building a Vision for the Future of Case Management

The case manager of the future will need to meet a number of new demands:

- Be flexible enough to work in developing organizational structures and meet the changing healthcare needs of society
- Participate in lifelong learning and be committed to continued professional development
- Network at every level—local, state, and national levels
- Be "proactive"—anticipating and communicating changes in technologies and professional obligations
- Remain open to new paradigms for service delivery

Markle (2004) claimed that CM has repeatedly demonstrated its ability to reduce healthcare costs, while maintaining quality for the benefit of patients. CM will continue to evolve as changes in the healthcare system occur but will remain a means to identify healthcare and patient care issues, and to obtain and evaluate the use of resources. Put simply, it will continue to have a positive impact economically on the U.S. healthcare system.

MAINTAINING QUALITY

Nursing Education

Kuric and White (2005) conducted a study to identify the current CM curriculum content in schools of nursing. Although CM is considered an essential function within the current healthcare environment as a means to provide high-quality, cost-effective care, CM content in nursing education programs remains limited. Table 1-11 lists content areas that should be included in the CM curriculum in schools that do teach case management.

According to Kuric and White (2005), CM should be integrated into all levels of nursing education, including ADN, BSN, and MSN programs. These authors

TABLE 1-11 Curricular Content Related to Case Management

- Client identification (e.g., chronically ill, repeated admissions, high risk for complications, frequent use of emergency department services)
- Family-centered care
- Planning and monitoring
- Collaboration
- Roles and models
- Quality of care
- Evaluation and outcomes management
- Legal and ethical issues
- Advocacy
- Resource management

also suggest that graduates who have a better understanding of CM functions are better able to serve as advocates for the patient and family. When nurses understand CM, they can fully use the case manager as a resource. Graduates who have a minimum of CM skills could provide basic CM services to patients.

Standards of Practice

CMSA wrote its first set of **standards of care** in 1995. These standards, which were most recently updated in 2002, are the foundation from which ethical principles for practice were developed. The Standards of Practice and Ethics Statements are both available from the CMSA national organization (Moreo & Lamb, 2003b). The standards list the acts that are expected to be performed and may not be omitted by an ordinary, prudent case manager, who is held to these standards by law. When these standards are not met, then the practitioner is considered to have committed a legally wrongful act. Words commonly used to characterize standards of care or standards of practice include "average, prudent, and reasonable" (Banja, 2006, p. 20). Standards of care provide guidelines for care by a case manager and outline his or her responsibilities. They are intended to identify and address the knowledge and skills of a case manager in today's healthcare environment (Moreo & Lamb, 2003a). In both an ethical and legal sense, standards of care guide practice (Banja, 2006).

Certifications/Credentialing

Certification is a means of validating to the public that a professional has achieved a given level of experience, education, and expertise. Certification is professionally and financially beneficial to the case manager's practice (Boling & Severson, 2005; Tahan, 2005; Wiser, 2003). The certification exam for case managers was developed based on a national study across disciplines, settings, and geographical areas, which identified activities, role relationships, knowledge, skills, and abilities of case managers (Tahan, Huber, & Downey, 2006). The Commission for Case Manager Certification (CCMC) not only conducted a national study, but also engaged in an ongoing dialogue with professional organizations to determine the integrity and validity of the CCMC exam. The exam addresses the roles and functions of a case manager, across disciplines and settings (CMSA, 2003; Huber & Tahan, 2004).

Certain requirements must be met to apply for certification, including licensure in the area of expertise, such as nursing or social work, and post–high

TABLE 1-12 Domains Tested on the Certification Exam

Activity Domains

- Case finding and intake
- Provision of case management services
- Outcomes evaluation and case closure
- Utilization management
- Psychosocial and economic issues
- Vocational rehabilitation

Knowledge Domains

- Case management principles and strategies
- Case management concepts
- Healthcare management and delivery; collaborations and interdisciplinary teams
- Healthcare reimbursement: managed care
- Psychosocial and support systems
- Vocational concepts and strategies

Source: Tahan, 2005; Tahan, Downey, & Huber, 2006.

school education or above in an accredited school, where the applicant majored in one of the healthcare disciplines. The ANA recommends at least a BSN degree for nurses. Other criteria include a minimum of 1 year of work experience that is supervised by a Certified Case Manager (CCM); or 24 months of working as a case manager, but not necessarily supervised by a CCM; or having worked as the director of a CM program, supervising other case managers for 12 or more months. Table 1-12 lists the core domains that are tested on the certification exam.

Through extensive research and analysis of findings, the roles, responsibilities, knowledge, and expertise of case managers have been identified (Tahan, 2006). The current certification exam is based on the most recent study, which was conducted to capture the current practice of case managers from different disciplines, settings, and geographical areas. The practice of CM spans the continuum of care and involves a variety of disciplines including nurses, social workers, rehabilitation counselors, physicians, and other allied health professionals (Tahan, 2006). Despite this wide variety of experience, there exists a core set of roles and activities based on knowledge of the CM process that is common to all case managers.

After analyzing the findings from the national study on roles and functions, Tahan, Downey, and Huber (2006) concluded that although case managers function in different settings across the healthcare continuum and the roles of the case managers are assumed by different disciplines, all case managers, regardless of the setting or professional discipline, share a core of knowledge that is necessary to meet the requirements of a case manager.

Requests for application or information regarding certification should be directed to the following groups:

Commission for Case Manager Certification
1835 Rohlwing Road, Suite E
Rolling Meadows, IL 60008
Phone: 847-818-0292
www.ccmcertification.org

Case Management Society of America
8201 Cantrell Road, Suite 230
Little Rock, AR 72227-2448
Phone: 501-225-2229
www.cmsa.org

Multistate Licensure

CMSA supports multistate licensure, noting that a lack of multistate licensure puts case managers in telehealth settings in legal jeopardy for violating state licensure laws. State licensing boards' goals are to protect the public's health, but in today's healthcare system, these agencies sometimes impede the delivery of CM services using telehealth strategies. The following states are "compact states" that have agreed to multistate licensing: Arizona, Arkansas, Delaware, Idaho, Iowa, Maine, Maryland, Mississippi, Nebraska, New Hampshire, New Mexico, North Carolina, North Dakota, South Carolina, South Dakota, Tennessee, Texas, Utah, Virginia, and Wisconsin. By the time this book is published, other states may have joined the compact as well. CMSA encourages case managers and their employers to work aggressively with state licensing boards to join the other compact states in advocating multistate licensing, so that it can be implemented in all states (Mueller, 2006). The benefit of membership in a compact state is that the case manager/disease manager is protected (i.e., covered by nursing legislation in both states) if he or she provides services via technology to a patient who resides in a state that is different from the provider's home state.

■ SUMMARY

This chapter reviewed the evolution of case management, its characteristics, and the roles, knowledge, and skills that are necessary for providing high-quality, cost-effective health care. Terminology was defined, because the language of managed care, case management, and disease management may be new for some nurses. Steps in the CM process were identified and compared with the nursing process. Methods for maintaining quality performance were addressed as well.

Now that you have finished the introduction, you should have a broad view of nursing case management. The following chapters will add more depth to your knowledge.

■ CASE STUDIES

If you were to become a director of case management, which issues in your organization would you prioritize and why?

■ DISCUSSION QUESTIONS

1. Define case management in your own words. What do the various definitions have in common?
2. List five of the most important characteristics of case management.
3. Compare the case management process to the nursing process by identifying the steps that are different in the two processes.
4. List three driving forces that affected health care and encouraged the establishment of case management.
5. What do you think about multistate licensure? Are you supportive or not?

■ CLASSROOM EXERCISES

With your classmates, discuss your experiences (personal or professional) with case management. Specifically, discuss the role of a case manager in the care delivered to a family member, friend, or colleague. Did it change their health outcome? Would this person's recovery or ability to cope with a chronic diagnosis have been different without the involvement of a case manager?

■ RECOMMENDED READINGS

Banja, J. D. (2006, July/August). Ethics, case management, and the standards of care. *Case Manager, 17*(4), 20–22.

Birmingham, J. (1996). How to apply CMSA's Standards of Practice for Case Management in a capitated environment. *Journal of Case Management, 2*(5), 9–22.

Lessard, M. J. (2007). Alphabet soup in case management. *Professional Case Management, 12*(2), 117–123.

Terra, S. M. (2009). Regulatory issues: Recovery Audit Contractors and their impact on case management. *Professional Case Management, 14*(5), 217–222.

▪ REFERENCES

The American Case Management Association [ACMA]. (2002). *Definition of case management.* Retrieved from http://www.acmaweb.org/section. asp?sID=4&mn=mn1&sn=sn1&wpg=mh

American Institute of Economic Research (AIER). (2005, March 14). *Newsletter, LXXII*(5).

Arbuckle, M., & Herrick, C. (2006). *Child and adolescent mental health: Interdisciplinary systems of care.* Sudbury, MA: Jones and Bartlett.

Ball, R. S. (2000). Nurse case managers and the Internet. *Lippincott's Case Management, 5,* 174–183.

Banja, J. D. (2006, July/August). Ethics, case management, and the standards of care. *Case Manager, 17*(4), 20–22.

Birmingham, J. (1996). How to apply CMSA's Standards of Practice for Case Management in a capitated environment. *Journal of Case Management, 2*(5), 9–22.

Boling, J., & Severson, M. (2005). Credentialing for case management. In C. L. Cohen & T. G. Cesta (Eds.), *Nursing case management: From essentials to advanced practice applications* (4th ed., pp. 296–322). St. Louis, MO: Elsevier Mosby.

Bower, K. (1992). *Case management.* New York: National League for Nursing.

Brown, N. J., & Magilvy, J. K (2001). Parish nursing as community-focused case management. In E. L. Cohen & T. G. Cesta (Eds.), *Nursing case management. From essentials to advanced practice applications* (3rd ed., pp. 155–164). St. Louis, MO: CV Mosby.

Carver, T. (2001). www.alternativecasemanagement.now: Looking for solutions to managing high-risk patients? Cyberspace may be the perfect place. *Nursing Management, 32*(8), 33–35.

Case Management Society of America (CMSA). *Philosophy, certification.* Retrieved August 2003, from www.cmsa.org

Case Management Society of America (CMSA), Piedmont Chapter State Convention (2006, September). *Delivering the magic of case management.* State Convention Center, Winston-Salem, NC.

Case Management Society of America (CMSA), Piedmont Chapter State Convention (2009, September). *Follow the yellow brick road: The road to health care reform and bills before Congress.* The Hawthorne Inn, Winston-Salem, NC.

Cohen, E. L., & Cesta, T. G. (2005). *Nursing case management: From essentials to advanced practice applications* (4th ed., pp. 3–26, 250–262). St. Louis, MO: Elsevier Mosby.

Commission for Case Management Certification (CCMC). (2003). *Definitions, case management philosophy and the certification program: Certification guide.* Retrieved August 2003, from http://www.ccmcertification.org

Del Togno-Armanasco, V., Olivas, G., & Harter, S. (1989). Developing an integrated nursing case management model. *Nursing Management, 20*(10), 26–29.

DiCenso, A., Guyatt, G., & Ciliska, D. (2005). *Evidence-based nursing: A guide to clinical practice.* St. Louis, MO: Elsevier Mosby.

Disease Management Association of American [DMAA]. (2004). Definition of disease management. Washington, DC: DMAA. http://www.dmaa.org/dm_definition.asp

Erkel, E. (1993). The impact of case management in preventive services, *Journal of Nursing Administration, 23*(1), 27–32.

Finkelman, A. W. (2001). *Managed care: A nursing perspective.* Upper Saddle River, NJ: Prentice Hall.

Finkelman, A. W. (2006). *Leadership and management in nursing.* Upper Saddle River, NJ: Pearson//Prentice Hall.

Flarey, D. L., & Blancett, S. S. (1996). *Handbook of nursing case management.* Gaithersburg, MD: Aspen.

Furman, R., & Jackson, R. (2001). Wrap-around services. An analysis of community-based mental health services for children. *Journal of Child and Adolescent Psychiatric Nursing, 15*(3), 124–130.

Girard, N. (1994). The case management model of patient care delivery. *AORN, 60*(3), 403–415.

A grand 2004! And predictions of issues affecting case managers in 2005 [editorial]. (2004). *Lippincott's Case Management, 9*(6), 247–249.

Hampton, D. (1993). Implementing a managed care framework through care maps. *Journal of Nursing Administration*, 23(5), 21–27.

Handron, D. S., Dosser, J. R., McCammon, S. L., & Powell, J. Y. (1998). "Wrap-around" the wave of the future: Theoretical and professional practice implications. *Journal of Family Nursing, 4*(1), 65–86.

Herrick, C. A. (2008, Fall). *Learning module I: Introduction to nursing case management* (NUR 541) [unpublished manuscript]. Greensboro, NC: University of North Carolina School of Nursing.

Herrick, C. A., & Bartlett, R. (2004). Psychiatric nursing case management: Past, present and future. *Issues in Mental Health Nursing, 25*(6), 589–602.

Howe, R. (2005). *The disease manager's handbook.* Sudbury, MA: Jones and Bartlett.

Huber, D. L. (2005). Overview of disease management and case management. In D. L. Huber (Ed.), *Disease management: A guide for case managers* (pp. 1–13). St. Louis, MO: Elsevier Saunders.

Huber, D. L., & Tahan, H. A. (2004). Managing forces of change: Commission for Case Manager Certification looks to the future. *Lippincott's Case Management, 9*(2), 57–60.

McKesson. (2010). *InterQual decision support: The gold standard in evidence-based clinical decision support.* Retrieved from http://www.mckesson.com/en_us/ McKesson.com/Our%2BBusinesses/McKesson%2BHealth%2BSolutions/ Solution%2BAreas/InterQual%2BDecision%2BSupport/ InterQual%2BDecision%2BSupport.html

Joers, D. M. (2001). Case management: Ripe for technology. *Advance Nurses, 3*(19), 25–26.

Kersbergen, A. L. (1996, August). Case management: A rich history of coordinating care to control costs. *Nursing Outlook, 44*(4), 169–172.

Kibbe, D. C. (2001, September/October). Physicians, care coordination, and the use of web-based information systems to manage chronic illness across the continuum. *Case Manager, 12*(5), 56–61.

Kuric, J. L., & White, A. H. (2005). Case management curriculum in nursing education. *Lippincott's Case Management, 10*(2), 102–107.

Lamb, G. S., & Zazworsky, D. (2005). The Carondelet community-based nurse case management program. In E. L. Cohen & T. G. Cesta (Eds.), *Nursing case management: From essentials to advanced practice applications* (4th ed., pp. 580–589). St. Louis, MO: Elsevier Mosby.

Lessard, M. J. (2007). Alphabet soup in case management. *Professional Case Management, 12*(2), 117–123.

Lind, P. H. (2005). Disease management: Applying systems thinking to quality patient care delivery. In E. L. Cohen & T. G. Cesta, (Eds.) *Nursing case management: From essentials to advanced practice applications* (4th ed., pp. 38–51). St. Louis, MO: Elsevier Mosby.

Markle, A. (2004, July/August). The economic impact of case management. *Case Manager, 15*(4), 54–58.

Moreo, K., & Lamb, G. (2003a). Providing relevant guidelines for case management practice: Revised CMSA Standards of Practice for case management. *Lippincott's Case Management 8*(3), 122–124.

Moreo, K., & Lamb, G. (2003b). CMSA updates standards of practice for case management. *Case Manager, 14*(3), 54.

Mueller, L. S. (2006). Legal and ethical forum: CMSA supports compliance with multistate licensure law. Nursing compact states reach 20. *Lippincott's Case Management, 11*(3), 124–126.

Mullahy, C. M. (2010). *The case manager's handbook* (4th ed., pp. 1–24). Sudbury, MA: Jones and Bartlett.

Park, E. J. (2006). Telehealth technology in case/disease management. *Lippincott's Case Management, 11*(3), 175–182

Sowell, R. L., & Meadows, T. M. (1994). An integrated case management model: Developing standards, evaluation and outcomes criteria. *Nursing Administration Quarterly, 18*(2), 53–64.

Swansburg, R. C., & Swansburg, R. J. (1998). The nurse manager's guide to financial management. In L. Roussel, R. Swansburg, & R. Swansburg (Eds.), *Management and leadership for nurse administrators* (4th ed., p. 297). Rockville, MD: Aspen.

Swansburg, R. (2002). Introduction to managed care. In R. Swansburg (Ed.), *Introduction to management and leadership for nursing managers* (3rd ed., pp. 7–21). Sudbury, MA: Jones and Bartlett.

Tahan, H. A. (1998). Case management: A heritage more than a century old. *Lippincott's Case Management, 3*(2), 55–62.

Tahan, H. A. (1999). Clarifying case management. What's in a label? *Nursing Case Management, 4*(6), 268–278.

Tahan, H. A. (2005). Clarifying certification and its value for case managers. *Lippincott's Case Management, 10*(1), 14–21.

Tahan, H. A. (2006, May/June). Essential activities and knowledge domains of case management: New insights from the CCMC roles and functions study. *Case Manager, 17*(3), 45–48.

Tahan, H. A., Downey, W. T., & Huber, D. L. (2006). Case managers' roles and functions: Commission for Case Manager Certification's 2004 research, Part II. *Lippincott's Case Management, 11*(2), 71–89.

Tahan, H. A., Huber, D. L., & Downey, W. T. (2006). Case managers' roles and functions: CCMC's 2004 research, Part I. *Lippincott's Case Management, 11*(1), 4–22.

Terra, S. M. (2009). Regulatory issues: Recovery Audit Contractors and their impact on case management. *Professional Case Management, 14*(5), 217–222.

Thurkettle, M. A., & Noji, A. (2003). Information management as a process and product of case management. *Lippincott's Case Management, 8*(3), 117–121. Retrieved May 27, 2004, from http://gateway2.ovid.com/ovidweb.cgi

Trinidad, E. A. (1993). Case management: A model of CNS practice. *Clinical Nurse Specialist, 7*(4), 221–223.

Wiser, S. (2003, July/August). Behind the scenes: Creating the CCM examination. *Case Manager, 14*(4), 56–57.

Zander, K. (2002). Nursing case management in the 21st century: Intervening where margin meets mission. *Nursing Administration Quarterly, 26*(5), 58–67.

Zander, K. (1988a). Managed care within acute care settings: Design and implementation via nursing case management. *Health Care Supervisor, 6*(2), 24–43.

Zander, K. (1988b). Nursing care management: Strategic management of cost and quality outcomes. *Journal of Nursing Administration, 18*(5), 23–30.

Appendix to Chapter 1
Nursing Case Management

DEFINITIONS

Algorithm A chronological delineation of steps for the patient's care to be applied as they relate to specific conditions or situations.

Authorization The approval for payments prior to the delivery of service, which is necessary in a capitated system; also known as preauthorization.

Balanced Budget Act (1997) Legislation that established the Medicare Plus Choice program. Among the choices were preferred provider organizations (PPOs) or provider-sponsored organizations (PSOs). Other changes included redistribution of payments between rural and urban areas. Hospital administrators have complained that the restricted reimbursements have necessitated cutbacks in personnel.

Benchmarking A method to identify "best practices" that allows healthcare organizations to compare their performance both within the organization and with other organizations that are comparable in size and organizational structure and provide services to similar populations. The purpose is to improve performance. The benefits of benchmarking are listed below:

- Identifying performance gaps
- Getting ideas from other organizations and identifying opportunities for change
- Developing consensus
- Applying new ideas to yield better outcomes in order to improve services.

Benefit The amount the insurance company will pay to the beneficiary, according to the insurance contract.

Broker of Services The healthcare provider who acts as case manager for the client, and who identifies the client's needs, matching the necessary resources to meet the healthcare needs, on a case-by-case basis across the continuum of care. The broker of services advocates for the client and family to receive necessary services.

Cap The maximum dollars that are allowed by the insurance company for a particular service.

Capitated Healthcare System A system of healthcare delivery in which providers receive a fixed amount of money, allocated per person for healthcare expenses. Providers receive a fixed amount of money over a specific period of time, regardless of the number of services provided (Mullahy, 2004).

Capitation A payer contracts with a provider for specific services. The third-party payer pays the provider a set amount of money on the basis of the number of enrolled members in the payer's organization. Capitation is a type of risk sharing in which the providers in a network receive fixed payments periodically for healthcare services rendered to the members of a particular healthcare plan.

Care Map (CMP) Depicts the multidisciplinary staff's interventions against a timeline. It also is a description of the indicators that measure quality. Care Maps are an excellent means by which physicians, nurses, and other healthcare professionals can monitor the quality of care for particular patients. CMP goes beyond the traditional critical path in that it identifies outcomes and includes quality descriptors and key interventions provided by the interdisciplinary team. It analyzes variances from the plan of care. A Care Map has also been described as a blueprint because it depicts practice patterns. It also documents the following:

- The length of stay (LOS)
- Nursing diagnosis
- A problem list
- Expected clinical outcomes
- Tasks assigned to each discipline in order to achieve the expected outcomes.

Carve Out Services excluded from a provider contract that may be covered through arrangements with other providers. Providers are not financially responsible for services carved out of their contact, but the subcontract does provide for services from another healthcare provider.

Case Mix Index The sum of all diagnostically related group (DRG) relative weights, divided by the number of cases.

Case Management (CM) There are a number of definitions for case management that can be found throughout the literature. Case management can be operationalized differently depending on the setting, the target population, and the specific discipline providing service. The definitions of CM cover a broad range of patient care activities, some of which are listed below:

- CM is a collaborative process of assessment, planning, facilitation and coordination, advocacy, and monitoring the patient's progress and the services he or she receives
- It is a healthcare delivery model that focuses on the quality of the care as well as the costs of care
- The practice can vary from setting to setting, depending upon the population served and the discipline involved in administering the CM services
- The case manager or care coordinator assess the patient's needs and matches healthcare resources to the person to meet his or her needs

According to Mullahy (2010), the Commission for Case Manager Certification (CCMC) defines case management as a "collaborative process that assesses, plans, implements, coordinates, monitors and evaluates the options and services required to meet an individual's health needs, using communication and available resources to promote quality, cost-effective outcomes" (p. 11).

The components of case management include:

1. Assessing
2. Planning
3. Implementing and coordinating care across the continuum
4. Evaluating to determine the effectiveness of the interventions
5. Measuring outcomes and changing the plan of care as needed
6. Collaborating with the patient, the family and the interdisciplinary team
7. Integrating services

Zander (19898a), the pioneer in CM, defined it as a model for managing an episode of a patient's illness to determine a set of strategies; this is done to manage costs and the quality of care and to determine the outcomes of a clinician's interventions throughout an illness.

COBRA The Consolidated Budget Reconciliation Act included in the Omnibus Reconciliation Acts of 1986, 1987, and 1988. The legislation modified reimbursements to providers in the prospective payment system.

Collaboration The cornerstone of case management and managed care. The multidisciplinary team manages the client's care according to the expertise of each discipline in an effort to improve access, enhance quality, ensure protection of the patient's rights, and reduce costs.

Collaborative Practice The establishment of an interdisciplinary team whose members work together to ensure quality care in a cost-effective manner, using the expertise of each member of the team. Good communication is the key to an effective collaborative practice.

Community Rating A practice in which insurance costs are the same for everyone in a geographic area, instead of varying based on age, health, or company size.

Continuity of Care A coordinating system of healthcare delivery that includes various settings that care for patients from the hospital to community health centers. Continuity of care requires professionals from different disciplines and different agencies to collaborate together for the benefit of the patient and his or her family.

Continuous Quality Improvement (CQI) A component of managed care that focuses on quality assessments and improvements. Variance analysis and trends are examined as part of this process. CQI involves rigorous, systematic, organization-wide processes intended to achieve ongoing improvement in the quality of products, services, and operations, and the elimination of waste. CQI programs focus on both outcome and the process of care.

Continuum of Care An integrated healthcare system including inpatient and outpatient services that address people of all ages from womb to tomb. Continuum of Care includes primary care, sub-acute care, ambulatory care, home health care, preventative mental health care for both inpatient and outpatient, and rehabilitation and long-term care.

Co-pay A co-payment; the amount for which the client is responsible for paying directly. It is *usually* 20% of the total payment. The insurer pays 80%. Also known as *cost sharing.*

Cost Containment Formal, active attempts to control healthcare costs through such efforts as improved efficiency, utilization review, claims review, prospective review, rate negotiations, and rate reviews.

Cost-Effectiveness The allocation of resources in an effort to maximize outcomes and minimize costs.

Credentialing The process of checking a practitioner's references and documenting his or her credentials, including training, experience, demonstrated ability, licensure verification, and adequate malpractice insurance. The purpose of credentialing is to ensure that only qualified practitioners with current demonstrated competence have practice privileges (Mullahy, 2004).

Critical Pathway (CP) Provides a guide for healthcare personnel to provide interventions along with the sequencing and timing for those interventions. The CP is especially helpful for patients who need complex care from multiple providers. The CP guides the practitioners to coordinate their care for patients with complex needs in order to achieve specific outcomes; it is developed by an interdisciplinary team for all healthcare providers to use as a guide to practice. Functions of the CP:

- Collaborative care
- Continuity of care
- Necessary resources
- Identification of variances to include factors that interfere with timely and effective outcomes
- Identification of a proposed discharge date
- Reduction of unnecessary services and barriers to achieving outcomes
- Variances are identified to enhance problem resolution
- Expected outcomes

After the CP has been developed, an interdisciplinary team of developers must provide in-service educational programs to educate the staff of professionals, so that all members of the team know when the critical incidents should occur, what interventions each member of the team is expected to provide to the patient, and what the expected outcomes are.

Deductible The initial amount that the consumer pays, before the health insurer pays for the rest of the costs of healthcare services.

Disability Benefit A payment that arises because of a total or permanent disability of an insured person. A provision may be added to a policy that specifies a waiver of the premium in case of total and permanent disability.

Disease Management (DM) & the Disease Manager Coordinates the healthcare interventions for a specific population who have similar conditions or characteristics. The emphasis is on teaching to prevent the exacerbation of systems of the disease, educating patients and families for self-care, using empowerment strategies. The focus is on the whole patient. The goals are to:

- Identify high-risk populations
- Improve compliance through monitoring and education
- Improve the patient's health status
- Minimize complications
- Eliminate unnecessary medical utilization
- Prevent repeated hospitalizations
- Obtain the best outcomes possible

The target populations are those people with chronic diseases, such as patients with diabetes, cancer patients, first-time mothers who live in poverty, etc. Disease management regimens are not only population based, but they also are founded on evidence-based medicine, which is research based.

Economic modeling The process by which a disease manager determines if the medical/nursing, disease management program makes economic sense so that the viability of a program is ensured (Howe, 2005).

e-Health The use of electronic technologies and telecommunications to practice clinical health care, patient and professional health-related education, public health, and health medicine. It includes the fields of telemedicine, telehealth, medical informatics, electronic patient records, supply chain management, and biotechnologies (Mullahy, 2010).

Evidence-Based Practice The guidelines or pathways that have been developed by expert opinion or clinical trials regarding decisions about patients' care to support "best practice" (DiCenso, Guyatt, & Ciliska, 2005).

Fee-for-Service A contractual arrangement in which physicians and hospitals are paid a "reasonable or customary" fee for a unit of services. The practitioner is paid directly for the particular service rendered. Fee-for-service is the "traditional" payment reimbursement system.

Gatekeeper A primary care provider who authorizes referrals to specialists (Mullhay, 2004).

Healthcare Systems in the United States include:

- Healthcare institutions such as hospitals, nursing homes, community health centers, physician practices, and public health departments. These institutions create a complex mix of healthcare providers.
- Professional make up includes different types of personnel from different disciplines. Each discipline governs its own members and provides its own standards of practice.
- Medical technology, electronic communication, and new drugs fuel rapid changes in the delivery of health care.
- The method of funding health care is considered dysfunctional and expensive. Keeping costs under control is a major issue. Personal health

insurance is funded by employers for their employees. If one loses his or her job, he or she loses health care.

■ Millions of Americans are not currently funded for health care, but Congress and the President are attempting to alleviate the problem of citizens lacking health insurance.

Health Insurance Portability and Accountability Act (HIPAA) Federal legislation that mandates:

■ Standards to protect patient's privacy and health information
■ Requires national standards to identify systems of health care for patients, providers, plans and employers
■ Case managers and disease managers must develop HIPAA compliance strategies
■ Healthcare providers should work with a compliance officer
■ Provide avenues for patient's complaints
■ Ensure that patients have access to their medical records
■ Release only minimal information with the patient's written consent to other agencies
■ HIPAA website will provide additional information (www.cms.hhs.gov/hipaa)

Health Maintenance Organization (HMO) A comprehensive healthcare financing and delivery organization, which provides or arranges for the provision of healthcare services to enrollees within a geographical area through a panel of providers. Four types of HMO models are commonly observed:

■ **Staff Model:** The physicians are salaried employees of the HMO.
■ **IPA Model:** The organization contracts with an independent practice association (IPA), which in turn contracts with independent physicians, who practice in their own offices.
■ **Group Model:** The organization contracts with multispecialty physician group practices.
■ **Network Model:** The organization contracts with two or more independent group practices and /or IPAs.

Characteristics of the HMO include the following:

■ Shifts utilization risks from payer to provider
■ Competes for consumers by offering less costly services
■ Serves a defined population
■ Provides for contracted services
■ Receives fixed annual or monthly payments for services rendered
■ May link each enrollee to a primary care provider (PCP)
■ Is an integrated delivery system (IDS)
■ Integrates service and financial systems
■ Balances between primary and specialty care
■ Uses primary care physicians and nurse practitioners at fixed salaries

- Uses gatekeepers to control referrals to specialists and decide whether procedures are necessary
- Centralizes resources
- Has a preventive care and wellness orientation
- Emphasizes complete patient care, disease management, and education for self-care
- Encourages physicians to be business-oriented practitioners

The HMO provides health care for a geographical area or a population and accepts the responsibility to deliver care to include an agreed-upon set of services to the members who are enrolled in the HMO. The reimbursement for the services rendered amount to a predetermined payment, paid in advance on behalf of the individual member of the HMO.

Indemnity The security against a potential loss or damage for a predetermined amount in the event that there is a loss.

Independent Practice Association (IPA) An HMO contracts with physicians to see patients in their own private offices. Physicians then can be reimbursed on a capitated or a fee-for-service basis, according to the agreement between the HMO and the physician. The IPA may act as an intermediary between the healthcare provider and the third-party payer.

Integrated Delivery System (IDS) Consists of a group of healthcare organizations that collaborate together to provide a full range of healthcare services, coordinating these services across the healthcare continuum.

InterQual A nationally accepted resource that includes criteria to determine the appropriateness of a patient's admission and continuing care based on the level and intensities of the care in relation to the severity of the illness. There are guidelines to review care provided to a particular population.

Key Players Usually include the consumer (patient and family) the third-party payers and the healthcare providers.

Life Care Planning An assessment of a person with a catastrophic illness or injury that results in a long-term rehabilitation plan, including the cost of care to meet the patient's needs over a lifetime. The purpose is to predict the impact of the illness or injury. Long-term needs are matched with cost estimates. Standards of practice, assessments that are comprehensive, and data analysis and research are included in the plan of care over the predicted lifetime of the patient. LCPs are written guidelines to maintain the best possible health of the patient.

Managed Care (MC) A capitated payment system that has become the predominant means of reimbursement to pay for the health care of individuals. The goal is to improve the delivery of services while containing costs. Managed Care Organizations (MCOs) distribute healthcare dollars, determine the use of healthcare services, and provide access to healthcare reimbursements. MCOs integrate the financing with the delivery of health care.

The advantages:

- Diminished spiraling of healthcare costs
- Limited use of expensive procedures
- Ensures that new mothers can stay in the hospital for 48 hours.
- Monitors physician's practices
- Keeps consumers informed

The disadvantages:

- Healthcare choices are limited.
- Many procedures are only partially paid for. The patient must provide copayment or the bill may go unpaid.
- Approvals and denials of health care may be made by nonprofessionals.
- Cancellations of coverage may occur if a new life threatening illness has been diagnosed. The new healthcare plan just approved by the Congress and the President may restrict these actions by a third-party payers.
- HMOs often do not cover mental health or substance abuse. Again, the new healthcare plan may soon cover these expenses.

Managed Care Organization (MCO) A health maintenance organization, preferred provider organization, other provider-sponsored network, or other health plan model that integrates the financing and delivery of health care.
Advantages of MCOs include the following:

- MCOs have held back the inflationary spiral of healthcare costs for a time.
- They provide fast-track treatment for life-threatening conditions.
- Expensive procedures are limited in number.
- By law, new mothers must stay in the hospital for 48 hours.
- MCOs are accountable for outcomes.
- MCO plans have received better report cards than traditional indemnity insurance plans.
- Physicians' practices are more closely monitored.
- Consumers are better informed.
- Conservative treatments are the focus.

Disadvantages of MCOs include these considerations:

- "The heart of the managed care revolution is money, not medicine" (Swansburg, 2002, p. 11). "Business people do not take the Hippocratic Oath" (p. 7). Economic decisions may take precedence over patient care decisions.
- Healthcare choices are limited.
- Many procedures are only partially paid for and must then be reimbursed by the patient or may go uncollected by the provider.
- MCOs conduct less research.
- Decisions about care are often made by a nonphysician, including approvals and denials.
- Members with rare diseases may not get the treatment they need.

- Patients are moved through the system by nonmedical personnel.
- Plans tend to examine statistical averages, which ignore individual outliers.
- HMOs do not fund mental health or substance abuse care appropriately.

Managed Competition A situation in which insurance plans compete for business from individuals as a way to keep costs down.

Medicaid A federal public assistance program that is funded, administered, and operated by participating state and territorial governments. Medicaid provides medical benefits to eligible low-income recipients who need health care, regardless of age. Eligible groups include persons who are aged, blind, disabled, or pregnant, as well as families with dependent children. The person's resources must be insufficient to pay for health care. Criteria for eligibility were established under Title XIX under the Social Security Act of 1986 (Mullahy, 2010).

Medical Savings Plans As defined by the American Institute of Economic Research (2005), arrangements with employers whereby the employees are allowed to contribute pretax dollars to medical savings accounts that can be used to pay for health expenses. A portion of the money can be used to purchase a health insurance policy of the employee's choice. These accounts encourage consumers to be more knowledgeable and take more responsibility for decisions about their medical care.

Medicare A federally administered health insurance program for persons aged 65 and older and also for disabled people younger than 65 years old. Created in 1965 under Title XVII of the Social Security Act, Medicare covers the cost of hospitalization, medical care, and some related services for eligible persons without regard to income. It has two parts:

- **Part A** (inpatient): Hospital insurance that is compulsory and covers inpatient hospital costs (currently reimbursed using the prospective payment system) and posthospital care. Medicare also pays for pharmaceuticals provided in the hospital, but not for drugs provided in outpatient settings.
- **Part B** (outpatient): A supplementary medical insurance program that covers medically necessary physicians' services, outpatient hospital services (currently it reimburses caregivers retrospectively), and a number of other medical services and supplies not covered by Part A. Participation in Part B is voluntary; enrollee is eligible for a premium regardless of income.

Medicare Prescription Drug Improvement and Modernization Act of 2003 (Part D) Federal legislations provides prescription drug benefits for patients who are covered by Medicare. Assistance in helping elderly patients to select a plan can be found on several websites: (http://acute.hsag.com/hprp_042004; www.medicare.gov). Case Managers should search the websites prior to advising patients. The greatest disadvantage for patients is the doughnut hole. After the patient uses a set dollar amount of resources the patient is no longer offered coverage until he or she spends a set amount of money, using their own resources, before coverage will begin again.

Medicare Supplement Policy/Medigap Policy/Medicare Wrap A health insurance policy for an individual who has Medicare but wishes to obtain supplemental insurance policy that provides additional funds for deductibles and co-payments, and that provides additional funds for non-Medicare-covered services such as outpatient care, vision and hearing care, and therapies whose costs exceed a predefined benefit limit.

Peer Review Organization (PRO) A federal program established by the Tax Equity and Fiscal Responsibility Act of 1982 (TEFRA), which monitors the medical necessity and quality of services provided to Medicare and Medicaid beneficiaries under the prospective payment reimbursement system. PROs also validate the provider coding assignments that affect Medicare reimbursement.

Play or Pay A business option in which the employer either provides health insurance for workers or pays into a government fund that would.

Point of Service (POS) A managed care plan in which members are given a choice from among two or more options at the point when certain services are needed; also called an open-ended health maintenance organization (HMO).

Preexisting Condition Any medical condition that has been diagnosed within a specified period immediately preceding the covered person's effective date of coverage under the group health insurance plan. Insurance companies use this term when identifying a person's medical history, and may exclude the individual from coverage because of a previous medical condition.

Preferred Provider Organization (PPO) A type of managed care plan that contracts with independent providers (e.g., hospitals, physicians, ancillary providers) for negotiated discounted fees for services provided to plan members.

Premium The rate that a plan's subscriber pays for coverage of healthcare services.

Prospective Payment System (PPS) A pay scale used to compensate hospitals and other providers for Medicare or other government-funded healthcare services. The pay scale is based on diagnostically related groups (DRGs). Under this system, Medicare pays a fixed amount for the patient's procedure or service, regardless of the actual cost incurred by the provider. The PPS is designed to encourage providers to deliver services in a cost-effective manner.

Provider-Sponsored Organization (PSO) A network of physicians and hospitals that are owned by those providers. In such a system, healthcare providers focus on treating patients. By comparison, health maintenance organizations (HMOs) are really insurance companies that invest in stocks, bonds, and other assets. PSOs offer less risk to providers than do HMOs because providers receive only part of their income from the PSO.

Quality The degree to which healthcare services for individuals or a population increase the likelihood of desired healthcare outcomes and are consistent with current professional knowledge. Quality of care takes into account all medical/nursing services, technical competence, humanitarian treatment, and appropriateness.

Recovery Audit Contractors (RACS) Medicare auditors review documents and processes found within hospital claims related to a variety of services to include equipment used for the patient, inpatient and outpatient services, skilled nursing services are all examined to determine medical necessity (Scott, P. Dec, 2009/Jan 2010).

Relative Weight An assigned weight that is intended to reflect the relative resource consumption associated with each diagnostically related group (DRG). The higher the relative weight, the greater the payment to the hospital.

Risk Management The process of minimizing losses that cannot be prevented through legal methods and public relations. A risk management program identifies, evaluates, and takes corrective action against risks that may lead to patient or employee injury, or to property loss or damage, with resulting financial loss or legal liability.

Self-Insurance A type of health insurance in which a company chooses to provide benefits to its employees financed entirely by the company (the employer). In this form of private coverage, the employer—rather than an insurance company— assumes the risks of the costs of health care for its employees. The company may employ a third-party administrator to manage the plan.

Single-Payer System A nationally administered healthcare system in which the government runs the system. Everyone pays into a fund that is administered by the government; the government, in turn, provides universal coverage for all citizens. The government collects the premiums and administers the healthcare benefits for everyone in the country.

Standards of Care Treatment modalities recognized by authorizing bodies or the medical community as safe and efficacious for the care of person with an illness or injury.

Target Utilization Rates Specific goals regarding use of medical services, usually included in risk-sharing arrangements between managed care organizations and healthcare providers.

Third-Party Administrator (TPA) An independent person or corporate entity that administers group benefits, claims, and administration for a self-insured company/ group. The company or group assumes all of the financial risks; the TPA does not assume any of them.

Third-Party Payer A public or private insurance provider that pays for health care, such as Medicaid or Blue Cross/Blue Shield or a health maintenance organization such as United Health Care.

Total Quality Management A management philosophy and system for continuously improving performance at every level of every business process by focusing on meeting or exceeding customer expectations.

Universal Coverage A national policy that ensures all citizens have some kind of healthcare insurance. In the United States, adoption of such a policy would extend healthcare insurance to the 37 million or more people who are currently not covered.

Usual and Customary A method of profiling fees for a geographic area and then reimbursing providers standard amounts based on these findings.

Utilization Management (UM) A process of integrating review and case management of services in a cooperative effort with other parties, including patients, employers, providers, and payers.

Utilization Review A process used by healthcare payers to evaluate and monitor all care and services rendered by healthcare providers for medical necessity, appropriateness, and efficiency. Review is also performed to ensure that neither overutilization nor underutilization occurs. Review techniques include prospective review, concurrent review, and retrospective review.

Variance Variables that interfere with the quality of care and impact the ability to save costs. They are deviations that may be related to a number of factors; the patient, the family, the caregiver or clinician, the hospital, or those factors that have to do with the healthcare system. Consequently, expected outcomes are not met.

Variance Analysis A systematic review that examines how or why outcomes are unexpected in relation to the patient or family, healthcare provider or practitioner, or healthcare agency or system. A crucial component of this analysis is comparing the delivery of care and the outcomes with an institution's standard of care. The purpose is to improve quality of care and contain costs. Attention to the outliers is paid to determine why the length of stay or other outcomes might exceed expectations.

Worker's Compensation The social insurance system for industrial and work-related injuries regulated in certain specified occupations by the federal government.

Worker's Compensation Law A statute imposing liability on employers to pay benefits and furnish care to employees who become injured, and to pay benefits to dependents of employees who are killed, in the course of and/or because of their employment (Mullahy, 2010).

ALPHABET SOUP OF MANAGED CARE

CM	Case management
CMP	Care map
CP	Clinical pathway; critical pathway
DM	Disease management
DRG	Diagnostically related groups
FFS	Fee-for-service
HCFA	Health Care Financing Administration, which oversees Medicare and Medicaid and is part of the U.S. Department of Health and Human Services (DHHS)
HIPAA	Health Insurance Portability and Accountability Act
HMO	Health maintenance organization
IDS	Integrated delivery system

IPA	Independent practice association
LOS	Length of stay
MCO	Managed care organization
POS	Point of service
PPO	Preferred provider organization
PPS	Prospective payment system
PRO	Professional review organization
PSO	Provider-sponsored organization
QA	Quality assurance/assessment
RACS	Recovery audit contractors
TEFRA	Tax Equity & Fiscal Responsibility Act of 1982; health plans contract with HCFA, which has defined the primary and secondary responsibilities for coverage under the Medicare Program
TPA	Third-party administrator
UM	Utilization management
UR	Utilization review

Cultural Competence

Jeanne B. Jenkins

2

■ OUTLINE

Introduction
Definitions
Cultural Competence Overview
Models of Cultural Competence
Cultural Competence and Communication
Cultural Issues Related to Health Care

■ OBJECTIVES

1. Describe the importance of cultural competence among nurse case managers.
2. Discuss models for developing cultural competence among nurse case managers.
3. Identify essential demographic changes among minority populations in the United States that are the driving forces to increasing cultural competence among healthcare professionals.

INTRODUCTION

Minorities currently make up nearly one-third of the U.S. population and are expected to be the majority by 2042 (U. S. Department of Commerce [DOC], U.S. Census Bureau, 2008). Nevertheless, minorities continue to receive fewer healthcare services in general and suffer more severe health problems than the majority population (Brach & Fraser, 2000). Cultural competence has become a priority for healthcare professionals, for numerous reasons, including evidence that cultural bias and prejudice among healthcare professionals contributes to health disparities among minorities (Brach & Fraser, 2000; Dreachslin, 2007; Taylor, 2005). Also, rising medical costs, limited resources, and increasing numbers of uninsured individuals have created numerous disparities in the quality of care provided to individuals of various racial/ethnic groups, resulting in poor health outcomes for minority patients (Taylor, 2005).

For nurse case managers to be effective care agents in this changing demo-graphic society, they must recognize the importance of providing culturally appropriate care (Giger & Davidhizar, 2008). Nurse case managers must work to identify existing cultural, social, and economic barriers that might prevent patients from seeking and receiving quality health care. They must also strive to be culturally aware through introspectively examining their own values and cultural heritage that may influence their relationship with culturally different individuals and families for which they are providing care (Muñoz, 2001). All aspects of the care provided to an individual of a different culture must be adapted to the individual's cultural, educational, and socioeconomic needs if it is to be effective (Giger & Davidhizar, 2008).

This chapter provides an overview of the concepts and implications of cultural competence and suggests practical applications of this knowledge for the nurse case manager.

DEFINITIONS

Culture

All too often, discussions of culture and cultural competence are omitted from textbooks geared toward nurse case managers or the concepts are mentioned only briefly, within the context of another subject such as ethical issues. In reality, the recognition of culture and its influence on health is critical to the nurse case manager's ability to provide efficient health care that is fair and equitable to all individuals.

Numerous definitions of culture can be found in the literature. Unfortunately, these definitions are often too general and risk omitting important aspects of the concept. Leininger (1991) defines culture as the learned and shared norms, beliefs, lifestyles, and values of a certain group of individuals that guides, in a patterned method, decision making, thought processes, and actions. Spector (2004) compares culture to a set of luggage that contains the beliefs, practices, norms, customs, and rituals of an individual, and that is collected over a life-time and passed to later generations. Giger and Davidhizar (2008) define culture as an imprinting of the mind that occurs over time; that is shaped by beliefs, values, norms, and practices; that guides thoughts and actions; and that is passed from one generation to the next. Andrews and Boyle (2008) contend that culture provides a guide for an individual's values, beliefs, and practices and is the manner in which one perceives, behaves, and evaluates the external environment.

Common to all of these definitions of culture is the idea that each culture has values that demonstrate the unique expressions acceptable to the culture, which consequently determines how individuals process, believe, and act (Giger & Davidhizar, 2004; Spector, 2004). Of course, culture is more than just a social interaction (Leininger & McFarland, 2006). Culture is the process through which individuals learn to interpret their environment from those persons around them, such as family, friends, and community. As healthcare providers, and particularly as nurse case managers in an increasingly global society, we must understand the values, attitudes, and behaviors of others and avoid holding onto personal stereotypes and biases that may undermine or inhibit our efforts to deliver quality care (Luna, 2002).

Cultural Awareness

Cultural awareness is the conscious act of examining oneself for personal biases, prejudices, assumptions, and stereotypes (Andrews & Boyle, 2008; Campinha-Bacote, 2009; Leonard & Plotnikoff, 2000). Nurse case managers must be aware of their own biases and prejudices toward certain racial or ethnic groups so that they can avoid delivering unequal treatment and care. Many times nurses believe that they must accept another individual's cultural belief system to be culturally competent, but this is not the case. Rather, the nurse case manager must be willing and open to treat each individual as a unique human being who is deserving of equal and fair treatment (Campinha-Bacote, 2009). Many argue that we will not be successful in achieving equality in health outcomes for all individuals until there is a partnership between social justice and cultural competence (Brach & Fraser, 2000; Giddings, 2005; Stacks, Salgado, & Holmes, 2004).

Nurse case managers must also be aware of the potential for racism to arise in the healthcare delivery system and in their own practice (Broome & McGuinness, 2007). Some also contend that disparities in the quality of care provided to individuals of various ethnic and racial groups may in part be due to racial prejudices (Broome & McGuinness, 2007; Smedley, Stith, & Nelson, 2002). To provide culturally competent care, all nurse case managers must be willing to search their own attitudes and beliefs for potential biases and prejudices and rid themselves of racial attitudes that may impede their ability to provide culturally competent care that is equal and fair to all.

Cultural Encounters

Given the ever-changing demographic make-up of the U.S. population, healthcare providers, including nurse case managers, will inevitably be involved in cultural encounters on a daily basis. A cultural encounter is the interaction of the healthcare professional with an individual or family from another culture

(Taylor, 2005). Cultural encounters should be viewed as potential opportunities to gain insight and understanding of patients' cultural values and beliefs that drive many of the decisions related to their health care. Approaching cultural encounters in this manner and with a positive mindset will allow the nurse case manager to establish a trusting and open relationship with the patient and family with whom he or she is working.

Cultural Competence

To become culturally competent, the nurse case manager must have knowledge, skill, and acceptance of the diversity found among the individuals requiring healthcare services (Luna, 2002). Achieving cultural competence for the nurse case manager depends on the personal philosophy and ethics that drive an individual's specific practices and actions (Luna, 2002). Over the past several years, a consistent effort has been made to improve the level of cultural awareness among healthcare providers so as to improve cultural competence in healthcare delivery (Muñoz, 2001). Achieving this level of cultural competence will allow the nurse case manager to exhibit attitudes, beliefs, and behaviors that show respect and acceptance of diverse cultures.

Providing culturally appropriate care has increasingly become a priority across many health services disciplines, such as medicine, physical therapy, social work, and pharmacy, and has become a standard of care for individuals and families. Organizations seeking state and national accreditation must now demonstrate that they provide culturally competent care to their patients. It is important to note, however, that cultural competence is an ongoing process that seeks to continually improve interactions and relationships so as to provide quality health care to all individuals of various racial and ethnic backgrounds.

Cultural Skill

Cultural skill is the ability of the nurse case manager to accurately perform a culturally based assessment of the individual to gain culturally relevant information (Campinha-Bacote, 2009). It allows the nurse case manager to ask open-ended questions in a culturally sensitive manner, thereby gathering useful information related to the individual's perspective of his or her illness. Cultural skill requires that the nurse case manager be able and willing to critically think through the assessment of the individual and to realize that different assessment skills are necessary for persons from different cultures.

Cultural Knowledge

To be effective in dealing with individuals from many different cultures, nurse case managers must have a desire to become more culturally competent. Campinha-Bacote (2009) describes this cultural desire as the energy and foundation for the cultural competence journey. Such a desire consists of a genuine attempt to be open and flexible to others, willing to learn from others, and accepting of different attitudes (Taylor, 2005). Attempts to develop cultural competence as a result of job requirements or professional responsibility will not be successful; instead, nurse case managers must take on a attitude of humility and evince a deep desire to uncover and learn about the attitudes and beliefs of persons who are different from them (Campinha-Bacote, 2009).

Ethnocentrism

Ethnocentrism, according to Thiederman (1986), refers to the belief that the values and norms of one culture are the best or the only acceptable ones. Nurse case managers must be able to accurately interpret their ethnocentric behaviors and responses to patients and families and recognize how these actions affect their care. Nurse case managers should not expect individuals of diverse cultures to change or conform to their practices or beliefs. Rather, the interventions or approach to care should be altered to meet the cultural needs of each individual. To guard against ethnocentrism, the nurse case manager must have a clear understanding of his or her own culture. Otherwise, there may be distortions related to the nurse case manager's perception of the patient and family that go beyond the lack of knowledge related to the patient's culture (Thiederman, 1986).

Bias and Stereotyping

Despite years of interventions, personal biases and stereotypes persist in our society today. Many individuals, including healthcare providers, may not be aware of these biases and the ways in which they affect a provider's interactions with patients. Nurse case managers must be willing to identify the sources of their personal biases or discrimination through self-reflection (Cohen & Cesta, 2005). Personal biases and stereotypes may have either a positive or a negative effect on nurse case managers' interactions with the patient or family for whom they are providing care. In some cases, the provider may not be aware of the effects on the relationship. For example, the nurse case manager might have personal biases related to the consumption of resources and the burden of care imposed by individuals who are illegal immigrants to the United

States (Carr, 2006). These biases may influence how that nurse case manager perceives, relates to, and cares for individuals from a certain culture. Although these biases and stereotypes may go undetected by the nurse case manager, they may have critical effects on the patient and family and severely inhibit the nurse case manager's relationship with the patient and family (Cohen & Cesta, 2005). For all these reasons, personal biases and stereotypes must be identified early and dealt with by the individual before cultural competence can be achieved.

Stigmatization

Stigma generally refers to negative attitudes that may be detrimental to an individual's interpersonal interactions (Paterson, Backmund, Hirsch, & Yim, 2007). These attitudes may take various forms; for example, ridicule, stereotyping, and name calling are all verbal forms of stigma. Stigma may result in discrimination, such as when healthcare providers refuse to accept and treat individuals based on their socioeconomic status or their ability to pay for services.

Vulnerable groups are at risk of stigmatization by society in general. For example, healthcare providers may hold the stigma that all individuals with hepatitis C are drug users who acquired the disease by injecting drugs (Paterson et al., 2007). As a result, these patients may be viewed as irresponsible and unimportant by the healthcare provider. This type of stigmatization may cause an individual with a disease to withhold important information and avoid further testing or treatment, resulting in depression and isolation for the individual with the disease (Paterson et al., 2007).

Another example of stigmatization occurs in children and adolescents and is related to body weight. Obesity in children and adolescents is increasingly becoming a public health issue, and this trend is disproportionately affecting children of Hispanic and African American cultures (Margulies, Floyd, & Hojnoski, 2008). Owing to their relationship with overweight and obesity, the incidence and prevalence of diseases such as diabetes, asthma, and hypertension have also begun to rise in younger age groups (Obesity Society, 2009). Stigma and biases have negative effects on the emotional well-being of a child, which may result in the child developing low self-esteem, depression, and social isolation (Obesity Society, 2009).

As nurse case managers working with vulnerable populations, it is imperative to approach these individuals with sensitivity, free of judgments and criticisms. The healthcare environment should be supportive of all individuals and not contribute to the negative attitudes that may be prevalent in the larger society. Healthcare providers, including nurse case managers, must be willing to change their attitudes and behaviors toward stigmatized populations. Further research is needed to explore whether the current healthcare and social systems are continuing to contribute to the negative practices and approaches of healthcare providers in relation to these vulnerable populations.

CULTURAL COMPETENCE OVERVIEW

"Cultural competence" has become a more widely used term as our awareness of the demographic differences within the larger society continues to evolve. Despite their best intentions, healthcare professionals, including nurse case managers, sometimes fail to change or modify their approaches to practice in response to the cultural needs of their patients and families (Taylor, 2005), which may result in actions that are perceived as culturally offensive or disrespectful. Nurse case managers may achieve cultural competence by striving for a more sophisticated level of thinking, attitudes, and personal beliefs (Giger & Davidhizar, 2004). This practice will, in turn, allow the nurse case manager to better manage and effectively design interventions that will optimize individual health, regardless of the person's cultural background. The manner in which individuals are viewed and care is provided is highly influenced by culture. It is important for nurse case managers to understand and realize this influence and to view each person as culturally unique. To do so, they must be able to discern their own cultural values and worldviews and not to attempt to impose them on the individual receiving the care.

MODELS OF CULTURAL COMPETENCE

Transcultural Nursing and the Cultural Care Model

Cultural competence is not a new concept to nursing. The idea of transcultural nursing was first introduced by Dr. Madeleine M. Leininger in the mid-1950s when she began to realize that culture and caring were two dimensions missing among healthcare services, including nursing (Leininger & McFarland, 2006). The goal of transcultural nursing is to use culturally based research as the foundation for delivering culturally appropriate care to individuals of varying cultural backgrounds (Leininger, 1991). After many years of study and research, Leininger developed the theory of "culture care diversity and universality" and the Sunrise Enabler to Discover Culture Care model (Leininger & McFarland, 2006). This theory and model provide nurses and nurse case managers with an effective guide for thinking, practice, and research (Leininger & McFarland, 2006).

The model of "culturally congruent care" (Schim, Doorenbos, Benkert, & Miller, 2007) builds on the work by Leininger and includes concepts at the provider and patient level. Schim and colleagues (2007) describe four constructs as the components necessary for the healthcare provider to achieve culturally congruent care: (1) cultural diversity, (2) cultural awareness, (3) cultural sensitivity, and (4) cultural competence. In this model, cultural diversity is evident in all aspects of life and society and varies depending on the demographic changes. This construct takes into consideration the effects of the cultural changes in society and the associated needs of the diverse cultural groups. Cultural awareness, according to this model, refers to the cognitive recognition of differences between groups. Cultural sensitivity is the attitudinal construct that refers to an individual's openness to acquiring knowledge related to diverse cultures. Finally, cultural competence is the behavioral response of the provider to the other three components of the model. For example, the nurse case manager may demonstrate an increase in knowledge related to diverse cultural groups and adapt the care provided as needed (Schim et al., 2007).

The Cultural Competence Model

Another model for cultural competence is known as "the process of cultural competence in the delivery of healthcare services" (Campinha-Bacote, 2002). According to this model, cultural competence is a dynamic process of five interrelated constructs: (1) cultural awareness, (2) cultural knowledge, (3) cultural skill, (4) cultural encounter, and (5) cultural desire (Campinha-Bacote, 2002; Campinha-Bacote & Muñoz, 2001). No matter where the nurse case manager enters the process, all five constructs must be experienced for cultural competence to be achieved (Campinha-Bacote & Muñoz, 2001). As the nurse case manager becomes more culturally aware, he or she will be less likely to label certain groups or attach negative stigmas to members of these groups. Rather, the nurse case manager will begin to critically think about which health services are needed to meet the particular needs of that cultural group and how the nurse case manager may facilitate meeting those needs (Campinha-Bacote & Muñoz, 2001).

As the nurse case manager seeks to gain cultural knowledge or to find information related to a specific culture, it is important to focus on the culture's health-related beliefs and values. This step includes understanding the culture's worldviews related to health and illness and discovering how these views guide the decision-making process employed by the members of the cultural group (Campinha-Bacote & Muñoz, 2001). The more knowledge the nurse case manager has regarding a particular culture, the less likely he or she will be to misinterpret certain actions, especially in conjunction with ethically related issues such as death and dying. Another key factor related to cultural knowledge is the importance of understanding disease prevalence, incidence, and differences in medication effectiveness among certain cultural groups (Campinha-Bacote & Muñoz, 2001).

The nurse case manager must also develop cultural skill so that he or she can obtain an appropriate cultural assessment of an individual and family. Being aware of how an individual's biological, physiological, and physical variations influence the physical examination is essential for the nurse case manager (Campinha-Bacote, 1999). For example, culturally related variations in body structure, skin color, hair texture, and facial features are important to recognize (Campinha-Bacote & Muñoz, 2001). Cultural skill also requires proper communication between the nurse case manager and the individual. To meet this goal, interpreters should be used as needed to ensure effective communication.

The nurse case manager should view each cultural encounter as an opportunity to learn more and to become more culturally competent. Of course, just because a nurse case manager has cared for several individuals from the same cultural background, it does not mean that the healthcare provider is culturally competent in that culture. Becoming culturally competent is much more complex, and the nurse case manager must continue to seek to learn more about the diverse cultures he or she encounters during the journey to becoming culturally competent.

The Cultural Development Model

Wells (2000) has developed the cultural development model (CDM), which proposes that cultural development goes beyond cultural awareness, cultural sensitivity, and cultural competence. This CDM consists of a continuum of six stages, divided into cognitive and affective phases, which require change within the healthcare professional and his or her institution. The cognitive phase consists of cultural incompetence, cultural knowledge, and cultural awareness stages; the focus of this phase is on learning about the culture (Wells, 2000). The affective phase consists of cultural sensitivity, cultural competence, and cultural proficiency. During this phase, the nurse case manager focuses on changing attitudes and actions by applying the knowledge gained in the cognitive phase (Wells, 2000). The first challenge of this and other models of cultural competence is examining oneself and creating change as needed.

The Transcultural Assessment Model

Giger and Davidhizar (2004) describe cultural competence as a dynamic, fluid, continuous process by which healthcare providers develop effective strategies for healthcare delivery that are based on the cultural attitudes, beliefs, and behaviors of the individuals receiving the care. The goal of transcultural nursing is to discover culturally relevant facts about the individual and family receiving the care and to use those facts as a guide for assessing, planning, implementing, and evaluating the care needed in a culturally appropriate manner (Giger & Davidhizar, 2004). The transcultural assessment model (Giger & Davidhizar, 2004, 2008) provides a method for assessing individual cultural variables and their effects on health behaviors. It contends that individuals are culturally unique. As such, the model identifies six cultural phenomena that affect health and should be included in a cultural assessment: (1) time orientation, (2) space, (3) social organization, (4) environmental control, (5) biological variation, and (6) communication (Giger & Davidhizar, 2002, 2004).

Each cultural group has *a time orientation* component that may vary among the members of the group. The time focus of a culture may be past, present, or future (Giger & Davidhizar, 2002). For example, cultures with a future orientation focus on long-range goals and engage in measures to prevent disease and illness in the future. These types of cultures are very schedule oriented and use appointments to organize activities (Spector, 2004). Other cultures are oriented more to the present and not as much to the future; thus they may be less concerned with long-range planning. Therefore, conflicts may arise with healthcare providers, as individuals with this type of time orientation may be consistently late to appointments and less concerned with long-term planning. As the nurse case manager works with patients and families from different cultures with various time orientations, it becomes important to ask patients about their expectations related to time (Spector, 2004). It is also critical that the case manager explain his or her expectations of time and the importance of scheduled appointments or meetings. This discussion may help to eliminate confusion in the future related to time and scheduled appointments.

The use of personal *space* is influenced by an individual's cultural group, but also varies among individuals within diverse groups. Nurse case managers should be sensitive and respectful of an individual's personal space. Four zones of interpersonal space have been defined: (1) intimate space (up to 1.5 feet); (2) personal distance (up to 4 feet); (3) social distance (between 4 and 12 feet); and (4) public distance (more than 12 feet) (Spector, 2004). Nurse case managers must be aware of the implications of space within a culture and take care not to violate a patient's intimate space, as doing so may create an uncomfortable situation for the individual.

Social organization refers to the immediate and extended family unit that influences the individual's cultural identification (Spector, 2004). The social environment shapes an individual's cultural behavior and determines what is acceptable in certain social situations. Patterned cultural behaviors are internalized through enculturation—that is, the process of acquiring knowledge and values by observing the life experiences of those within the social environment (Giger & Davidhizar, 2004).

Environmental control refers to the complex traditional health beliefs of a culture and the use of folk medicine and traditional healers as a method to direct or control environmental factors. This factor plays an important role in individuals' responses to illness and health and their use of healthcare resources (Giger & Davidhizar, 2002; Spector, 2004). Further discussion of alternative health practices appears later in this chapter.

Biological variation refers to the physical and genetic characteristics of individuals belonging to a particular culture (Giger & Davidhizar, 2004). For example, certain cultural groups may respond differently to medications, have different food preferences and nutritional needs, and be more susceptible to certain diseases, such as sickle cell disease in African Americans (Giger & Davidhizar, 2004). As previously discussed, the nurse case manager must possess cultural skill in assessment of individuals from diverse cultures.

Communication is often the most significant obstacle for individuals of diverse cultures and healthcare providers, including nurse case managers (Giger & Davidhizar, 2004). Language differences may create cultural barriers and result in a negative experience for the patient. Nurse case managers should avoid becoming frustrated with individuals who speak different languages and take steps to ensure that the communication is understood and effective. This task may be accomplished with the use of a competent, skilled interpreter (Giger & Davidhizar, 2004; Spector, 2004). The impact of communication and cultural competence is discussed further in the next section.

CULTURAL COMPETENCE AND COMMUNICATION

According to the 2000 U.S. Census, nearly 47 million people in the United States—or one in five persons age 5 and older—speak a language other than English at home (U.S. DOC, Census Bureau, 2003). According to Andrews and Boyle (2008), the term "cultural competence" implies that the nurse case manager has developed certain psychomotor or behavioral skills such as using effective communication methods for non-English-speaking individuals and families. Communication is an essential part of the healthcare provider–patient relationship, and open communication must be facilitated in an effective manner (Muñoz, 2001). Establishing trust through appropriate communication is essential to the success of the relationship and implies that the nurse case manager understands the individual's cultural needs related to his or her health care (Muñoz, 2001).

Two forms of communication are distinguished: verbal and nonverbal. Effective verbal communication or oral language comprises an exchange process between the nurse case manager and the patient (Muñoz & Luckmann, 2005). Unfortunately, language barriers may create frustration and distrust among individuals of diverse cultures. Ensuring that a properly trained interpreter is used when communicating with patients and families will help to decrease the potential for confusion and misunderstanding. The nurse case manager should avoid using family members and especially children as translators, however, as this increases the potential for miscommunication and errors.

Nonverbal or body language is the second form of communication. Many times the impact of nonverbal communication, such as eye contact, touch, and silence, is overlooked in relation to cultural competence. Eye contact is a nonverbal communication tool that is viewed differently among cultures. In some cases, nurse case managers may have been taught to always maintain eye contact with the individuals with whom they are speaking; however, this behavior may be perceived by other cultures as disrespectful or aggressive. For example, Native Americans may look toward the floor during discussions to demonstrate their attentiveness to what the speaker is saying (Andrews & Boyle, 2008). Eye contact in many cultures is also related to respect for the elders in the family, as in the Hispanic cultures.

While touch is a vital component of holistic nursing, careful consideration should be given to the use of touch with individuals from different cultures (Spector, 2004). Some cultures have strict values and beliefs related to touch, especially for children and women. For example, in many Hispanic and Arabic cultures, women may refuse assessment by a male healthcare provider (Andrews & Boyle, 2008). It is important for the nurse case manager to be aware of this information when assisting patients and families with follow-up appointments with healthcare providers. Also, the nurse case manager should always ask permission of all patients prior to touching them for an examination, as this practice demonstrates respect for their personal (intimate) space and their cultural values. Nurse case managers are also in a pivotal position to educate and inform others in the healthcare setting about an individual's views and beliefs regarding nonverbal communication, which may in turn improve and build trust within the patient–provider relationship.

In some cultures, such as Native Americans, silence is viewed as an important part of understanding and respect, indicating that the information provided deserves thoughtful consideration (Andrews & Boyle, 2008). Other individuals find silence to be uncomfortable. In traditional Asian cultures, such as Chinese and Japanese cultures, silence provides a time for the listener to focus on the content provided by the speaker before moving on with the conversation (Andrews & Boyle, 2008). The nurse case manager should be aware of how silence is perceived by the cultural group to which the patient belongs and respect those practices during the cultural encounter.

Effective cultural competence and communication requires awareness, sensitivity, and knowledge of cultures (Muñoz, 2001). Nurse case managers must understand and appreciate the importance of language and culture and the effects of effective communication on healthcare delivery. They must also have a willingness to engage in open communication with patients and families regardless of any differences in language. As the demographic characteristics of the United States continue to change, it is not appropriate to assume that all individuals who seek healthcare services will be proficient in the English language. Indeed, such an assumption creates many challenges and barriers to effective care as these individuals and families attempt to navigate the highly complex U.S. healthcare system. Nurse case managers must be advocates for these individuals and strive to break down these barriers that create these disparities in care. Effective communication ensures an accurate health history, gathers information about the patient's health beliefs and attitudes, and leads to the development of an acceptable plan of care (Muñoz, 2001). It also develops trust between the nurse case manager and the individual and family, which in turn may result in better adherence to the plan of care and improved healthcare outcomes.

CULTURAL ISSUES RELATED TO HEALTH CARE

As part of the *Healthy People 2020* initiative, one of the overarching goals is to eliminate health disparities among different groups of the U.S. population (U.S. Department of Health and Human Services, 2008). Significant disparities in health outcomes continue to exist among minority groups in the United States. For example, the mortality rate from heart disease is 40% higher in African Americans than in Caucasian Americans (American Heart Association [AHA], 2009), and the rate for prostate cancer is more than double in African American males (Centers for Disease Control and Prevention [CDC], 2009b).

Many times healthcare professionals may fail to recognize the ineffectiveness of their interventions due to a lack of cultural awareness and an inability to alter their approach so as to provide culturally appropriate care. For example, healthcare facilities often provide informational brochures related to certain illnesses and diseases, but these brochures may not always be available in languages other than English. The need for cultural competence in health care is clear, yet most healthcare professionals find it quite challenging to achieve (Taylor, 2005). Many professionals, including nurse case managers, may lack the awareness, knowledge, skills, and time needed to become effective as culturally competent providers (Taylor, 2005).

Relationship Between Health Beliefs and Culture

Culture influences individual expectations and perceptions regarding health outcomes and disease (Giger & Davidhizar, 2008). These influences help to shape our worldviews of health and illness, which includes the assumptions, beliefs, and explanations regarding life events that are specific to a particular cultural group (Andrews & Boyle, 2008). This health belief system or worldview is often shared among similar culture groups and may differ from that of the nurse case manager.

An example of a health belief system is the use of folk or traditional healers as a method of seeking care for a disease or illness. It is important for the nurse case manager to recognize and accept these traditional healers as part of the care for the individual. Allowing personal biases to interfere with care and cause judgments to be made may result in distrust and miscommunication between the case manager and the patient (Andrews & Boyle, 2008). Instead, the nurse case manager should be respectful and listen to the traditional healer, as he or she may be able to provide insightful information related to the culture and the patient receiving the care. Many times the folk healer may use spiritual healing as part of the remedies, or there may be a separate spiritual leader involved in the individual's life (Andrews & Boyle, 2008). With an increasing level of cultural awareness and cultural competence, the nurse case manager will feel more comfortable in allowing such a traditional healer to be a part of the care of the individual and to work together with healthcare providers to provide quality care that is respectful of the individual's culture.

Complementary and alternative medicine (CAM) therapies are also important for the nurse case manager to understand, in terms of both their impact and the influence of culture on these therapies. While the safety and efficacy of many of these therapies are not well established, CAM is widely used and accepted in many cultures. Such therapies include practices such as acupuncture, aromatherapy, massage, Reiki, Therapeutic Touch, and meditation, among many others. The nurse case manager must remain open to the patient's use of these therapies and include them in the plan of care as appropriate (Andrews & Boyle, 2008).

Diverse Cultures in United States

The nurse case manger should understand and realize that in many cases certain demographic factors contribute to the racial health disparities that exist in our society today. Such factors may include socioeconomic status (education, employment, and poverty), lifestyle choices (physical activity and alcohol consumption), social environment (economic opportunities, racial/ethnic discrimination, and communities), and access to health promotion services (cancer screening and vaccination) (Williams, Neighbors, & Jackson, 2003). As a consequence of these factors, the nurse case manager must understand and realize that the interventions and strategies used with an African American male with hypertension, for example, will not be the same as those used with a Hispanic male with the same condition.

The African American population in the United States is projected to increase from 41.1 million people in 2008 to 65.7 million people by 2050 (U.S. DOC, U.S. Census Bureau, 2008). It is impossible to characterize all African American individuals as sharing the same characteristics, because this is a very diverse group within itself. Some African Americans view illness as an imbalance in the individual's life, whereas others believe that every event has an opposite event that occurs. For example, for every illness diagnosis, there is a cure for someone else (Giger & Davidhizar, 2008). This cultural belief is important for the nurse case manager to understand and recognize, because it may influence the individual's willingness to seek medical care or engage in preventive interventions. Nevertheless, there are certain commonalities that are important for the nurse case manager to be aware of and to take into consideration when planning and coordinating care for this cultural group. For example, in most African American families, the focus is on the woman or mother, who is seen as being responsible for ensuring the health of the family (Giger & Davidhizar, 2008).

Some African Americans look only at the current situation (present time focused) and are not future time oriented. Many view time as flexible, in which case it is important that the nurse case manager work with the individual and family members to understand the importance of taking medications on time and not skipping a dose (Giger & Davidhizar, 2008). Many African Americans may believe that if they forget their medications today, it is acceptable to take double doses the next day to catch up. In this situation, the nurse case manager should educate the individual on proper medication administration while maintaining respect for the cultural differences demonstrated by this belief system.

African Americans remain over represented among populations with life-threatening illnesses such as cancer and cardiovascular disease. African American males continue to have extraordinarily high death rates from myocardial infarction—higher than the rates found among any other group in the United States (AHA, 2009). African Americans are also at a disproportional risk of death from stroke (AHA, 2009) and HIV/AIDS; they account for nearly half of all HIV/AIDS cases in the United States, for example (CDC, 2007). Although other factors, such as lifestyle choices, socioeconomic status, and genetics, influence African Americans' increased incidence of these diseases, it is important for the nurse case manager to work with each individual to identify specific barriers to health promotion and prevention.

The Hispanic American population in the United States is projected to nearly triple in coming years, from 46.7 million in 2008 to 132.8 million in 2050 (U.S. DOC, Census Bureau, 2008). By 2050, one in three U.S. residents will be Hispanic (U.S. DOC, Census Bureau, 2008). Due to disparities among demographic factors such as educational level and socioeconomic status, many Hispanic Americans currently lack health insurance coverage; indeed, they may not understand why insurance is needed (Giger & Davidhizar, 2008). Many Hispanic Americans continue to rely on their cultural-based traditional remedies as the primary method of meeting their healthcare needs.

Spanish is the common language among Hispanic Americans; however, it may be spoken in several dialects depending on the origin of the individual. This diversity creates challenges for communication and illustrates the need to use properly trained interpreters. Hispanic Americans may be hesitant to reveal information about themselves to strangers (Giger & Davidhizar, 2008). Consequently, it is important for the nurse case manager to develop a trusting relationship with the individual and family to elicit the most information related to the person's health and cultural practices. Hispanic Americans are also very respectful and value courtesy. They may not follow through on tasks or arrangements, however, owing to a lack of understanding of the importance of the task (Giger & Davidhizar, 2008).

Within the Hispanic culture, family is highly valued. Generally, families are large and several families may reside together in the same home. Traditionally, the male is considered the decision maker and the authority figure in the family (Giger & Davidhizar, 2008; Spector, 2004). Hispanic Americans are present time oriented and may not be willing to make appointments or commitments for the future. Health beliefs among members of this cultural group vary, with some believing health is a result of good luck or a reward from God, and others viewing health as representing a state of balance within the universe (Giger & Davidhizar, 2008; Spector, 2004). Like African Americans, Hispanic Americans often rely on traditional remedies for healing and health.

The leading causes of death among Hispanic Americans are heart disease, cancer, and unintentional injuries or accidents (CDC, 2009a). Diabetes is another growing health concern among the Hispanic American population. According to the CDC, the prevalence of diabetes among this population is more than double that among the non-Hispanic American population (CDC, 2004). Nurse case managers should carefully assess the dietary habits of the individuals with whom they are working and provide culturally appropriate information related to healthy food choices. They should also discuss factors such as accessibility to healthy food options, which may continue to create barriers to optimal health for Hispanic Americans.

Asian Americans are among the many minority groups that are subject to wide disparities in health care. The Asian American population within the United States is expected to grow from 15.5 million people (5.1% of the total U.S. population) in 2008 to 40.6 million (9.2%) by 2050 (U.S. DOC, U.S. Census Bureau, 2008). Heart disease, cancer, and stroke are among the leading causes of death for this population (CDC, 2008). The Asian culture believes that health is a state of balance or harmony between spirit and physical concerns. Members of this culture typically value nutrition as a method of maintaining health, along with daily exercise (Spector, 2004). Asian Americans also often use CAM as a method to control pain and other symptoms. For example, acupuncture is widely used for the treatment of pain by members of this culture, and herbal remedies are a widely practiced tradition of the ancient healers (Spector, 2004).

Language barriers that may prevent effective communication are prevalent in the Asian American population. These individuals typically feel isolated when they are in the hospital setting. Indeed, a hospitalization presents many challenges for Asian American patients, including food preferences, communication, and general confusion regarding the practices and procedures (Spector, 2004). In general, the Asian Americans do not complain about their hospital experiences. Instead, they may sit quietly in their room, not eating, and not able to communicate. Unfortunately, many healthcare providers who lack cultural competence and are not sensitive to patients' cultural beliefs and practices may interpret this behavior as indicating satisfaction with the care provided (Spector, 2004).

Ethical Issues

In today's healthcare settings, nurse case managers will face multiple ethical challenges related to diversity. Ethical dilemmas occur when culturally based moral practices conflict with the ethics of human rights (Donnelly, 2000). Issues may arise in determining which values are right or wrong. For example, finding the balance between financial responsibility and adequate care has raised many questions about the motivations underlying decisions made by healthcare professionals and their services provided to individuals of diverse cultures (Mullahy, 1999). The increase in the number of undocumented immigrants to the United States has also raised concerns among all healthcare providers as they struggle to meet the needs of these patients. Nurse case managers, for example, may be faced with the ethical dilemma of coordinating care for individuals who have entered the United States without proper documentation (Carr, 2006). In all circumstances, nurse case managers must uphold the tenets of ethical practice while respecting the patient's dignity and autonomy (Donnelly, 2000).

Ultimately, each nurse case manager must strive to become culturally competent by acknowledging the differences among individuals, advocating for those culturally diverse groups who are marginalized by the current healthcare system, and maintaining zero tolerance for biases and prejudices that might lead to inequality in care (Meleis, 1999). Clinical expertise, combined with the knowledge of resources related to cost, and a caring focus, has in many situations put the nurse case manager in the position of being the ethical link in the solution (Mullahy, 1999). The one-size-fits-all approach is no longer acceptable. The nurse case manager has the opportunity to lead the way in evaluating decisions that are made in a stereotypical manner (Mullahy, 1999) and striving to remain culturally up-to-date.

▪ SUMMARY

Providing culturally competent care is essential to nurse case managers as we strive to remove the barriers that result in disparities in care provided to minority populations. Increasing cultural awareness, both on an individual level and within the profession as a whole, is the first step in this process to improve the quality of health care provided. Increased understanding of the multiple facets of cultural competence and a focus on improving cultural skills will allow the nurse case manager to proceed with a more efficient cultural encounter with patients and families of different racial and ethnic backgrounds. Various cultural competence models provide a framework to guide the process of improving cultural competence both within the individual healthcare professional and within the institution.

Nurse case managers who respect the cultural values and beliefs of others will be more effective in establishing trust and effective communication. Trust and communication are essential factors to forming a positive relationship between the nurse case manager and the patient and family. Effective communication provides an avenue for developing trust between the nurse case manager and the individual, which in turn demonstrates the nurse case manager's understanding of the influence the individual's culture has on his or her healthcare beliefs and decisions. As the demographics of the U.S. population continue to change, nurse case managers must strive to provide culturally competent health care and set an example for other healthcare professionals within their institutions in an effort to improve care for all people.

■ CASE STUDIES

The first step to becoming culturally competent is to know yourself and your own heritage, including your values and beliefs that may be based on your culture, your social interactions, and your life experiences. Because our society is becoming more diverse, both nurses and nurse case managers must address issues of cultural awareness and sensitivity.

Ask yourself the following questions:

1. What is my personal ethno-cultural heritage, and how deeply do I identify with it?
2. How deeply do I identify with my personal and professional heritage?
3. What is my own cultural blindness, bias, or prejudice?
4. What are some examples of my stereotyping a group of people?
5. What have I learned about health in the context of my personal heritage and from my education as a healthcare professional?
6. Think about the fact that the nursing profession has its own cultural heritage, which may not always be in synchrony with the patient's or family's cultural beliefs and expectations. As nurses, we are socialized into a system of beliefs. What are some examples of beliefs or values that we adhere to? Describe a case in which your own beliefs and values were called into question.

■ DISCUSSION QUESTIONS

1. Why is culturally competent care an essential ingredient for quality care?
2. What is the role of a case manager on an interdisciplinary case management team?
3. Why is communication so important to building effective partnerships?
4. What are the keys to establishing good patient communication?
5. Why does a positive vision help to empower families to try to participate in their own care?
6. Define each of the following terms:

   a. Prejudice
   b. Bias
   c. Discrimination
   d. Stereotyping
   e. Stigmatization

■ CLASSROOM EXERCISES

1. Working with your fellow students, assess the degree of successful collaboration among different ethnic groups within your present organizations.
2. How effective is the organization in developing programs to meet the needs of a diverse population?
3. How do the services that focus on culture differ from the usual services provided?
4. Identify a group in your geographical area whose members you realize have been stereotyped and stigmatized. Analyze how this has happened and which factors contributed to this process.
5. Define the culture of poverty. Did poverty contribute to the stigmatization of the group identified in Exercise 4? How does powerlessness affect the group's ability to access care?

■ RECOMMENDED READINGS

Brach, C., & Fraser, I. (2000). Can cultural competency reduce racial and ethnic health disparities? A review and conceptual model. *Medical Care Research and Review, 57*(Suppl. 1), 181–217.

Broome, B., & McGuinness, T. (2007). A CRASH course in cultural competence for nurses. *Urologic Nursing, 27*(4), 292–304.

Campinha-Bacote, J. (1999). A model and instrument for addressing cultural competence in health care. *Journal of Nursing Education, 38*(5), 203–207.

Campinha-Bacote, J. (2002). The process of cultural competence in the delivery of healthcare services: A model of care. *Journal of Transcultural Nursing, 13*(3), 181–184.

Campinha-Bacote, J. (2009). A culturally competent model of care for African Americans. *Urologic Nursing, 29*(1), 49–54.

Campinha-Bacote, J., & Muñoz, C. (2001). A guiding framework for delivering culturally competent services in case management. *Case Manager, 12*(2), 48–52.

Donnelly, P. L. (2000). Ethics and cross-cultural nursing. *Journal of Transcultural Nursing, 11*(2), 119–126.

Dreachslin, J. L. (2007). Diversity management and cultural competence: Research, practice, and the business case. *Journal of Healthcare Management, 52*(2), 79–86.

Margulies, A. S., Floyd, R. G., & Hojnoski, R. L. (2008). Body size stigmatization: An examination of attitudes of African American preschool-age children attending Head Start. *Journal of Pediatric Psychology, 33*(5), 487–496.

Meleis, A. I. (1999). Culturally competent care. *Journal of Transcultural Nursing, 10*(1), 12.

Taylor, R. (2005). Addressing barriers to cultural competence. *Journal for Nurses in Staff Development, 21*(4), 135–142.

Thiederman, S. B. (1986). Ethnocentricism: A barrier to effective health care. *Nurse Practitioner, 11*(8), 52–59.

■ REFERENCES

American Heart Association (AHA). (2009). *Heart disease and stroke statistics.* Retrieved July 2, 2009, from http://www.americanheart.org/downloadable/heart/1240250946756LS1982%20Heart%20and%20Stroke%20Update.042009.pdf

Andrews, M. M., & Boyle, J. S. (2008). *Transcultural concepts in nursing care* (5th ed.). Philadelphia, PA: Wolters Kluwer/Lippincott Williams & Wilkins.

Brach, C., & Fraser, I. (2000). Can cultural competency reduce racial and ethnic health disparities? A review and conceptual model. *Medical Care Research and Review, 57*(Suppl. 1), 181–217.

Broome, B., & McGuinness, T. (2007). A CRASH course in cultural competence for nurses. *Urologic Nursing, 27*(4), 292–304.

Campinha-Bacote, J. (1999). A model and instrument for addressing cultural competence in health care. *Journal of Nursing Education, 38*(5), 203–207.

Campinha-Bacote, J. (2002). The process of cultural competence in the delivery of healthcare services: A model of care. *Journal of Transcultural Nursing, 13*(3), 181–184.

Campinha-Bacote, J. (2009). A culturally competent model of care for African Americans. *Urologic Nursing, 29*(1), 49–54.

Campinha-Bacote, J., & Muñoz, C. (2001). A guiding framework for delivering culturally competent services in case management. *Case Manager, 12*(2), 48–52.

Carr, D. D. (2006). Implications for case management: Ensuring access and delivery of quality health care to undocumented immigrant populations. *Lippincott's Case Management, 11*(4), 195–204.

Centers for Disease Control and Prevention (CDC). (2004, October 15). Prevalence of diabetes among Hispanics: Selected areas, 1998–2002. *Morbidity and Mortality Weekly Report, 53*(40), 941–944.

Centers for Disease Control and Prevention (CDC). (2007). *HIV and African Americans.* Retrieved July 12, 2009, from http://www.cdc.gov/hiv/topics/aa

Centers for Disease Control and Prevention (CDC). (2008). *Asian American populations.* Retrieved July 10, 2009, from http://www.cdc.gov/omhd/Populations/AsianAm/AsianAm.htm

Centers for Disease Control and Prevention (CDC). (2009a). *Health of Hispanic or Latino population.* Retrieved July 12, 2009, from http://www.cdc.gov/nchs/fastats/hispanic_health.htm

Centers for Disease Control and Prevention (CDC). (2009b). *Prostate cancer rates by race and ethnicity.* Retrieved July 12, 2009, from http://www.cdc.gov/cancer/prostate/statistics/race.htm

Cohen, E. L., & Cesta, T. G. (2005). *Nursing case management: From essentials to advanced practice applications* (4th ed.). St. Louis, MO: Elsevier Mosby.

Donnelly, P. L. (2000). Ethics and cross-cultural nursing. *Journal of Transcultural Nursing, 11*(2), 119–126.

Dreachslin, J. L. (2007). Diversity management and cultural competence: Research, practice, and the business case. *Journal of Healthcare Management, 52*(2), 79–86.

Giddings, L. S. (2005). Health disparities, social injustice, and the culture of nursing. *Nursing Research, 54*(5), 304–312.

Giger, J. N., & Davidhizar, R. E. (2002). The Giger and Davidhizar transcultural assessment model. *Journal of Transcultural Nursing, 13*(3), 185–188.

Giger, J. N., & Davidhizar, R. E. (2004). *Transcultural nursing: Assessment and intervention* (4th ed.). St. Louis, MO: Mosby.

Giger, J. N., & Davidhizar, R. E. (2008). *Transcultural nursing: Assessment and intervention* (5th ed.). St. Louis, MO: Mosby Elsevier.

Leininger, M. M. (1991). The theory of culture care diversity and universality. In M. M. Leininger (Ed.), *Culture care diversity and universality: A theory of nursing* (pp. 5–68). New York: National League for Nursing Press.

Leininger, M. M., & McFarland, M. R. (2006). *Cultural care diversity and universality: A worldwide nursing theory* (2nd ed.). Sudbury, MA: Jones and Bartlett.

Leonard, B. J., & Plotnikoff, G. A. (2000). Awareness: The heart of cultural competence. *AACN Clinical Issues, 11*(1), 51–59.

Luna, I. (2002). Diversity issues in the delivery of healthcare. *Lippincott's Case Management, 7*(4), 138–146.

Margulies, A. S., Floyd, R. G., & Hojnoski, R. L. (2008). Body size stigmatization: An examination of attitudes of African American preschool-age children attending Head Start. *Journal of Pediatric Psychology, 33*(5), 487–496.

Meleis, A. I. (1999). Culturally competent care. *Journal of Transcultural Nursing, 10*(1), 12.

Mullahy, C. M. (1999). Case management: An ethically responsible solution. *Case Manager, 10*(5), 59–62.

Muñoz, C. C. (2001). Addressing the linguistic and cultural needs of case management clients. *Case Manager, 12*(6), 58–62.

Muñoz, C., & Luckmann, J. (2005). *Transcultural communication in nursing* (2nd ed.). Clifton Park, NY: Thomson Delmar Learning.

Obesity Society. (2009). *Obesity, bias, and stigmatization.* Retrieved July 10, 2009, from http://www.obesity.org/information/weight_bias.asp

Paterson, B. L., Backmund, M., Hirsch, G., & Yim, C. (2007). The depiction of stigmatization in research about hepatitis C. *International Journal of Drug Policy, 18*(5), 364–373.

Schim, S. M., Doorenbos, A., Benkert, R., & Miller, J. (2007). Culturally congruent care: Pulling the puzzle together. *Journal of Transcultural Nursing, 18*(2), 103–110.

Smedley, B., Stith, A., & Nelson, A. (2002). *Unequal treatment: Confronting racial and ethical disparities in healthcare.* Washington, DC: National Academy Press.

Spector, R. E. (2004). *Cultural diversity in health and illness* (6th ed.). Upper Saddle River, NJ: Pearson.

Stacks, J., Salgado, M., & Holmes, S. (2004). Cultural competence and social justice: A partnership for change. *Transitions, 15*(3), 4–5.

Taylor, R. (2005). Addressing barriers to cultural competence. *Journal for Nurses in Staff Development, 21*(4), 135–142.

Thiederman, S. B. (1986). Ethnocentricsm: A barrier to effective health care. *Nurse Practitioner, 11*(8), 52–59.

U.S. Department of Commerce (DOC), U.S. Census Bureau. (2008, August 14). *An older and more diverse nation by midcentury.* Retrieved July 2, 2009, from http://www.census.gov/PressRelease/www/releases/archives/population/012496.html

U.S. Department of Commerce (DOC), U.S. Census Bureau. (2003, October 8). *Nearly 1-in-5 speak a foreign language at home.* Retrieved July 2, 2009, from http://www.census.gov/Press-Release/www/releases/archives/census_2000/001406.html

U.S. Department of Health and Human Services (DHHS), Office of Disease Prevention and Health Promotion. (2008, December 11). *Healthy people 2020.* Retrieved March 28, 2010, from http://www.healthypeople.gov/HP2020/Advisory/PhaseI/summary.htm#_Toc211942897

Wells, M. I. (2000). Beyond cultural competence: A model for individual and institutional cultural development. *Journal of Community Health Nursing, 17*(4), 189–199.

Williams, D. R., Neighbors, H. W., & Jackson, J. S. (2003). Racial/ethnic discrimination and health: Findings from community studies. *American Journal of Public Health, 93*(2), 200–208.

Managed Care: Examining Today's Healthcare System

Jie Hu
Charlotte A. Herrick

3

■ OBJECTIVES

1. Examine the current healthcare system and healthcare reform.

2. Describe managed care and managed care plans as part of the healthcare system.

3. Evaluate the effects of managed care on health care in terms of costs and quality of care.

4. Describe the roles of nurse case managers in managed care and their evolution within the current healthcare system.

5. Discuss the reasons why nurse case managers need to understand the "business" of healthcare financing.

INTRODUCTION

Managed care is a healthcare delivery system that coordinates the financing of health care with the twin goals of controlling costs while maintaining the quality of care (Huber, 2006). Managed care is based on the traditional U.S. healthcare system, which consists of employer-based, indemnity insurance and fee-for-service (FFS) payments for health care (Sekhri, 2000). Escalating costs and the declining quality of care, combined with the effects of the current economic recession, are the primary issues being addressed in the ongoing debate about health-care reform. The never-ending increases in healthcare spending and the escalating costs of health insurance premiums have created great challenges for the healthcare industry (Mays, Claxton, & White, 2004). It is imperative that nurse case managers understand the healthcare system and the changes that healthcare reform may bring for managed care.

This chapter describes managed care and summarizes the issues in healthcare reform. It presents an overview of the U.S. healthcare system and the issues surrounding reform of that system. Managed care, including its relationship with case management, is addressed as well. The role of the nurse case manager in managed care and the potential changes in that role as a result of health reform will be explored. Finally, the business of healthcare financing and the components of insurance coverage are examined.

THE U.S. HEALTHCARE SYSTEM

The U.S. healthcare system relies on the private and public sectors for financing, purchasing, and delivering healthcare services (Brown, 2008; Sekhri, 2000). In addition, it constitutes what is called "the safety net," which includes public and voluntary hospitals, community health centers, public health clinics, and free clinics with services donated by private physicians (Brown, 2008). The majority of healthcare expenditures in 2007 were derived from private insurance (35%).

Other funding sources included Medicare and the State Children's Health Insurance Program (SCHIP) (15%), Medicaid (15%), out-of-pocket payments from private citizens (12%), and other public (12%) and private (5%) resources. Spending on health care includes expenditures for hospital care (31%); nursing home care (8%); prescription drugs (10%); other spending, such as outpatient clinics (25%); physicians' services (21%); and the administrative costs on programs after expenses (i.e., net costs) (7%) (Centers for Medicare and Medicaid Services, Office of the Actuary, National Health Statistics Group, 2009a).

In 2007, the United States' total health expenditures reached $2.2 trillion. Each person averaged $7,421 in medical expenses. The United States spends 16.2% of its gross domestic product (GDP) on health care compared to 8.7% spent in other nations (Centers for Medicare and Medicaid Services, Office of the Actuary, National Health Statistics Group, 2009b; World Health Organization [WHO], 2009). It is projected that health expenditures will increase to 20.3% of U.S. GDP by 2018 (Sisko et al., 2009).

U.S. expenditures on health are the highest in the world (WHO, 2009); even so, the United States is the only wealthy, industrialized country that does not medically insure all of its citizens (Institute of Medicine, National Academy of Sciences, 2004). Currently approximately 47 million Americans lack health insurance and, therefore, have limited access to healthcare services (U.S. Census Bureau, 2009). Furthermore, according to a report prepared by Families USA (2009), 86.7 million Americans (approximately 33.1% of the total population) younger than age 65 were uninsured at some point between 2007 and 2008. In addition, tens of millions of people face the prospect of eroding coverage and the potential loss of healthcare insurance due to unemployment during the current economic recession (Keepnews, 2009). Given all of these factors, healthcare reform is essential to address the issues of coverage, costs, and the quality of care.

HEALTHCARE REFORM

The debate about healthcare reform has focused on the rights of all Americans to health care, including those related to access to care, coverage, efficiency, cost-effectiveness, and quality of care. The key question is, What should be the extent of government's involvement?

The cost and quality of care are also important elements in healthcare reform. While the United States has extraordinarily high healthcare costs, spending more than twice as much as other nations, it lags behind other industrialized countries in terms of infant mortality rates and life expectancy (Roehr, 2008). In terms of life expectancy, the United States ranks 42nd in the world, and 50th after the European Union (WHO, 2006). The U.S. healthcare system ranks last in 37 measures in terms of access to care, quality of health care, and health outcomes compared to 19 other industrialized countries (Roehr, 2008). One of the most important factors contributing to the low performance by the U.S. healthcare industry in terms of quality, access, equity, efficiency, and health outcomes is the lack of universal coverage (Davis, Guterman, Collins, Stremikis, Rustgi, & Nuzum, 2009). However, Hadley and colleagues (2008) argue that covering all uninsured people will result in an increase in medical spending by $122.6 billion, which would increase healthcare spending by 5% (0.8% of GDP).

In 2009, the Obama administration proposed comprehensive healthcare reform legislation that would expand healthcare coverage, make health care affordable, and introduce essential reforms in the health insurance market (White House, 2009). On November 7, 2009, the House of Representatives passed a health insurance reform bill titled "The Affordable Health Care for America Act." As of January 2010, "The Patient Protection and Affordable Care Act" was under consideration in the Senate (Kaiser Family Foundation, 2009a, 2009b). The goals of both bills are to improve health outcomes and the quality of care, increase efficiency, and decrease the total health system costs, which have greatly affected the overall costs of health care for all Americans—and made health insurance unaffordable for many citizens, thereby swelling the ranks of the uninsured or underinsured (Davis et al., 2009). The House and Senate bills would affect providers' financial incentives, alter the organization and delivery of healthcare services, and invest in prevention and population health so as to provide the best health care and achieve the best health outcomes for all (Davis et al., 2009). On March 21, 2010, the House of Representatives held a historic vote and passed healthcare reform legislation.

Understanding the healthcare system and healthcare reform will enable nurse case managers to provide the best advice to their clients and coordinate the most appropriate care on their client's behalf.

THE DEVELOPMENT OF MANAGED CARE

The concept of managed care used in the U.S. healthcare system dates back to 1929, when the first health insurance plan was started by physicians to provide essential healthcare coverage for blue-collar workers in Los Angeles. In 1933, Dr. Sidney Garfield established a prepaid healthcare delivery system, known as Kaiser Permanente; this California managed care health plan provided health care to workers who were not able to afford healthcare insurance (Verheijde, 2006). The Kaiser Permanente Health Care plan still exists today.

Under traditional indemnity insurance, patients chose their own healthcare providers, and providers and hospitals received reimbursements based on a fee-for-service arrangement. With traditional indemnity insurance, over utilization was a fact of life. In the 1960s, prepaid group practice plans were recognized as a mechanism that might be able to control the rising costs of health care. In 1973, the U.S. Congress passed the Health Maintenance Organization Act to authorize using federal funds for the development of health maintenance organizations (HMOs) (Finkelman, 2001; Gerardi, 2005).

Economic pressures and medical waste were well-recognized contributors to rising costs, which were the major factors in promoting the evolution of managed care (Verheijde, 2006). Prior to the advent of managed care, the costs of health care were so excessive that they were crippling American industry, bankrupting local and state governments, and adding to the federal deficit, severely limiting the funds available for other services. Major factors driving the rapid increase in healthcare costs during the 1980s included the rising costs for medical services, increasing numbers of diagnostic procedures, development of medical technology, increasing pharmaceutical costs, and the growing number of older Americans with chronic conditions. Fraud throughout the system was another factor contributing to the high costs of health care.

Indemnity insurance carriers struggled to control the escalating costs under FFS plans, which resulted in increased premiums for consumers. Given this environment, managed care became even more attractive, evolving into the dominant model for the delivery of health care by the late 1980s (Verheijde, 2006).

Managed care allows healthcare managers to intervene between physicians and patients to ensure that the care delivered to patients is appropriate and at the lowest cost. Today, most healthcare insurers, including many public-funded programs, use some form of managed care in an attempt to control healthcare costs. With the passage of the Balanced Budget Act of 1997, for example, Medicare made a strong entrance into the managed care arena. This federally funded program has the following primary responsibilities:

- Provide health care to plan members, who are in their sixties or older,
- Ensure that members have access to covered healthcare services,
- Ensure that services are appropriate and of good quality,
- Reimburse providers for services rendered,
- Provide health care on a prepaid basis,
- Restrict care for members only,
- Ensure that case management services are in place, and
- Provide for utilization reviews and ensure that quality monitors have been established (adapted from Rossi, 2003)

In summary, the driving forces for changes in the healthcare delivery system over the last several decades include the following trends:

- Consumer demands for quality care that is cost-effective,
- Proliferation of new discoveries in medical science and technology,
- Increasing government regulations,
- Greater market competition,
- Spiraling healthcare costs and the demand for economic restraints by employers and the federal and state governments,
- A shift from hospital care to community practice,
- An aging population,
- An increasing prevalence of chronic diseases,
- A fragmented healthcare delivery system characterized by duplication of services,
- A lack of accountability,
- A shift in the government's payment strategies from retrospective payment mechanisms to prospective payment systems,
- Changes in healthcare structures from hierarchical organizations to integrated delivery systems,

- Increasing numbers of uninsured persons,
- Greater emphasis on prevention rather than cure,
- "Voices" such as that of the Institute of Medicine, which has called for interdisciplinary education and practice,
- Greater numbers of patients with multiple healthcare needs who also have social and family problems,
- As a consequence of the emphasis on quality, a focus on certification as a means to ensure that case managers are competent to provide quality case management services,
- Over-utilization of emergency room services,
- Increasing emphasis on prevention, and
- Changes from FFS funding to a capitated delivery system

Traditional	Capitation
Patient centered	Population based
Illness/curative	Illness prevention/wellness
Tracking beds and admissions	Tracking health status and outcomes
Service use generates revenue	Service use increases costs
Institutional care	Community care
Episodic care	Continuum of care
Individual healthcare providers	Collaborative interdisciplinary teams

WHAT IS MANAGED CARE?

Managed care is a delivery system that controls the financing and delivery of healthcare services across the continuum of care (American Heart Association [AHA], 2009). It has been defined as a system that combines the delivery of health care with the payments for health care, influencing the utilization of services. Managed care employs management techniques that are designed to promote the delivery of cost-effective care (Department of Health and Human Services [DHHS], 2009). Such a healthcare system integrates the financing and delivery of healthcare services to covered individuals by contract with selected institutional and professional providers, who furnish a comprehensive set of healthcare services. The goals of managed care are to ensure that the health care provided via the system will be of high quality, that costs are controlled, that the care is appropriate for patient's condition, and that the care is provided by the appropriate provider (AHA, 2009).

Managed care has continued to rapidly evolve over the past several decades. In recent years, the trend has been away from inpatient hierarchical structures and toward a continuum of care model that integrates inpatient and community systems of care. In many cases, managed care organizations are recommending flexibility. (Carneal & Andrea, 2001). Structures are changing to seamless systems of care in which services are coordinated and integrated into an overall healthcare delivery system across the continuum of care. Seamless systems have the following components:

- linkages between all levels of the system
- open communication pathways
- informational support systems
- clinical integration across the continuum of care
- multifocal decision making
- interprofessional partnerships
- interdisciplinary team approaches
- changes in organizational structures that support integrated systems of care, whereby healthcare structures evolve from large hierarchical structures to more horizontal and integrated systems with a broader scope of practice

Managed care has also changed the way healthcare services are paid for, shifting from the traditional FFS arrangement to a system with varying mechanisms and fee structures to manage costs. The emphasis is on cost containment. Because the policies set by managed care organizations (MCOs) directly affect nursing practice, it behooves nurses to understand the various healthcare structures and the ways in which health care is financed.

A survey conducted in 2001, Brzytwa, Copeland, and Herwson found that many nurses are not knowledgeable about the financial aspects of nursing and healthcare delivery, including case management. Nurse leaders in states with a high percentage of MCOs have expressed concerns about this deficiency, believing that if nurses are to actively participate in decisions about healthcare services that affect their practice, they must be knowledgeable about the "business" aspects of nursing and healthcare delivery. According to these opinion leaders, more research is needed to determine the best approaches to teaching managed care principles and competencies, which directly affect nursing practice. It is especially important that nurse case managers understand the financial implications of their decisions when coordinating healthcare services for patients and families.

MCOs within the healthcare system deliver care that is determined by the standards set by each MCO regarding the selection of providers, the services that are covered, and the outcomes that are monitored by mechanisms that the MCO has established for quality assurance and utilization review. The MCO provides financial incentives for patients to use specific providers, who are associated with each specific plan.

MANAGED CARE PLANS

Managed care plans are "health insurance plans that contract with specific health care providers and medical facilities to provide care for their members at reduced costs" (AHA, 2009). A managed care health plan is a combination of interdependent systems of care, whose responsibilities include the financing and delivery of healthcare services. Managed care plans incorporate the following components:

- arrangements with selected providers to furnish a comprehensive set of healthcare services to members
- explicit standards for the selection of healthcare providers (which must be established and addressed by the larger group)
- programs for ongoing quality assurance and utilization review
- financial incentives for members to use the plan's providers and the procedures associated with the managed care plan

The HMO is the traditional managed care model, which generally provides healthcare insurance through a network of hospitals, physicians, and contracted healthcare providers for a fixed, prepaid fee. The goal of managed care programs is to provide high-quality healthcare services within a network of healthcare providers so as to reduce costs. With HMOs, a primary benefit is a reduction in healthcare costs for the plan's members. Members are required to select providers within the network; the plan will not pay for care rendered by providers outside the network, unless it is preauthorized or an emergency. HMOs are the most restrictive type of health plan, in that they restrict members' ability to select a healthcare provider and limit the use of primary care physicians (PCPs) as the point of referral for specialist care and for diagnostic or surgical services. In other words, authorization by the HMO is necessary to access a specialist, a hospital, or any other costly medical service. Perhaps because of these restrictions, HMOs provide health benefits that require the lowest out-of pocket expenses for their members (AHA, 2009). HMOs are also engaged in care management activities for the management of chronic illnesses and provide care for members with comorbidities (Scanlon, Swaminathan, Chernew, & Lee, 2006).

The most popular managed care plan is the preferred provider organization (PPO), which allows patients greater freedom in choosing their providers. The PPO combines characteristics of the traditional indemnity health insurance plan (FFS) with managed care. This health insurance plan is similar to the HMO in that the payment consists of a fixed premium and the member receives medical healthcare benefits within the network. Compared with the HMO, however, the PPO provides members with more choices of healthcare providers, including specialists. Members may seek medical care outside the network, and they may visit a specialist without a referral. On the one hand, members receive financial incentives to stay within the network, including lower deductibles, lower co-payments, and higher reimbursements when using a specialist from within the network. On the other hand, PPO members pay more out-of-pocket expenses compared to members of HMOs. For example, if a PPO member visits a family physician from outside the network, he or she may have to pay as much as 50% of the total bill out of his or her own pocket (AHA, 2009).

Point-of-service (POS) plans allow their members to choose an HMO or PPO each time they visit a healthcare provider. This type of arrangement is referred as an HMO/PPO hybrid. POS plans offer more flexibility and freedom of choice than HMOs and have become a popular healthcare plan option. The POS plan has a contracted provider network, but does not enforce any restrictions on members in selecting a PCP. The PCP must make the referral to a specialist, however. Members who do not use PCPs for referrals but seek care on their own, even within the network, have higher co-pays and deductibles. POS members can seek care outside of the network, but incur a higher co-pay or higher deductible for going this route (AHA, 2009).

Since the HMO Act of 1973, enrollment in managed care plans in the United States has grown dramatically, increasing from 27% of all employees with employer-based insurance in 1998 to 97% in 2007 (Kaiser Family Foundation, 2009b). By 2009, 124.6 million people were enrolled in managed care plans in the United States, with HMOs having the largest enrollment (64.5 million), followed by PPOs (61.9 million) (Managed Care On Line [MCOL], 2009). Employer-sponsored insurance is the leading source of health insurance in the United States, covering approximately 159 million non elderly people. Employers offered approximately 60% of the total insurance coverage available in this country in 2009, compared to 63% in 2008 (Kaiser Family Foundation, 2009b).

Historically, managed care plans have controlled their costs by relying on limiting provider networks and using PCPs as gatekeepers, thereby limiting members' access to specialty services. Their medical authorization policies enabled MCOs to limit authorization for expanded specialty services resulting in cost containment for employees and others. (Draper, Hurley, Lesser, & Strunk, 2002). More recently, managed care plans have faced mounting pressures from marketplace forces, with consumers demanding more choices and fewer restrictions on access to care. As a consequence, the distinction between the HMO and the PPO has become less marked in terms of benefits and limitations over time. HMOs now offer a wide range of provider networks with no gatekeepers, and their premiums are similar to those charged by PPOs. All types of managed care plans have faced similar issues related to their ability to control costs while loosening their restrictions, which may result in increased premiums. Consequently, the U.S. market for health care is now characterized by fewer affordable insurance options available for employees and an increasing number of uninsured and underinsured people (Draper et al., 2002).

MANAGED CARE AND COST SAVINGS

Managed care plans provide financial incentives to prevent healthcare providers from overtreating patients and overusing medical procedures with poor surgical outcomes (Halm, Press, Tuhrim, Wang, Rojas, & Chassin, 2008). Unlike traditional indemnity FFS plans, managed care plans contract with physicians at lower prices, monitor providers, and change providers' incentives; these measures have effectively reduced healthcare expenditures while maintaining the quality of care (Chernew, Hirth, Sonnad, Ermann, & Fendrick, 1998; Sekhri, 2000). Managed care has also decreased the rate of increase in health expenditures on hospital care, physician services, and prescription drugs by using practices such as provider networks, provider risk contracting, primary care gatekeeping, and utilization review. The impact of managed care on healthcare premiums is also evidenced by a decline in the double-digit inflation that caused medical costs to skyrocket between 1993 and 1997 (Mays et al., 2004; Sekhri, 2000). With the current economic recession and a new increase in healthcare costs, however, health plans have now begun to consider other cost-containment strategies for managing health care (Mays et al., 2004).

Managed care plans have directly reduced the number of hospital admissions through an improvement in primary care for Medicare-insured patients. A recent study using hospital discharge data from 2001 for elderly patients who were enrolled in Medicare HMOs in New York, Pennsylvania, Florida, and California found that there were fewer hospitalizations for preventable conditions among older Medicare enrollees in HMOs compared to those elders in traditional FFS Medicare plans. The findings of this study suggest that managed care provisions for primary and preventive care may have better outcomes than traditional Medicare programs for older adults in these states (Basu & Mobley, 2007). Controlling healthcare costs has also been achieved through higher HMO penetration in some geographic areas (Sari, 2002).

MANAGED CARE AND QUALITY

As MCOs have continued growing rapidly, quality of care has become a central concern of the public. Questions have been raised about the quality of care provided by managed care plans, which by definition take responsibility for both financial risk and the delivery of care (Scanlon, Rolph, Darby, & Doty, 2000). Government regulations, quality improvement methods, and market competition are the major approaches that have been used to drive improvements in the quality of managed care. The National Committee for Quality Assurance, The Joint Commission (formerly the Joint Commission on Accreditation of Healthcare Organizations), and the Foundation for Accountability are the major organizations that evaluate the quality of managed care plans (Hellinger & Young, 2005).

More recently, the Centers for Medicare and Medicaid Services (CMS) have developed a new program to evaluate Medicare patients and the outcomes of their care (i.e., the quality of their care), called Recovery Audit Contractors (RAC). The RAC program will identify improper Medicare payments in an attempt to prevent fraud, waste, and abuse in the Medicare program (CMS, 2009a; Terra, 2009). Consequently, Medicare patients will be closely monitored in terms of their treatment and outcomes and the charges for their treatment. Quality of care evaluation methods generally include three different criteria:

- The input of quality as measured by staffing and equipment
- The process of quality, as measured by the length of stay, the number of procedures, the number of tests performed, and the number of follow-up visits
- The output of quality, as measured by the outcome of treatment (Sari, 2002)

National surveys, such as the Medical Expenditure Panel Survey and the National Health Interview Survey, have also been used to examine managed care organizations (Liang, Phillips, & Haas, 2006).

Analysis of multiple indicators of the performance of managed care plans over time has suggested that MC plans do demonstrate high-quality performance (Swaminathan, Chernew, & Scanlon, 2008). Although the role of managed care and its effectiveness in controlling costs have been well established on a broad scale, the findings have been mixed depending on which categories and populations were considered. An early study reported that managed care has not decreased the overall effectiveness of health care in the United States (Hellinger, 1998). Nevertheless, many studies have found that hospitals and physicians have improved their efficiency in providing healthcare services as a result of managed care–driven practices (Sekhri, 2000). Managed care plans have also demonstrated a strong causal relationship between preventive care and the health of the HMO enrollees (Rizzio, 2005). HMOs have played a significant role in quality improvement by restructuring healthcare interventions so as to achieve the goal of quality improvement, by developing the necessary technical abilities to implement quality improvement activities (Scanlon et al., 2000).

Researchers have also examined the satisfaction levels of various populations of HMO enrollees regarding the quality of their managed care. An early study reported that members of HMOs were less satisfied with their care, believed they had received poor care, and felt they had more problems accessing specialized care. In this research, young people with a high socioeconomic status and individuals with fewer health problems were notably more satisfied with their healthcare plans than older adults, people with a lower socioeconomic status, and persons who had more health problems (Hellinger, 1998).

Despite the fact that managed care has had positive outcomes in terms of cost savings and has improved the quality of care, healthcare disparities still exist among minority populations in managed care settings. Studies have reported that managed care may have negative effects on the health care delivered to vulnerable populations, including members of racial minorities and other ethnic groups. Many minorities, particularly Hispanics and Asian Americans, have long experienced barriers to accessing health care (Phillips, Mayer, & Aday, 2000). Even today, racial and ethnic minorities in managed care settings are often under diagnosed and under treated (Keen & Overstreet, 2007).

Several studies have pointed to deficiencies in the quality of care delivered by MCOs for the elderly, the poor, mentally ill persons, diabetic patients, and patients with hypertension. Also, researchers have found deficits involving preventive care for these groups. For example, many elderly patients do not receive pneumococcal vaccinations when they are enrolled in managed care plans (McGlynn, Adams, Keesey, Hicks, DeCristofar, & Keer, 2003; Swansburg, 2002). Contradicting these negative findings, a study on the quality of managed care and the choice of care plans in New York involving SCHIP indicated that low-income parents who chose managed care plans received better quality of care, as measured by the Consumer Assessment to Health Plans Survey (CAHPS) (Liu et al., 2009).

Market forces associated with managed care have affected the quality of health care and access to care, and have contributed to declines in healthcare costs in recent years. Competition has improved the quality of care provided by hospitals (Encinosa & Hagan, 2006). However, a recent study on the relationship between competition and the quality of care reported that increased HMO penetration was not associated with improved quality of care (Scanlon, Swaminathan, Lee, & Chernew, 2008). In another study, hospital competition and HMO penetration did not affect the safety net of hospitals that serve the poor and the more vulnerable populations (Scanlon, Chernew, Swaminathan, & Lee, 2006). An adverse relationship was found between competitive managed care plans and quality of care in the New York SCHIP market (Liu & Phelps, 2008).

Escarce and colleagues (2006) examined the effect of hospital competition and HMO penetration on rates of mortality after hospitalization for a heart attack, hip fracture, stroke, gastrointestinal hemorrhage, congestive heart failure, or diabetes in three states (New York, California, and Wisconsin). They found that a high HMO penetration rate was associated with decreased deaths in California but had no effect on death rates in New York.

The effect of managed care on quality of care among Medicare patients enrolled in a Medicare Choice Managed Care plan who were undergoing carotid endarterectomies was examined by Halm and colleagues (2008). According to these researchers, patients covered by the managed care plan were less likely to use surgeons or hospitals than patients who were enrolled in traditional FFS healthcare plans. Halm and colleagues concluded that Medicare managed care plans did not positively affect the referral patterns or outcomes of patients undergoing carotid endarterectomies.

Zwanziger and Khan (2006) have examined the effect of managed care and market forces on the "safety net" hospitals. They found that these hospitals were not likely to be members of managed care networks and were less competitive with hospitals that served disadvantaged (i.e., more vulnerable) populations.

Managed care plans have dramatically influenced medical practice by restricting physicians' professional and clinical autonomy through the use of gatekeepers for referrals, utilization reviews, treatment guidelines, drug formularies, and preauthorization procedures. One study found that physicians' perceptions of managed care were related to their involvement with managed care plans and their particular practice setting. Some studies have revealed that physicians generally perceive the effect of managed care on the quality of care as neutral to negative, while others have reported that physicians are satisfied or very satisfied with the quality of care that they provide to patients who are insured by these plans. Primary care physicians are more satisfied than other physicians with the effect of managed care on treatment and outcomes. Physicians consistently report strong negative perceptions about the impact that managed care has had on patients' access to specialists (Christianson, Warrick, & Wholey, 2005).

Managed care and the quality of care have also been examined from patients' perspectives. In one study, patients in more managed plans generally rated their primary physicians as providing lower quality of care than those physicians in a less managed care environment. (Grembowski, Patrick, Williams, Diehr, & Martin, 2005). In another study, Hayes (2003) found that nurse practitioners had negative attitudes toward managed care.

The negative effects of managed care, including the cost-containment strategies associated with this approach, have raised some concerns about managed care's influence on physician–patient relationships. However, in a recent study, patients reported that they trusted their physicians despite the conflicts of interest that physicians may have because of the financial arrangements designed to limit the use of some therapeutic procedures (Keating, Landrum, Landon, Ayanian, Borbas, & Guadagnoli, 2007).

In summary, managed care and the quality of health care are issues that have increased the public's concerns and sparked debate about healthcare reform among healthcare providers, policymakers, and the general public. Inconclusive evidence has shown that the quality of health care has not been compromised by the widespread adoption of managed care, despite the key role played by cost-containment strategies in managed care. Overall, managed care has had a positive impact on controlling the escalating costs of health care without producing any negative effects on the quality of care provided to patients (Sekhri, 2000). Young and wealthy populations are especially satisfied with managed care, whereas vulnerable populations, chronically ill individuals, and older adults with low incomes have experienced some disadvantages as a result of the trend toward managed care services.

NURSE CASE MANAGEMENT IN A CHANGING HEALTHCARE SYSTEM

Nurse case managers face many challenges as they seek to provide quality, cost-effective care in a managed care environment. Healthcare reform is as controversial among nurse case managers as it has been among the public, as demonstrated by the heated debates seen in the reform-related "town meetings" held by senators and representatives during the summer of 2009.

In the future, changes in the U.S. healthcare system will continue to have a profound impact on the growth of nursing case management. Today nurse case managers can be found in almost every setting (Yamamoto & Lucey, 2005). The American Case Management Association (ACMA) and the Case Management Society of America (CSMA) will continue to expand their memberships as the demand grows for healthcare professionals to coordinate and integrate care across the healthcare continuum. Case management has the following goals:

- Provide continuity of care, by developing a system of care around the patient and family
- Optimize self-care, by educating patients and families about the illness and the necessary home care,
- Enhance the patient's quality of life,
- Decrease the length of stay (LOS) in hospitals,
- Increase provider and patient satisfaction,
- Promote cost-effective use of healthcare resources by coordinating resources to ensure quality and to reduce costs,
- Focus on prevention,
- Implement cost-efficient mechanisms to achieve the best outcomes.

As healthcare plans have begun to shift their focus from cure to care, case management has grown in importance owing to the new emphasis on identifying and addressing the healthcare needs of high-risk patients, thereby ensuring both cost savings and better clinical outcomes. New approaches in case management need to be addressed and customized to care for patients and families, especially those with chronic healthcare conditions (Mays et al., 2004). Nursing case management (NCM) practice delivers health care to clients that is client and family centered, and targeted to improving the quality of care. Nurse case managers must continue to promote the patient's and family's autonomy, by providing patient education that enables individuals and families to successfully navigate the complex, fragmented, and often confusing healthcare delivery system (Carter, 2009). To do so, nurse case managers will need to perfect their collaborative skills, thereby ensuring that they can work effectively with caregivers in different disciplines in a variety of settings. Key responsibilities for this role will include the coordination of care, advocacy, assessing and monitoring the plan of care, and facilitating follow-up care after discharge to ensure that the quality of aftercare is appropriate for the patient and family and is being provided by the right healthcare professional (Yamamoto & Lucey, 2005).

Nurse case manager leaders must have a thorough understanding of healthcare financing, must be knowledgeable about evidence-based practice, and should document how case management affects the quality of care for patients as well as how case management practice reduces costs. Outcome measurements document the effectiveness of nursing case management and should be reported on a regular basis to nursing administration.

Case managers must understand the financial implications of each patient's insurance policy (i.e., the "business of health care") as necessary to develop a plan of care. Each case manager must understand the components of the patient's insurance policy, including the following elements:

- The types of services covered,
- Number of days covered,
- Specific treatment restrictions,
- Restrictions on specific healthcare providers, especially if they are out of the network, and
- The maximum amount of dollars covered during a period of time or per illness (Yamamoto & Lucey, 2005).

The nurse case manager should work closely with the insurer to facilitate the delivery of the services that are necessary to meet the patient needs and that are appropriate, cost-effective, and of high quality.

Nurse administrators and case managers need to balance patient care responsibilities and financial considerations as part of their goal to provide quality care. They must be experts at negotiating contracts, planning new ventures, using human resources, and empowering staff to provide quality, cost-effective care to ensure good outcomes for patients, while remaining vigilant in terms of costs. Administrators must support case management services to ensure that there is continuity of care for the patient, from the hospital to the community, and that quality is maintained even during the transition from hospital to the next level of care. The nurse case manager will play a pivotal role in ensuring a smooth transition across the healthcare continuum.

▪ SUMMARY

The U.S. care system consists of private and public sectors for financing, purchasing, and delivering healthcare services. Managed care is a system of healthcare delivery that controls costs and maintains quality of care. Managed care and quality of health care have increased public health concerns and sparked debate. Healthcare reform legislation will expand healthcare coverage, make health care affordable, and introduced reforms in the health insurance market. Managed care plans include HMO, PPO, and POS. Managed care has reduced number of hospital admissions and improved quality of care. Managed care has also decreased the rate of increase in health expenditures on hospital care, physician services, and prescription drugs. Nurse case managers might face challenges as they seek to provide quality, cost-effective care in a managed care environment. Nurse case manager leaders must have a thorough understanding of healthcare financing, must be knowledgeable about evidence-based practice, and should document how case management affects the quality of care for patients as well as how case management practice reduces costs.

■ CASE STUDIES

You are an acute care case manager on a medical/surgical unit. Mrs. D. has been diagnosed with colon cancer and was admitted 3 weeks ago for a colectomy. She has been struggling at home with ostomy care and proper nutrition. She has been admitted today with severe dehydration. According to utilization guidelines, this patient meets the criteria to be admitted at a 24-hour observation status. As a nurse case manager, you know that Mrs. D. will need to be in the hospital longer than 24 hours and may need temporary placement while she recovers from the surgery. Given that Mrs. D. is insured by a managed care organization and your hospital's utilization rate is scrutinized daily, which alternative plans might you suggest as a compromise with the insurance provider that would assure Mrs. D. has enough time to recover?

■ DISCUSSION QUESTIONS

1. What is the ultimate goal of case management?
2. What are the benefits of prospective payment? What are the drawbacks?
3. Describe the paradigm shift from disease to wellness over the last 20 years.
4. Discuss the current healthcare reform legislations.
5. What are the benefits of reforming the current healthcare system?

■ CLASSROOM EXERCISES

Along with your fellow students, select different roles (social worker, physician, nurse case manager, insurance company representative) to play in the following case scenario. The various roles should bring differing perspectives to the scenario. Working together, try to negotiate a compromise to facilitate the best outcome for Mr. C.

Mr. C. is a 61-year-old male who has been diagnosed with early-stage Alzheimer's disease. He lives alone, with the occasional help of an elderly next-door neighbor. His ex-wife lives in the same town, as does his daughter, to whom he has not spoken in 15 years. Mr. C. is currently covered under a national HMO insurance plan.

Mr. C. was admitted to the hospital after a neighbor found him wandering around the neighborhood looking through trashcans. He stated that "he was at the grocery store getting some food for dinner." The neighbor tried to call his ex-wife but she did not answer. He took Mr. C. to the hospital, where he is being admitted for 24-hour observation.

The goal of this exercise is to ensure Mr. C.'s safety and continued treatment.

■ RECOMMENDED READINGS

Basu, J., & Mobley, L. R. (2007). Do HMOs reduce preventable hospitalizations for Medicare beneficiaries? *Medical Care Research and Review, 64*(5), 544–567.

Brown, L. D. (2008). The amazing noncollapsing U.S. health care system: Is reform finally at hand? *New England Journal of Medicine, 358*(4), 325–327

Carter, J. J. (2009). Finding our place at the discussion table: Case management and healthcare reform. *Professional Case Management, 14*(4), 165–166.

Centers for Medicare & Medicaid Services. (2009). *Recovery audit contractor.* Retrieved from http://www.cms.hhs.gov/RAC

Christianson, J. B., Warrick, L. H., & Wholey, D. R. (2005). Physicians' perceptions of managed care: A review of literature. *Medical Care Research & Review, 62*, 635–675.

Hadley, J., Holahan, J., Coughlin, T., & Miller, D. (2008). Covering the uninsured in 2008: Current costs, sources of payment, and incremental costs. *Health Affairs, 27*, w339–w415.

Keepnews, D. M. (2009). U.S. health reform: A continuing imperative. *Policy, Politics, & Nursing Practice, 10*, 92–93.

Roehr, B. (2008). Health care in US ranks lowest among developed countries. *British Medical Journal, 337*, doi:10.1136/bmj.a889.

■ REFERENCES

American Heart Association (AHA). (2009). *Managed health care plans.* Retrieved from http://www.americanheart.org/presenter.jhtml?identifier=4663

Basu, J., & Mobley, L. R. (2007). Do HMOs reduce preventable hospitalizations for Medicare beneficiaries? *Medical Care Research and Review, 64*(5), 544–567.

Brown, L. D. (2008). The amazing noncollapsing U.S. health care system: Is reform finally at hand? *New England Journal of Medicine, 358*(4), 325–327

Brzytwa, E., Copeland, L., & Herwson, M. (2001). Managed care education: A needs assessment of employers and educators of nurses. *Journal of Nursing Education, 39*, 197–204.

Carneal, G., & Andrea, G. (2001). Defining the parameters of case management in a managed care setting. *Managed Care Quarterly, 9*, 55–60

Carter, J. J. (2009). Finding our place at the discussion table: Case management and healthcare reform. *Professional Case Management, 14*(4), 165–166.

Centers for Medicare and Medicaid Services, Office of the Actuary, National Health Statistics Group. (2009a). *Breakdown of health costs in US, 2007.* Retrieved from http://www.cms.hhs.gov/NationalHealthExpendData/downloads/PieChartSourcesExpenditures2007.pdf

Centers for Medicare and Medicaid Services, Office of the Actuary, National Health Statistics Group. (2009b). *The nation's health dollar, calendar year 2007: Where it came from, where it went.* Retrieved from http://www.cms.hhs.gov/ NationalHealthExpendData/02_NationalHealthAccountsHistorical.asp

Chernew, M. E., Hirth, R. A., Sonnad, S. S., Ermann, R., & Fendrick, A. M. (1998). Managed care, medical technology, and health care cost growth: A review of the evidence. *Medical Care Research & Review, 55,* 259–288.

Christianson, J. B., Warrick, L. H., & Wholey, D. R. (2005). Physicians' perceptions of managed care: A review of literature. *Medical Care Research & Review, 62,* 635–675.

Davis, K., Guterman, S., Collins, S. R., Stremikis, K., Rustgi, S., & Nuzum, R. (2009). *Starting on the path to a high performance health system: Analysis of health system reform provisions of reform bills in the House of Representatives and Senate, the Commonwealth Fund, December 2009.* Retrieved from http://www. commonwealthfund.org/Content/Publications/Fund-Reports/2009/Nov/Starting-on-the-Path-to-a-High-Performance-Health-System.aspx?page=all

Department of Human Health Services (DHHS). (2009). *Managed care terminology.* Retrieved from http://aspe.os.dhhs.gov/progsys/forum/mcobib.htm

Draper, D. A., Hurley, R. E., Lesser, C. S., & Strunk, B. C. (2002). The changing face of managed care. *Health Affairs, 21,* 11–23.

Encinosa, W., & Hagan, M. (2006). Introduction: AHRQ research on health care markets. *Medical Care Research & Review, 63*(6S), 3–8.

Escarce, J. J., Jain, A. K., & Rogowski, J. (2006). Hospital competition, managed care, and mortality after hospitalization for medical conditions: Evidence from three studies. *Medical Care Research & Review, 63,* 112S–140S.

Families USA. (2009). *Americans are at risk: One in three uninsured.* Retrieved from http://www.familiesusa.org/assets/pdfs/americans-at-risk.pdf

Finkelman, A. W. (2001). *Managed care: A nursing perspective.* Upper Saddle River: NJ: Prentice Hall.

Gerardi, T. (2005). The managed care market: Nurse case management as a strategy for success. In E. Cohen & G. Cesta (Eds.), *Nursing case management: From essentials to advanced practice applications* (4th ed., pp. 210–218). Philadelphia: Elsevier Mosby.

Grembowski, D. E., Patrick, D. L., Williams, B., Diehr, P., & Martin, D. P. (2005). Managed care and patient-related quality of care from primary physicians. *Medical Care Research & Review, 62,* 31–55.

Hadley, J., Holahan, J., Coughlin, T., & Miller, D. (2008). Covering the uninsured in 2008: Current costs, sources of payment, and incremental costs. *Health Affairs, 27,* w339–w415.

Halm, E. A., Press, M. J., Tuhrim, S., Wang, J., Rojas, M., & Chassin, M. R. (2008). Does managed care affect quality? Appropriateness, referral patterns, and outcomes of carotid endarterectomy. *American Journal of Medical Quality, 23,* 448–456.

Hayes, E. F. (2003). Nurse practitioner self-confidence and attitudes regarding managed care. *Journal of the American Academy of Nurse Practitioners, 15,* 501–508.

Hellinger, F. J. (1998). The effect of managed care on quality: A review of recent evidence. *Archives of Internal Medicine, 158,* 833–841.

Hellinger, F. J., & Young, G. J. (2005). Health plan liability and ERISA: The expanding scope of state legislation. *American Journal of Public Health, 95,* 217–223.

Huber, D. L. (2006). *Leadership and nursing care management* (3rd ed.). St. Louis, MO: Saunders/Elsevier.

Institute of Medicine, National Academy of Sciences. (2004). *Insuring America's health: Principles and recommendations.* Retrieved from http://www.iom.edu/Reports/2004/Insuring-Americas-Health-Principles-and-Recommendations.aspx

Kaiser Family Foundation. (2009a). *Kaiser and Health Research and Educational Trust employer health benefits 2009 summary of findings.* Retrieved from http://www.kff.org/insurance

Kaiser Family Foundation. (2009b). *Summaries of coverage provisions in House and Senate reform legislation.* Retrieved from http://www.kff.org/healthreform/8023.cfm

Keating, N. L., Landrum, M. B., Landon, B. E., Ayanian, J. Z., Borbas, C., & Guadagnoli, E. (2007). The influence of cost containment strategies and physicians' financial arrangements on patients' trust and satisfaction. *Journal of Ambulatory Care Management, 30,* 92–104.

Keen, C., & Overstreet, K. M. (2007). Disparities in depression care in managed care settings. *Journal of Continuing Education in the Health Professions, 27,* S26–S32.

Keepnews, D. M. (2009). U.S. health reform: A continuing imperative. *Policy, Politics, & Nursing Practice, 10,* 92–93.

Liang, S.-Y., Phillips, K. A., & Haas, J. S. (2006). Measuring managed care and its environment using national surveys: A review and assessment. *Medical Care Research & Review, 63*(6S), 9–36.

Liu, H., & Phelps, C. E. (2008). Nonprice competition and quality of care in managed care: The New York SCHIP market. *Health Services Research, 43,* 971–987.

Liu, H., Phelps, C. E., Veazie, P. J., Dick, A. W., Klein, J. D., Shone, L. P., et al. (2009). Managed care quality of care and plan choice in New York SCHIP. *Health Services Research, 44,* 843–861.

Managed Care On Line (MCOL). (2009). *Managed care fact sheet from MCOL. Health reform: Impact on health plans and Medicare.* Retrieved from http://www.mcareol.com/factshts/factnati.htm

Mays, G. P., Claxton, G., & White, J. (2004). Managed care rebound? Recent changes in health plans' cost containment strategies. *Health Affairs, W4,* 427–436.

McGlynn, E. A., Asch, S. M., Adams, J., Keesey, J., Hicks, J., DeCristofaro, A., et al. (2003). The quality of health care delivered to adults in the United States. *New England Journal of Medicine, 348,* 2635–2645.

Phillips, K. A., Mayer, M. L., & Aday, L. (2000). Barriers to care among racial/ethnic groups under managed care. *Health Affairs, 19,* 65–75.

Rizzio, J. A. (2005). Are HMO's bad for health maintenance? *Health Economics, 14,* 1117–1131.

Roehr, B. (2008). Health care in US ranks lowest among developed countries. *British Medical Journal, 337,* doi:10.1136/bmj.a889.

Rossi, P. A. (2003). Managed care. In P. A. Rossi (Ed.), *Case management in health care* (2nd ed., pp. 61–105). Philadelphia: Saunders.

Sari, N. (2002). Do competition and managed care improve quality? *Health Economics, 11,* 571–584.

Scanlon, D. P., Chernew, M., Swaminathan, S., & Lee, W. (2006). Competition in health insurance markets: Limitations of current measures for policy analysis. *Medical Care Research & Review, 63*(6S), 37–55.

Scanlon, D. P., Rolph, E., Darby, C., & Doty, H. E. (2000). Are managed care plans organizing for quality? *Medical Care Research & Review, 57,* 9–32.

Scanlon, D. P., Swaminathan, S., Lee, W., & Chernew, M. (2008). Does competition improve health care quality? *Health Research and Educational Trust.* DOI: 10.1111/j.1475-6773.2008.00899.x. 1931–1951.

Scanlon, D. P. S., Swaminathan, S., Chernew, M., & Lee, W. (2006). Market and plan characteristics related to HMO quality and improvement. *Medical Care Research & Review, 63*(6S), 56–89.

Sekhri, N. K. (2000). Managed care: The US experience. *Bulletin of the World Health Organization, 78,* 830–844.

Sisko, A., Truffer, C., Smith, S., Keehan, S., Cylus, J., Poisal, J. A., et al. (2009). Health spending projections through 2018: Recession effects add uncertainty to the outlook. *Health Affairs, 28,* w346–w357.

Swaminathan, S., Chernew, M. E., & Scanlon, D. P. (2008). Persistence of HMO performance measures. *Health Services Research, 43,* 2033–2037.

Swansburg, R. (2002). Introduction to managed care. In R. S. R. Swansburg (Eds.), *Introduction to management and leadership for nursing managers* (3rd ed., pp. 7–21). Sudbury, MA: Jones and Bartlett.

Terra, S. (2009). Recovery audit contractors and their impact on case management. *Professional Case Management, 14,* 217–223.

U.S. Census Bureau. (2009). *Income, poverty, and health insurance coverage in the United States: 2008.* Washington, DC: Author. Retrieved from http://www.census. gov/Press-Release/www/releases/archives/income_wealth/014227.html

Verheijde, J. L. (2006). *Managing care: A shared responsibility.* Dordrecht, The Netherlands: Springer.

White House. (2009). *Remarks by the President to a joint session of Congress on health care.* Retrieved from http://www.whitehouse.gov/the_press_office/ Remarks-by-the-President-to-a-Joint-Session-of-Congress-on-Health-Care

World Health Organization (WHO). (2006). *The world health report 2006: Working together for health.* Retrieved from http://www.who.int/whr/2006/whr06_en.pdf

World Health Organization (WHO). (2009). *World health statistics 2009.* Retrieved from http://www.who.int/whosis/whostat/2009/en/index.html

Yamamoto, L., & Lucey, C. (2005). Case management "within the walls": A glimpse into the future. *Critical Care Nursing, 28,* 162–178.

Zwanziger, J., & Khan, N. (2006). Safety-net activities and hospital contracting with managed care organizations. *Medical Care Research & Review, 63*(6S), 90–111.

Case Management: An Overview of Roles, Skills, and Functions

Laura J. Fero
Charlotte A. Herrick

4

■ OBJECTIVES

1. List the various roles of a healthcare coordinator or nurse case manager.

2. Relate the roles to the overall goals of care coordination.

3. Describe functions and the skills that are necessary to implement the various roles of the healthcare coordinator/nurse case manager.

INTRODUCTION

The roles and functions of a healthcare coordinator/case manager can vary depending on the setting in which the case management process takes place, the model to which the institution subscribes, the goals of the program, and the population that is the focus of care. Individual institutions develop their own job descriptions and role titles depending on their organizational structure and operations, policies and procedures, and financial status; the goals of the healthcare program; and the model adopted to guide the practice of care coordination (Cohen & Cesta, 2001, 2005). Overall, the case manager or healthcare coordinator

TABLE 4-1 The Healthcare Coordinator/Case Manager's Roles

Assessor	Case finder	Planner	Liaison
Broker	Gatekeeper	Change agent	Facilitator
Coordinator	Monitor	Clinician/ practitioner	Administrator/leader/ manager
Communicator	Negotiator	Educator	Advocate
Consultant	Salesperson	Collaborator/ team builder	Entrepreneur
Utilization manager	Record keeper/ documenter	Data analyst	Researcher
Discharge planner	Problem solver	Financial advisor	Resource manager

is considered the linchpin for the healthcare system. A linchpin is defined as a "central, cohesive element, a source of support and stability" (Herrick, Bartlett, Pearson, Schmidt, & Cherry, 2006, p. 139; Turkettle & Noj, 2003).

The following descriptions address some of the roles of the care coordinator or case manager, which are summarized in Tables 4-1 and 4-2. The role of consultant and entrepreneur will be discussed in Chapter 7, on private practitioners.

COMMUNICATOR

The role of communicator is an essential task of a care coordinator. One of the chief functions of care coordination is information management. It requires focused communication between the care coordinator/case manager and the referral sources, the physicians, the patient and family, the payer sources, vendors, and legal entities (Mullahy, 2010). Communication is a means of transmitting information and of establishing rapport linking two or more people in a collaborative relationship (Fattorusso & Quinn, 2007). Successful communication requires a bidirectional exchange. The purposes of communication in care coordination are to inquire, inform, negotiate, motivate, and persuade. It is up to the care coordinator/case manager to keep a dialogue going that is open and honest and to continually disseminate pertinent information to all stakeholders.

Care coordinators communicate in a variety of ways: by telephone, in person, and in writing though correspondence, case notes, emails, memos, and reports. Team members may not communicate directly with one another or

TABLE 4-2 The Roles of the Healthcare Coordinator or Nurse Case Manager to Meet the Goals of Healthcare Coordination

Goals of Care Coordination or Case Management	Roles of the Healthcare Coordinator or Nurse Case Manager
Integrate, coordinate care, and facilitate the delivery of healthcare services to ensure quality.	■ Care coordinator ■ Broker/manager/leader ■ Planner ■ Negotiator
Reduce the length of stay (LOS), thereby reducing costs, while simultaneously maintaining quality.	■ Monitor ■ Discharge planner ■ Financial adviser ■ Gatekeeper
Eliminate duplication of services and enhance the continuity of care across the healthcare continuum.	■ Negotiator ■ Facilitator ■ Coordinator ■ Resource manager
Facilitate access to care across the healthcare continuum.	■ Negotiator ■ Care coordinator ■ Broker
Reduce recidivism, especially among the mentally ill—eliminate the revolving door. Be sure the patient is ready for discharge.	■ Advocate ■ Assessor/monitor/evaluator ■ Liaison ■ Discharge planner/coordinator/facilitator
Focus on prevention and health promotion.	■ Educator ■ Communicator ■ Case finder ■ Change agent ■ Consultant
Improve the satisfaction among all stakeholders—patients, families, staff, and physicians.	■ Communicator/supporter ■ Mentor ■ Leader with the ability to enhance the empowerment of patients and their healthcare providers
Empower families for self-care and self-responsibility.	■ Educator ■ Supporter ■ Clinician/practitioner ■ Active listener
Improve models of care as new information and technologies appear on the horizon.	■ Researcher ■ Change agent

they may communicate ineffectively "on the run," a practice that makes clear communication difficult. The care coordinator is the pivotal person who communicates with all stakeholders about the care of the patient. In some cases, it may be necessary to call a group meeting to ensure that the healthcare team is on the same page in carrying out the care plan. The care coordinator puts mechanisms in place to assure effective communication takes place among all stakeholders. He or she uses established communication systems to receive and relay information both inside and outside the healthcare institution (Hogan & Nickitas, 2009).

The care coordinator is the communication specialist. He or she should communicate timely, complete, and essential information to all interested players, thereby keeping them up-to-date about the patient's progress. It is the responsibility of the care coordinator/case manager to make sure all parties have the information they need to make the best decisions. The care coordinator should assess how, in which form, when, and which information each stakeholder needs to develop the best patterns of communication (Birmingham & Anctil, 2002).

Another important strategy of the communicator role is translating the meaning of medical terminology to the patient and family members. Care coordinators must communicate clearly so that misconceptions can be avoided. Patients and family members need to fully understand the pertinent information so that they can make informed decisions.

Telephone-based disease management is rapidly becoming a popular case management strategy. It provides patients and families with ongoing support without requiring them to leave home. With this approach, the care coordinator/case manager is just a phone call away. The phone is a useful healthcare coordination tool because it provides a channel of communication without driving up costs. Documentation of phone conversations is important (Mullahy, 2004)! In addition, the care coordinator/case manager who is providing care coordination services by phone must have excellent listening and communication skills. Good assessment skills are necessary to detect what is true and what may be false and to determine the patient's progress or lack of progress. Open-ended questions are likely to tap into more information than questions that can be answered with a brief "yes" or "no." A rule of thumb is to first answer the patient's questions prior to discussing other treatment issues (Mullahy, 2010). (Telephone communication—telehealth—is discussed in more detail in Chapter 12.)

The healthcare coordinator must be a diplomat, who is able to communicate with many different groups and people on many different levels (Table 4-3). Unfortunately, as described in Table 4-4, the effectiveness of communication may be diminished by some of the barriers that are frequently occupational

TABLE 4-3 Skills Necessary for the Communication Specialist/Healthcare Coordinator

- Good interpersonal skills, active listening, and communication skills
- Cultural sensitivity
- Good writing skills for documentation and report writing
- The ability to deal with difficult people and situations (emotional intelligence, conflict resolution)
- Collaboration and group leadership/followership skills (servant leadership)
- Public speaking skills
- Good public relations skills
- Team building skills/collaboration skills
- Consultation skills

TABLE 4-4 Barriers to Good Communication

- People hear what they want to hear (selective hearing).
- People hear within a window of time.
- People hear only what they are capable of hearing.
- People hear what they think other people want them to hear (selective hearing).
- People may not attend to the message.
- Extraneous background noises may prevent understanding.
- Frequent interruptions may diminish communication.

Source: Fink-Samnick, 2004.

hazards, especially in the complex managed care environment (Finkelman, 2001). On some occasions, a person may not want to hear the message. Also, sometimes the problem cannot be fixed. Some messages may be so painful that the patient or family member goes into denial in an attempt to avoid the painful reality.

> **■ A Reminder**
>
> I know that you believe you understand what you think I said.
> But I am not sure you realize that what you heard is not what I meant.

Strategies to Overcome the Barriers to Good Communication

Assess the other person's mood. Is he or she open and able to listen intently to what the communicator has to say? To ensure clarity, use reflection and restatement to reinforce what was said. Be sure to separate miscellaneous "stuff" from the message, so it is precise and to the point. Providing feedback is an important communication strategy (Finkelman, 2001). Also, time spent now on communicating clearly will save time later.

The ability to identify communication barriers and deal with them effectively will allow the care coordinator to continue to provide quality services while keeping costs down (Fink-Samnick, 2004). As the communicator, the care coordinator/case manager must make sure that all channels of communication remain open for all stakeholders, thereby allowing caregivers to provide quality patient care.

BROKER

As a broker, the care coordinator manages cases one by one. He or she identifies individual needs and matches these needs with available resources and services. The care coordinator assists the physician, patient, and family to obtain needed resources, personnel, professionals, money, and equipment (Cohen & Cesta, 2005). As the broker, facilitating access to resources across the continuum of care is a continuing role for healthcare coordinators in all settings and models— "within the walls," "beyond the walls," and as part of the continuum of care. Table 4-5 summarizes the skills needed by the broker/care coordinator.

NEGOTIATOR

A healthcare coordinator also assumes the role of negotiator. Negotiation is necessary to find ways to achieve common goals and obtain the best outcomes. In this form of communication, two or more parties identify their common interests and reconcile their differences to achieve a mutually satisfactory objective or to solve a problem. Negotiation is a reciprocal process with the goal of reaching a satisfactory conclusion for both parties so that they are both winners. It is intended to provide a satisfactory solution to a conflict or reach an agreement to accomplish goals that are acceptable to both parties. The conclusion of the negotiating process should be a "workable and enduring" agreement (Fattorusso & Quinn, 2007, p. 53).

The negotiator first needs information about services, fees, providers' credentials, and the delivery of supplies or services before he or she can broker arrangements for services, supplies, and equipment and negotiate fees that will achieve the goals of cost-effectiveness and quality care (Fattorusso & Quinn,

TABLE 4-5 Skills Necessary for the Broker/Care Coordinator

- Assessment skills to identify needs and resources
- Negotiation skills
- Problem-solving skills
- Networking skills to contact community and professional agencies

2007, p. 55). This information should be provided for both the first choice and the best alternative. During the negotiating process, a strategy that might be necessary is BATNA—a mnemonic meaning "the best alternative to a negotiated agreement" that was introduced in 1981 by Fisher and Ury in *Getting to Yes* (cited in Fattorusso & Quinn, 2007, p. 56).

The Case Management Society of American (CMSA) has established national standards to guide case managers who negotiate with providers, payers, and patients and families to achieve the best possible outcomes. These standards are summarized in Table 4-6.

Healthcare professionals do not always agree or have the same opinions. To smooth over these disagreements, the care coordinator acts as a negotiator, using conflict management skills to facilitate a compromise between parties. Difficulty dealing with individual team members with different personalities within a large complex healthcare organization is a frequent occurrence that care coordinators/case managers must handle (Mullahy, 2010). Table 4-7 offers some suggestions that may facilitate this process.

TABLE 4-6 The CMSA Standards for Negotiation

- Advocate and strive to achieve consensus among all parties. When consensus cannot be achieved, review all the alternatives, while encouraging the healthcare team to respect the family's wishes.
- Discuss the consequences of alternatives with all stakeholders.
- Represent the patient's interests by advocating for the necessary funding, appropriate treatment, and best treatment alternatives.
- Educate the patient and family about treatment options, and assist them to access necessary and appropriate services.

Source: Lowrey, 2004.

TABLE 4-7 The Rules of Engagement: Suggestions for a Successful Negotiation

- Always negotiate on a case-by-case basis.
- Try to sell your ideas without imposing them. Use persuasion.
- Be assertive. Do not be aggressive.
- Use collaborative skills.
- Clarify the issues.
- Stay focused on the problem. Do *not* let feelings get in the way.
- Define the limits—time limits, financial resource limits, medical resource limits.
- Know your power—personal power, expertise, and your own limitations.
- Be aware of hidden agendas.
- Know when to walk away: What is the bottom line?
- Never take the first offer.
- Be ready to compromise if necessary so that each party can be a "winner."

The negotiation process generally follows the process outlined here:

1. Establish criteria (i.e., the rules of engagement).
2. Exchange information.
3. Reach a compromise.
4. If an impasse occurs, set aside the issue (park the problem) and concentrate on smaller issues to keep communication open for an eventual agreement.
5. Be aware of changes in both your own and your opponent's demeanor.
6. Read between the lines—read facial expressions and body language.
7. Do *not* assume that something will *not* work. Always assume that *it will work*.
8. Once you have reached a verbal agreement, *get it in writing*.

Table 4-8 suggests a process for obtaining the goal of negotiation: a win/win solution.

Expert negotiators can separate people from the problem and negotiate through a "collaborative lens." The negotiator is a continuing and necessary role for healthcare coordinators/case managers, who take on this responsibility as part of their quest to obtain resources on behalf of patients and families (Birmingham & Anctil, 2002). The care coordinator/case manager uses negotiation skills to facilitate and coordinate all levels of care, motivating all stakeholders to work together collaboratively (Table 4-9).

For a care coordinator to effectively deal with complex situations, including those involving payers, patients, and other professionals, he or she must

---

TABLE 4-8 Seven Steps to a Win/Win Negotiation

1. **Listen:** Encourage the other person to describe his or her thoughts, ideas, and feelings. Use door openers, encouragers, and open-ended questions.
2. **Provide feedback:** Let the other party know you understand. Your feedback should be factual, non emotional, and solution focused.
3. **Affirm:** Provide the other party with positive feedback about his or her thoughts, ideas, or feelings about a situation.
4. **Look for a need:** Behind problems are usually personal, professional, or institutional needs. Once you have discovered your opponent's need(s), reconfirm what you think the need(s) is, follow with a restatement of what you perceived as his or her need(s), and then state your need(s).
5. **Examine possible solutions:** Discuss the possible solutions and the consequences of each.
6. **Select the best solution:** The solution should meet each party's needs.
7. **Follow up:** Agree on a specific time period to try out the solution and then make a date for a follow-up meeting.

TABLE 4-9 Skills Necessary for the Negotiator

- Interpersonal, communication, and active listening skills
- Knowledge of the issues (clinical, findings, service requirements, models of case management, evidence-based practice, funding issues)
- Conflict resolution skills
- Negotiation skills
- Delegation skills
- Collaborative skills
- Critical thinking skills
- Ability to tolerate stress

have excellent communication, conflict resolution, delegation, and negotiation skills. An excellent memory also helps. Negotiating skills can be learned. Indeed, several books from the popular press describe how to develop negotiating skills, including *Getting to Yes* by Fisher and Ury (1981) and *Negotiating for Dummies* by Donaldson and Donaldson (1996).

Familiarity with available resources and healthcare delivery systems is important to obtaining a favorable outcome from the negotiating process. As a successful negotiator, the care coordinator/case manager must establish rapport with all stakeholders, which paves the way for negotiating with all parties. Problem solving can be accomplished through a collaborative process (Birmingham & Anctil, 2000). Once an agreement is achieved and documented in writing, the care coordinator should send copies of the written agreement to all of the stakeholders (Lowrey, 2004).

ADVOCATE

The role of an advocate is central to the role of case manager/care coordinator (Daniels & Ramey, 2005; Tahan, 2005). Advocacy involves speaking up for what is right for patients in the belief that the advocate will make a difference on their behalf (Feuer, 2003). To be an effective advocate, the care coordinator/case manager needs to be empathic and able to convey an understanding of the psychosocial issues related to the patient's illness or injury (Chalmers, 2009). Care coordinators/case managers must be able to envision themselves in another person's shoes. Put another way, they must demonstrate emotional intelligence. Emotional intelligence encompasses being both self-aware and aware of the feelings of others (Hogan & Nickitas, 2009). The care coordinator/case manager helps families and patients examine their thoughts and feelings so that they better understand themselves and the ways in which their illness or injury affects them, especially when working with difficult patients (Fattorusso & Quinn, 2007).

Traditionally, professionals who coordinate healthcare services have thought of themselves as patient advocates. Today, however, advocacy in healthcare coordination often involves multiple parties. Case managers frequently face ethical dilemmas because they must be loyal to more than one party, some with conflicting needs (Banja, 2007). Recognizing these conflicts, Owen and Schuetze (2006) describe advocacy in care coordination/case management as a balancing act. Patients need the right treatment, at the right time, from the right provider. Families need the right information to make appropriate decisions. Hospitals need to allocate the fewest possible resources for the best clinical outcomes to maintain financial stability. Insurers need to limit their financial risks while funding necessary treatments, and they are beholden to their stockholders. Employers need to curtail healthcare cost inflation, while providing workers with appropriate benefits. Employers must also have a margin of profit to stay in business. These are the conflicting interests with which care coordinators/case managers wrestle on a daily basis. Moreover, care coordinators/case managers must balance advocacy with objectivity (Banja, 2007).

Care coordinators/case managers may be expected to advocate for all of these stakeholders, including the third-party payer, the hospital or healthcare organization, the physician, the patient and the family, and sometimes other healthcare providers. As an advocate, he or she balances the needs of the various providers, healthcare agencies, and insurers, while focusing primarily on the patient, thereby providing patient-centered care (Tahan, 2005).

A Balancing Act

A balancing act where the care coordinator must advocate for all parties is illustrated in the following scenario. The goal of the advocacy in this case was related to cost containment, with the decision focusing on whether to move a patient who is deemed appropriate for transfer to a facility that provides a lower level of care. Moving the patient from a more expensive level of care to a lesser level of care would save money for the healthcare organization, the insurance provider, and the patient—but the family does not agree. The care coordinator educates the family in an effort to persuade them to accept the move. The care coordinator facilitates an agreement among all of the stake-holders (i.e., the institution's staff, the referral agency, the physician, the patient and the family), so that all agree that the move is in the best interests of everyone. The care coordinator acts an advocate for all of the stakeholders simultaneously, serving as an educator and a negotiator who balances the needs of all parties.

TABLE 4-10 Teaching Strategies Commonly Used in Advocacy

The advocate teaches:

- What the patient and family need to know about the illness and its treatment. They also need to know which resources they will need and how to get them and from whom.
- Which expectations are realistic and which are unrealistic, and which limitations the healthcare providers and payers are subject to. What patients and families expect may not always be possible.
- Which self-help books are available, such as *Your Medical Rights: How to Become an Empowered Consumer* by Charles B. Inlander and Eugene L. Pavalon and *Working with Your Doctor: Getting the Health Care You Deserve* by Nancy Keene (cited in Feuer, 2003, p. 26).
- Which support groups are available. The care coordinator/cases manager may refer the patient and family to a support group either in the community or online (Feuer, 2003).

The Advocate as Teacher

The healthcare coordinator/case manager acting as an advocate ensures that patient rights are respected, including the rights of informed consent, self-determination, and privacy (Hellwig, Yam, & Giguilio, 2003). He or she teaches the patient and family to be self-advocates—an important aspect of healthcare coordination in today's increasingly more complex healthcare environment. To do so, the care coordinator/case manager uses the teaching strategies outlined in Table 4-10.

The Advocate as a Support Person and Negotiator

The advocate not only shares information and guides the decision-making process, but also honors the patient's or family's decisions. The care coordinator advocates for their rights to make their own decisions (i.e., the right to self-determination). Advocacy during the current managed care era also means advocating for patient services with insurance companies, even in the face of denials. Coffman (2001) advises persistence accompanied by a positive attitude may win the day. Tahan (2005) has equated advocacy with counseling, suggesting that both require open communication, connection, honesty, respect, and trust. Attending, listening, responding, and supporting are also counseling skills used to fulfill the advocacy role. Table 4-11 lists skills necessary for an advocate.

Advocacy also entails speaking out publicly on behalf of patients' and families' healthcare needs. Tahan (2005) calls this practice "global advocacy focused on the community." For example, advocates may write letters to the editor on

TABLE 4-11 Skills Important for Advocacy

- Communication skills, especially conveying empathy and understanding
- Ethical decision-making skills
- Conflict resolution skills
- Teaching/counseling/coaching skills
- Writing skills
- Public speaking skills
- Brokering/negotiating skills (appealing denials)

behalf of those who cannot or do not advocate for themselves. They may lobby legislators or others who hold the purse strings for healthcare resources (e.g., health insurance for poor individuals who are ineligible for Medicaid). As an advocate, the care coordinator speaks out professionally and publicly to support the rights and needs of patients and to encourage others to improve the healthcare system. Advocacy in case management is broader than in direct nursing care. It encompasses all of the stakeholders, rather than focusing solely on the patient. The advocate negotiates solutions that support best practices among all of the care providers to ensure patients' and families' safety and well-being.

EDUCATOR

The healthcare coordinator/nurse case manager frequently is an educator, when working with all parties on the care management team. He or she is a knowledge and information broker. The care coordinator/case manager educates the patient and family about the medical condition, treatment options, and possible adverse side effects of medications and risks associated with medical procedures. Education is extremely important for the patient and family so that they can make informed decisions and eventually manage their own care. The healthcare coordinator/nurse case manager may pull representatives from all disciplines and services together to meet with the patient and family, discuss the plan of care, and explain it in such a way that it makes sense to the patient and family. Thus it is important for the care coordinator to understand not only family dynamics but also group dynamics if he or she is to be a successful educator. One of the goals of the educator is to empower the patient and family in decision making and in learning self-responsibility and self-care.

The Patient and the Health Coach/Educator

Table 4-12 outlines the skills needed to fulfill the role of educator. The health coach not only educates the patient about self-care but also, through the

TABLE 4-12 Skills Important to the Role of Educator

- Communication/interpersonal skills
- Family and group therapy skills
- Empowerment/motivational/persuasion skills
- Supervisory skills
- Health coach/motivational interviewing

process of motivational interviewing, motivates, encourages, and may even prod a patient to live a healthier lifestyle. He or she is persuasive, selling the patient on lifestyle changes such as losing weight, exercising more, and following a diabetic diet. Motivational interviewing includes listening, recognizing, and affirming that healthy behaviors are in the patient's best interest (Howe, 2005). Working together, the coach/case manager and the patient write goals to facilitate a change in the patient's daily life style so as to enhance the patient's ability to achieve optimal health. For example, the goal of the patient with chronic obstructive pulmonary disease should be to stop smoking.

The Physician and Nursing Staff

As an educator, the healthcare coordinator may provide the physician with information that the physician may not have. For example, suppose a nurse case manager conducted a home visit and discovered living conditions that would affect the plan of care upon discharge. The care coordinator/case manager would immediately inform the healthcare team and the discharge planner, including the physician, that the discharge plan is in need of a revision to better meet the patient's needs.

The healthcare coordinator/case manager also educates physicians and other healthcare providers about how care coordination services can be of assistance to them and what the benefits are. In addition, he or she teaches physicians about reimbursement issues and other information about managed care.

The focus of the care coordinator as an educator is not only the patient and the family, but also the physicians, nurses, and other healthcare providers, so that they clearly understand the role of the care coordinator/case manager as a "helper" (and not a threat). Although case management has a long history, it is a relatively recent development in many acute care hospitals. Therefore, educating other professionals about this role is required to win their support.

CHANGE AGENT

Care coordinators/nurse case managers play a major role in the change process and act as change agents within healthcare institutions. They answer questions

TABLE 4-13 The Skills of a Change Agent

- Communication/interpersonal skills
- Sales skills
- Motivational skills—the ability to energize other people
- Group management skills
- Public relations skills
- Persuasive skills
- The ability to combine ideas from unconnected sources—integrative thinking
- Flexibility and self-confidence
- Realistic
- Visionary

and address concerns regarding impending changes that seem to be an ongoing occurrence in today's healthcare system. They also act as salespersons, selling care coordination services to hospital personnel and community agencies. Change has always been a constant occurrence in the healthcare milieu. The difference is that today it is more rapid (Sullivan & Decker, 2009).

Care coordinators should expect resistance to change and should be prepared to deal with it when implementing new policies and procedures (Cohen & Cesta, 2005; Sullivan & Decker, 2009). They should enter the change process with the understanding that resistance is a coping mechanism and can be overcome by the use of good communication skills, education, good public relations, ongoing group support, and the support of leaders and managers. Keeping co-workers and others affected by the change informed is vital (Sullivan & Decker, 2009). Table 4-13 summarizes the skills needed by a change agent.

COORDINATOR AND CARE FACILITATOR

Traditionally, "case manager" has been the title for nurses and social workers whose roles are to be the coordinator of care. In fact, the terms "care coordinator" and "case manager" have been used interchangeably. More recently, both patients and professionals have begun using the term "care coordination" to describe this function: Patients do not want to be "cases that are managed." The response of case managers has been to honor that wish and have switched to the term "care coordinator" to signal their responsibility.

Actually, coordinating healthcare services is at the crux of case management. Coordination involves organizing, securing, integrating, and modifying the resources necessary to meet the patient's, family's, or community's healthcare needs. Case coordinators/case managers facilitate access to care. In the

TABLE 4-14 Skills Necessary for Coordinating Care

- Interpersonal, communication, and active listening
- Clinical skills
- Assessment skills
- Facilitative skills
- Organizational skills
- Collaboration skills
- Negotiation skills
- Broker skills
- Critical thinking/problem-solving skills
- Counselor/educator skills

hospital, they are responsible for coordinating the day-to-day tasks, tests and procedures, transitional plans for referral or discharge, and patient and family teaching. They are also responsible for carrying out these tasks in a timely manner. Care coordinators/case managers coordinate the care of the patient in an effort to reduce fragmentation or duplication of services and to promote collaboration among team members. When problems with the plan of care arise, these individuals are responsible for taking charge and planning different interventions. Working as a coordinator, these professionals communicate any change of plans to the other healthcare providers and try to prevent any delay in care. They monitor the patient's progress and the length of stay, and plan for a timely discharge (Woodall, 2005).

Care coordinators/case managers coordinate care across the healthcare continuum, working with professionals and agencies to pave the way for smooth transfers, thereby ensuring the delivery of continuing quality, cost-effective care across the healthcare continuum (Tahan, 2007). Birmingham (2007) acknowledges that case managers are often required to balance more than several roles—for example, coordinator, discharge planner, and utilization manager. She suggests that trends in hospital case management have emphasized fiscal interests regarding reimbursements, at the expense of the case manager's responsibilities for coordination and discharge planning. She warns case managers to guard against the pressure to focus on costs rather than the quality of patient care. Care coordinators/case managers must work at balancing quality and costs. Table 4-14 summarizes the skills needed to fulfill this task.

DISCHARGE PLANNER

An important subrole in coordinating care is discharge planning to ensure continuity of care (Table 4-15). Discharge planning is frequently the role of the

TABLE 4-15 Discharge Planning

Starting at admission, discharge planning entails the following responsibilities:
- Identifying patients who are at risk for adverse outcomes
- Ensuring that there is adequate discharge planning
- Assessing for post-acute needs
- Monitoring for changes in the discharge plan
- Ensuring the choice of post-acute providers is appropriate to the needs of the patient
- Counseling patients and families about the discharge plan
- Teaching the patient and family skills that they will need to know after discharge
- Implementing the discharge plan

Source: Birmingham, 2007.

care coordinator/nurse case manager, but may be assigned to a social worker who is a member of the care coordination team. Discharge planners make sure medical equipment and other support services are in place and available when the patient arrives home. The discharge planner ensures that the transition from one level of care to another, or from the hospital to another facility or home, is a smooth one for both the patient and the family.

During a single episode of an illness, care may be provided in several different settings. Even though there is the potential for system-based errors to occur during transitions, the care coordinator's or case manager's responsibility as the discharge planner is to ensure that the quality of care is maintained as the patient moves from one level of care to the next. It is up to the care coordinator/case manager to make sure that each transition involves the right care by the right provider so that all parties can achieve the right outcome (Tahan, 2007).

RESOURCE MANAGER, UTILIZATION MANAGER AND REVIEWER, GATEKEEPER, PAYER-BASED NURSE CASE MANAGER, AND FINANCIAL ADVISOR

One care coordinator/case manager may carry out all of these functions—resource manager (RM), utilization manager (UM) and reviewer (UR), gatekeeper, payer-based nurse case manager (PB-NCM), and financial advisor—along with other case management functions. However, in some settings, a financial specialist may serve as the resource manager and/or utilization manager. In other settings, it may be the responsibility of the entire case management team to carry out the functions of an RM or UM. The RM/UM determines the necessary resources that are to be used when planning patient care (Cohen & Cesta,

2005). He or she ensures that the right services are provided at the appropriate level of care by the right healthcare professional at the most competitive cost to meet the needs of the patient (Fattorusso & Quinn, 2007)

Resource Manager

The care coordinator, as a resource manager, plays a vital role in controlling the length of stay and the use of resources, and is responsible for limiting unnecessary costs by coordinating care appropriately. A care coordinator/case manager probably spends as much time negotiating for resources to provide the best care for the patient, either in the hospital or at home, as he or she spends trying to coordinate the resources to implement the plan of care. The care coordination team must guard against over- or under utilization of resources and allocate them wisely. The resource manager makes sure that the appropriate services are provided to the patient to maximize his or her recovery at the lowest cost and in a timely manner.

Utilization Manager and Reviewer

The UM examines the costs of services, the ways in which people access them, and the frequency and duration of their use. He or she identifies the most expensive procedures, providers, and patients by tracking services, patients, and costs. The UM also uses standards and criteria to authorize and manage service delivery, including approvals and denials. The healthcare coordinator and the UM/UR must collaborate closely to ensure that the best quality of care is provided, while still containing costs (Mullahy, 2000).

Knowledge of insurance contracts, especially claims and benefits, is essential for healthcare coordinators and nurse case managers, who must negotiate with insurance companies on behalf of patients. Monitoring the appropriate use of resources, along with their costs, and matching the needs of the patient with the available and appropriate resources enforce a policy of efficiency and cost-effectiveness, which provides for the stability of the organization (Mullahy, 2010).

The UM/UR conducts periodic utilization reviews and analyzes the data from the reviews. Utilization reviews are conducted to examine the appropriate use of resources. Reviews of admissions, length of stays, discharges, and services are conducted during preadmission, hospitalization, and readmissions. Unnecessary services, inefficient use of resources, and the incurred costs are examined to determine the link between quality of care and costs. At the end of a review, the data are studied by the director of the case management program, in conjunction with the UR, and later discussed with the staff.

The results are then fed to the chief executive officer (CEO) or the chief financial officer (CFO) and discussed with them by the director of the case management program. Plans are discussed to address and rectify issues of poor resource utilization (Cohen & Cesta, 2005). The resource manager and UM/UR, either embodied by one person or acting as a team, monitor the utilization of services in terms of supply and demand, over- or under utilization of resources, and overall spending, including the costs of services.

Gatekeeper

As the gatekeeper, the healthcare coordinator or case manager monitors payments for resources, keeping them within the parameters established by the managed care contract between the patient and the payer. It is up to the care coordinator to ensure that the use of necessary resources is completed within acceptable and reimbursable time frames. If costs are excessive or services are required beyond the time limits, then either alternative plans must be developed or services must be renegotiated. This is a function of all healthcare coordinators/case managers; they are responsible for all referrals and for coordinating all services in a timely and cost-effective manner (Finkelman, 2001; Gerardi, 2005). The gatekeeper stands at the gate guarding the agency's cash reserves and the insurance company's financial resources. He or she decides which services are required and when, and if they are available under the patient's managed care contract.

The Payer-Based Healthcare Coordinator/Nurse Case Manager/ Discharge Planner

This role—summarized by the acronym PB-NCM-DCP—is another financial role for care coordinators/case managers who are employed by third-party payers, such as an insurance company. In the Greensboro/High Point/Winston-Salem area of North Carolina, both United Health Care and Partners employ nurse case managers. The collaborative work of the triad of primary care provider, hospital nurse case manager or hospital social worker, and PB-NCM-DCP is extremely beneficial upon admission, but especially during the time of discharge. The PB-NCM-DCP can be a valuable resource in facilitating a patient's discharge. Note, however, that the care coordinator/nurse case manager, who represents the insurance company, is not legally responsible for the discharge plan. Instead, he or she guides the provider and the hospital discharge planner (either a nurse or a social worker) in planning the discharge. The three collaborate on developing the best, most cost-effective discharge plan. The PB-NCM-DCP researches the potential resources and costs, and then

TABLE 4-16 Skills Necessary for the Role of Payer-Based Healthcare
Coordinator/Nurse Case Manager/Discharge Planner

- Collaborative/interpersonal/communication skills
- Case finding/screening/assessment
- Critical thinking skills for problem identification and problem resolution
- Assessment of resources—current and future
- Knowledge about insurance claims administration and benefits
- Ability to track the patient's progress and monitor the cost and quality of care provided by healthcare providers
- Knowledge of insurance contracts, including claims and benefits
- Knowledge of community resources and their costs
- Knowledge of which providers are in the network and which are outside the network

provides information to the hospital discharge planner about options that are covered in the patient's health insurance contract.

The triad of primary care provider, hospital nurse case manager or hospital social worker, and PB-NCM-DCP work together to develop a plan for accessing the necessary services. They communicate with one another in a timely fashion to avoid unnecessary delays in discharging the patient. The PB-NCM-DCP knows the criteria necessary for the insurance company to pay for skilled nursing, home health, and other services that may be required after discharge. He or she assists the hospital nurse case manager and the primary care provider in the planning process. A smooth transition and good outcomes are the desired result of the collegial and collaborative relationships among the providers and payers. Table 4-16 summarizes the skills that facilitate this process.

The PB-NCM-DCP collaborates with the hospital case manager, social worker, primary care nurse, or primary care provider to identify needs, assesses the necessary resources, and determines coverage under the patient's healthcare contract with the third-party payer. Functioning as an assessor, analyst, and broker, this professional contacts future potential providers within the insurance company's network whose services may be needed to meet the patient's needs after discharge. He or she determines if the insurance contract contains the appropriate financial criteria to pay for each of the healthcare providers. The PB-NCM-DCP also provides the authorization for care.

Planning is essential in order for the PB-NCM-DCP and the primary care coordinator to work together to negotiate services and payments for the future. The nurse case manager, who works for the third-party payer, serves as the liaison between the insurance company and the provider(s). Collaboration among members of this triad team is never more important than during admission and discharge (Birmingham, 2007). A study conducted by Greenwald and

Jack (2009) revealed that it is difficult to identify the risks that might lead to rehospitalization, but a multidisciplinary team working together before and after discharge can reduce the incidence of rehospitalization.

Having knowledge about how health insurance plans work helps the discharge planner in arranging physician visits, referrals, and obtaining special equipment for the home (Mullahy, 2000, 2010). Working with the insurance case manager, as well as with the primary care provider, patient and family, and family's pharmacy, is of utmost importance at the time of discharge (Greenwald & Jack, 2009). Providing a smooth transition from one level of care to the next is an essential ingredient of effective case management (Birmingham, 2007).

Financial Advisor

As a financial advisor, the healthcare coordinator addresses the issues of cost versus quality. An understanding of evidence-based medicine, insurance reimbursements, and Medicare/Medicaid is required of the financial adviser (Table 4-17). It is also necessary to know about reimbursement strategies, such as diagnostically related groups (DRGs), capitated contracts, and coding. The care coordinator researches affordable healthcare clinics and pharmaceutical programs to meet the financial and healthcare needs of each patient (Scott, 2007). The financial advisor/case manager considers all options, examining both fiscal and quality matters.

When patients and families are faced with unplanned catastrophic costs, the initial step for the care coordinator is to refer them to the business office for assistance and then to recommend a financial counseling service (Scott, 2007). The care coordinator/case manager should also educate the family about opportunities to apply for food stamps and other government programs.

TABLE 4-17 Skills Necessary for the Resource Manager, Utilization Reviewer, and Financial Advisor

- Business and financial skills
- Assessment skills
- Data analysis skills
- Negotiation skills
- Advocacy skills
- Analytical skills
- Critical thinking skills/problem-solving skills
- Knowledge of managed care and third-party payers
- Counseling/advising skills

Business and financial skills are important for care coordinators, who are financial advisors because the goal of case management is to contain costs while maintaining quality. All care coordinators and nurse case managers who are in roles that require financial management must have skills in finance, contracting, and reimbursements; they must also know how to make cost comparisons. Care coordinators should be aware of the financial implications of different options. The care coordinator/nurse case manager must analyze all of these options, consider a decision in terms of its impact on the quality of care and financial impact, and then advocate for the best option.

ADMINISTRATOR/MANAGER/LEADER

The management and leadership role not only applies to the healthcare coordinator/nurse case manager who works as an administrator or director of a program (addressed in Chapter 1), but who is also a care coordinator or case manager. The latter professionals need leadership and management skills because they are responsible for facilitating, expediting, and coordinating care. The care coordinator/nurse case manager plans, coordinates, and organizes all treatments and resources, and is responsible for following through to make sure that they are correctly implemented. The manager/leader solves problems, sets goals and priorities, provides timelines, and collaborates with others to develop a plan of care. Once the plan of care is in place, the care coordinator/case manager supervises its implementation. Along the way, he or she may delegate certain responsibilities to other members of the interdisciplinary team. The manager/leader continually evaluates the overall plan of care, its implementation, the outcomes, and the effectiveness of the interdisciplinary healthcare team.

The care coordinator/nurse case manager as a leader/manager must have good working relationships with all types of people, including the patient and family, physicians, employers, insurers, dieticians, therapists, and social workers. He or she should inspire the healthcare team to strive to provide patient care that is satisfactory, effective, patient centered, timely, and efficient. To achieve these goals, the team members must collaborate successfully (Cohen & Cesta, 2005). Collaboration to achieve agreed-upon goals among professionals, the patient, and family members often is not an easy feat, so the leader/manager must be both patient and persistent. He or she must facilitate the collaborative activities of the team members to meet the stated goals of the group. (Collaboration is discussed in greater detail in Chapter 6.)

A nursing administration or an organizational dynamics course will provide an in-depth review of the skills, functions, and responsibilities of a leader/

TABLE 4-18 Leadership/Management Skills

- Leadership/management skills
- Delegation skills
- Supervisory skills (monitor/evaluator)
- Analytic skills
- Organizational skills
- Collaborative skills
- Excellent interpersonal skills
- Skill as a visionary
- Motivational skills

manager. Table 4-18 briefly summarizes the skills needed to fulfill this position.

RESEARCHER

Care coordinators/nurse case managers may conduct clinical research. As part of doing so, they may write grants and research proposals. The goal of such research is often to examine innovative approaches to the delivery of health care in an attempt to bridge the gap between theory and practice. To date, the majority of case management research has focused on outcome studies and has examined issues such as length of stay and costs. Lately, more studies have examined specific interventions that influence outcomes. Currently, care coordinators/nurse case managers are seeking frameworks to guide their practice, building on knowledge from the past and asking questions for the future.

More research manuscripts on case management topic are now being published by *Journal of Professional Case Management*. For example, the August 2009 issue included an article titled "Reducing Unnecessary Medicare Admissions," where the research was sponsored by the Centers for Medicare and Medicaid Services. The study comprised a six-state research project that was conducted by a research team of healthcare professionals, including Romero, Brown, Richards, Collier, Jantz, Michelman, and Davidson.

Some researchers have studied practice issues in terms of standards of care and evidence-based practice (Stanton & MacRobert, 2007). Evidence-based practice is the application of the best clinical interventions, where "the best" is based on scientific research evidence related to the patient's diagnosis or condition and the clinical situation (Sullivan & Decker, 2009). Evidence-based practice guides healthcare practitioners in selecting the best interventions based on clinically relevant outcome data (Finkelman, 2006). After implementation, the current outcomes are evaluated to support the nurse case manager's practice (Goode, 2005). Barriers to understanding evidence-based practice include the following obstacles:

- Lack of value for research and/or administrative support
- Lack of understanding regarding the structure of electronic databases
- Difficulty accessing research materials, especially in rural areas
- Lack of computer skills and/or research skills (Stanton & MacRobert, 2007)

The Internet has proven to be a great help in overcoming these barriers. The CMSA website, for example, identifies resources to guide case managers in conducting clinical research and implementing evidence-based practice. Evidence-based practice is an important component in improving the quality of health care.

Recent National Studies

The Commission for Case Management Certification (CCMC) conducted a series of national studies on the roles of case managers across the United States, in a variety of settings and disciplines, to determine the strategies used in each role. The impetus for this research was the need to develop a valid certification exam so that it would reflect the knowledge areas deemed important by case managers from across disciplines, settings, and geographical areas. The study contributed information about the domains of practice and the knowledge required for effective case management.

Another study carried out by CCMC reflected the changing dynamics of the field of case management and its continuing evolution. The conclusions of this study were that case managers function in different settings and that the role is performed by different disciplines. Even so, all case managers share a core body of knowledge necessary to effectively perform the role (Huber & Tahan, 2004; Tahan, Downey, & Huber, 2006; Tahan, Huber, & Downey, 2006).

Research Skills

Case management research remains in its infancy. Nursing case management needs to continue to develop measures that are reliable and valid and to perfect the case manager's research skills. Goode (2005) has emphasized the necessity of lifelong learning if a professional is to remain current as a researcher/case manager. The need for clinical research is growing, as the demand for reporting outcome data will undoubtedly be linked to third-party reimbursements to a greater extent in the future (Goode, 2005).

TABLE 4-19 Clinical Skills

The clinician/nurse case manager:
- Must have a wide range of skills and experience.
- Should have a broad knowledge about disease processes, therapeutic tests, practices, and procedures, across settings.
- Is a role model for other staff and should strive to demonstrate the highest level of clinical knowledge (Cohen & Cesta, 2005).
- Must acknowledge the limitations of his or her clinical expertise and work within these limitations, as well as understanding the scope of practice.
- Should attend continuing education courses, seminars, and workshops to keep current with the medical trends and treatments.
- Should have good writing skills. The case manager must carefully document outcomes, thereby illustrating that care coordination/case management is the strategy to achieve best practice, to contain costs, and to ensure that the patient receives quality care. Without good documentation supporting its value, a case management program can be eliminated at the drop of an administrator's hat.

CLINICIAN

All care coordinators/case managers are required to have expert clinical skills regardless of their role, the discipline, or the setting. Good clinical skills are pertinent to all care coordinators, whereas some other skills (e.g., financial skills) may be pertinent to some roles and not others. Nurse case managers involved in utilization management and review must have analytical and financial skills, for example.

All care coordinators/nurse case managers need to understand third-party reimbursements, but not all need to be financial experts. Put simply, the most essential role of a healthcare coordinator/nurse case manager is the role of clinician/practitioner, and all of these professionals need to be experts in nursing care (Table 4-19).

■ SUMMARY

Many skills required for the various roles filled by healthcare coordinators/case managers overlap, and several are basic to all of these roles. The debate about who is best qualified to be a care coordinator continues. Nurses can offer many skills and have attributes that other disciplines do not have. Currently, most healthcare coordinators are either social workers or nurses. Either embodied in one person or working together as a dyad team, personnel geared toward healthcare coordination effectively facilitate holistic care by contributing to a broad perspective of acute and community care. (The dyad team is discussed in detail in Chapter 6.) To demonstrate their effectiveness as part of the health-care delivery system, case managers should carefully document the outcomes that they achieve.

Care coordination or case management is practiced in many settings and by many disciplines. The goals of care coordination/case management are to contain costs while providing the highest-quality care to patients and families. Today, care coordination/case management is one of the fastest-growing medically related professions in the United States (Cohen & Cesta, 2005). This growth is expected to continue as long as the U.S. healthcare system remains fragmented, with providers functioning in a managed care environment that focuses largely on cost containment. Currently, we are grappling with how to reform this ungainly healthcare system. Until reform is accomplished, however, the need for care coordinators/case managers will persist.

■ CASE STUDIES

Mr. P. is an 88-year-old, recently widowed male who was admitted to the hospital following a fall outside his home on an uneven sidewalk. He has successfully undergone hip replacement surgery and is beginning his rehabilitation on the acute care surgical unit. Mr. P. has a 61-year-old son who is married and lives approximately one hour away. The son and daughter-in-law have visited frequently but will not be able to care for Mr. P. at discharge. The physical therapist does not believe that Mr. P. will do well enough at home to discharge independently.

1. What are three basic goals to achieve during your initial interview with Mr. P.?
2. Which negotiation skills could you use if Mr. P. is uncomfortable with the discharge plan?
3. Which arrangements should be made for Mr. P. at discharge?
4. Which communication skills would enhance the discharge planning process?

■ DISCUSSION QUESTIONS

1. Discuss three roles of the nurse case manager (including one in the community setting and one in the acute care setting).
2. How does each role assist the healthcare coordinator in meeting the goals of case management?
3. Describe the functions that are related to each of the roles.
4. Which skills are necessary to carry out each role?

■ CLASSROOM EXERCISES

With your fellow students, engage in a classroom discussion of the following topics:

1. As a manager or case manager, which strategies would you use to empower your staff and patients that would enhance their welfare? Give specific examples of what you may have done or may want to do in the future.
2. Which experiences have you had as a staff nurse (or patient) whereby another professional empowered you in terms of your own professional or personal growth and development? Describe the experience.
3. Discuss your experiences in collaborating with personnel from other disciplines or any experiences you may have had as a member of an interdisciplinary team.

RECOMMENDED READINGS

Feuer, L. (2003). Encouraging the advocacy role. *Case Manager*, *14*(4), 24–26.

Fink-Samnick, E. (2004, September/October). Was that fee or free? Managing communication barriers. *Case Manager*, *15*(5), 52–55.

Greenwald, J. L., & Jack, B. W. (2009). Preventing the preventable: Rehospitalization through coordination, patient-centered discharge processes. *Journal of Professional Case Management*, *14*(3), 135–140.

Lowrey, S. (2004, January/February). Negotiating for successful outcomes in case management practice. *Case Manager*, *15*(1), 70–72.

Owen, M., & Schuetze, K. (2006). Case managers face a "balancing act" of patient advocacy, demands from other parties. *Lippincott's Case Management*, *11*(4), 226–228.

Romero, A., Brown, C., Richards, F., Collier, P., Jentz, S., Michelman, M., et al. (2009). Reducing unnecessary Medicare admissions: A six state project. *Journal of Professional Case Management*, *14*(3), 143–150.

Tahan, H. A. (2007). One patient, numerous healthcare providers, and multiple care settings: Addressing the concerns of care transitions through case management. *Professional Case Management*, *12*(1), 37–46.

REFERENCES

Banja, J. (2007). Case managers and ethics: Balancing advocacy with objective evaluation. *Professional Case Management*, *12*(2), 68–69.

Birmingham, J. (2007). Case management: Two regulations with coexisting functions (utilization review and discharge planning–case management). *Professional Case Management, 12*(1), 16–24.

Birmingham, J., & Anctil, B. (2002). Managing the dynamics of collaboration. *Case Manager, 13*(3), 73–77.

Chalmers, L. (2009). From ethics violation remediation: A learning experience. *Journal of Professional Case Management, 14*(3), 151–153.

Coffman, S. (2001). Examining advocacy and case management in managed care. *Pediatric Nursing, 27*(3), 287–289.

Cohen, E. L., & Cesta, T. G. (2001). *Nursing case management: From essentials to advanced practice applications* (3rd ed.). St. Louis, MO: Mosby.

Cohen, E. L., & Cesta, T. G. (2005). *Nursing case management: From essentials to advanced practice* (4th ed.). St. Louis, MO: Elsevier/Mosby.

Daniels, S., & Ramey, M. (2005). *The leader's guide to hospital case management.* Sudbury, MA: Jones and Bartlett.

Donaldson, M. C., & Donaldson, M. (1996). *Negotiating for dummies.* Foster City, CA: IDG Books Worldwide.

Fattorusso, D., & Quinn, C. E. (2007). *A case manager's study guide: Preparing for certification* (3rd ed.). Sudbury, MA: Jones and Bartlett.

Feuer, L. (2003). Encouraging the advocacy role. *Case Manager, 14*(4), 24–26.

Fink-Samnick, E. (2004, September/October). Was that fee or free? Managing communication barriers. *Case Manager, 15*(5), 52–55.

Finkelman, A. W. (2001). Case management and collaborative care. In *Managed care: A nursing perspective* (pp. 123–148). Upper Saddle River, NJ: Prentice Hall.

Finkelman, A. W. (2006). *Leadership and management in nursing.* Upper Saddle River, NJ: Pearson/Prentice Hall.

Fisher, R., & Ury, W. (1981). *Getting to yes: Negotiating agreement without giving in* (2nd ed.). New York: Penguin Books.

Gerardi, T. (2005). The managed care market. In E. L. Cohen & T. G. Cesta (Eds.), *Nursing case management: From essentials to advanced practice applications* (4th ed., pp. 210–218). St. Louis, MO: Elsevier/Mosby.

Goode, C. J. (2005). Outcomes effectiveness and evidence-based practice. In E. L. Cohen & T. G. Cesta (Eds.), *Nursing case management: From essentials to advanced practice applications* (4th ed., pp. 572–579). St. Louis, MO: Elsevier/Mosby.

Greenwald, J. L., & Jack, B. W. (2009). Preventing the preventable: Rehospitalization through coordination, patient-centered discharge processes. *Journal of Professional Case Management, 14*(3), 135–140.

Hellwig, S. D., Yam, M., & Giguilio, M. (2003). Nurse case managers' perceptions of advocacy. *Lippincott's Case Management, 8*(2), 53–65.

Herrick, C. A., Bartlett, T. R., Pearson, G. S., Schmidt, C., & Cherry, J. (2006). System of care in nursing: Across the life span and across settings. In M. Arbuckle & C. Herrick (Eds.), *Child and adolescent mental health: System of care interdisciplinary practice* (pp. 129–157). Sudbury, MA: Jones and Bartlett.

Hogan, M. A., & Nickitas, D. M. (2009). *Nursing leadership and management: Reviews and rationales.* Upper Saddle River, NJ: Pearson/Prentice Hall.

Howe, R. (2005). Motivational interviewing. In *The disease manager's handbook* (pp. 81–82). Sudbury, MA: Jones and Bartlett.

Huber, D. L., & Tahan, H. A. (2004). Managing forces of change: Commission for case manager certification looks to the future. *Lippincott's Case Management, 9*(2), 57–60.

Lowrey, S. (2004, January/February). Negotiating for successful outcomes in case management practice. *Case Manager, 15*(1), 70–72.

Mullahy, C. M. (2000, March/April). The effective integration of utilization and case management. *Case Manager, 11*(2), 53–56.

Mullahy, C. M. (2010). *The case manager's handbook* (4th ed.). Sudbury, MA: Jones and Bartlett.

Owen, M., & Schuetze, K. (2006). Case managers face a "balancing act" of patient advocacy, demands from other parties. *Lippincott's Case Management, 11*(4), 226–228.

Romero, A., Brown, C., Richards, F., Collier, P., Jentz, S., Michelman, M., et al. (2009). Reducing unnecessary Medicare admissions: A six state project. *Journal of Professional Case Management, 14*(3), 143–150.

Scott, R. (2007, February/March). The essence of hospital case management. *Case in Point,* 10–11.

Stanton, M., & MacRobert, M. (2007). Putting the easy into evidence-based practice. *Professional Case Management, 12*(1), 5–13.

Sullivan, E. J., & Decker, P. J. (2009). Leading, managing, following. In *Effective leadership and management in nursing* (7th ed., pp. 43–65). Upper Saddle River, NJ: Pearson/Prentice Hall.

Tahan, H. A. (2005). Essentials of advocacy in case management. *Lippincott's Case Management, 10*(3), 136–145.

Tahan, H. A. (2007). One patient, numerous healthcare providers, and multiple care settings: Addressing the concerns of care transitions through case management. *Professional Case Management, 12*(1), 37–46.

Tahan, H. A., Downey, W. T., & Huber, D. L. (2006). Case managers' roles and functions. Commission for Case Management Certification 2004 research: Part II. *Lippincott's Case Management, 11*(2), 71–87.

Tahan, H. A., Huber, D., & Downey, W. (2006). Case managers' roles and functions. CCMC 2004 research: Part I. *Lippincott's Case Management, 11*(1), 4–22.

Turkettle, M. A., & Noj, A. (2003). Case management: A source of support and stability for the client and the health care system. *Lippincott's Case Management, 8*(2), 88–94.

Woodall, J. (2005). Case management. In E. L. Cohen & T. G. Cesta (Eds.), *Nursing case management: From essentials to advanced practice applications* (4th ed., pp. 55–67). St. Louis, MO: Elsevier/Mosby.

Models of Care

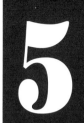

Laura J. Fero
Charlotte A. Herrick

■ OUTLINE

■ OBJECTIVES

1. Describe "within the walls" (acute care) case management models, "outside the walls" (community-based) case management models, and continuum-of-care case management models.

2. Identify the roles of the case manager and the case management team.

3. Describe the setting and the target population for each case management model.

4. Compare the goals and the outcomes for each case management model.

INTRODUCTION

A variety of models have been developed both "within the walls" (inpatient) and "beyond the walls" (community-based outpatient and continuum-of-care models). In this chapter, we use the term "case management" to describe all of these models, because most were developed as case management was evolving. Traditionally, the term most widely used was "case management" rather than the currently preferred "care coordination." Case management is an interdisciplinary healthcare delivery service that may take many forms depending on the discipline, the structure of the organization, the hospital's staffing patterns, the target population served, and the model selected to guide case management practice (Herrick & Bartlett, 2004; Huber, 2002).

Models have been developed to provide a framework for case management practice to meet the demands of both inpatient and outpatient settings. Continuum-of-care models span the boundaries of both inpatient and outpatient settings. As the number of patients with chronic diseases has grown, a chronic care model has been developed as well.

Although the chronic care model is primarily a community-based model, sometimes a designated person from the assigned case management team must follow the patient when he or she is hospitalized, working closely with the hospital case manager in preparation for discharge; thus this model spans the boundaries between the acute care and community settings.

This chapter describes the various models of case management. It provides a historical perspective on the development of the various models of case management.

"WITHIN THE WALLS" MODELS: ACUTE CARE

In acute care case management programs, the role of the case manager is an integrative one, beginning at the acute phase of the patient's illness and sometimes continuing beyond discharge (Scott, 2007). Inpatient models were developed as means to care for patients in acute care settings. The New England model was copied by many hospitals. Most inpatient case management programs emphasize utilization review (UR) and discharge planning (DCP) (Daniels & Ramey, 2005). Most hospital case management programs have included some or all of the following components:

- *Clinical models* include direct patient care responsibilities. Recently, this model has evolved into a disease management model, in an acute care setting.
- *Collaborative practice models* include a multidisciplinary team, using clinical pathways, variance reporting, patient teaching, and monitoring and evaluating care.
- *Population models* focus on an acute care episode, which includes UR services and DCP, based on a specific disease and a service line. The specific disease usually involves one that is associated with high costs.
- *Functional models* focus on acute care episodes, and include UR and DCP. Consolidation of services occurs when several departments are collapsed into one—for example, social work (MSW) and UR, or nursing (RN) and UR. This type of merger means that some positions can be eliminated in both departments, so costs are reduced.
- *Clinical resource management models* include disease management models that target high-risk populations and outcomes models that focus on data collection (UR and DCP) (Daniels & Ramey, 2005, pp. 94–96).

Many organizations have created their own unique models, combining elements of these components to better meet the needs of their patients in their specific settings. Daniels and Ramey (2005) label these models "hybrids" (p. 96). Whichever model is used, the role of the case manager in a "within the walls" model is to link the patient, the physician, the nursing staff, and the payer to meet the desired outcomes, notably cost containment and quality care.

The New England Model (Zander Model)

During the advent of managed care in the 1980s, managers at the New England Medical Center (NEMC) developed a case management approach that grew out of the model for primary care nursing. The impetus for developing the New England model was the implementation of regulations related to diagnostically related groups (DRGs), the prospective payment system, and other changes in the methods by which hospitals are reimbursed for services rendered.

In this primary care case management model, nurse case managers are responsible for coordinating the patient's care 24 hours per day, 7 days per week; they coordinate the interdisciplinary team to achieve this goal. Patients are assigned to a group practice composed of physicians and primary care and secondary care nurses, who are responsible for delivering the direct care. The case manager is also a part of the group practice. His or her authority extends over all units—wherever the patient is located in the hospital during the course of the patient's stay (Zander, 1988a, 1988b, 1991, 1992a, 1992b).

Clinical pathways (CPs) were developed at NEMC to monitor care delivery, the patient's progress, and measure outcomes. Multidisciplinary action plans (care MAPs) were developed based on the CPs, expanding on them to include standards of care, practices specific to a diagnostic type, continuous quality improvement, resource allocation, cost reimbursement, and patient care outcomes (Cohen & Cesta, 2005a, 2005b; Zander, 1998a, 1998b).

The Goals

Cost containment and reduction in the length of stay (LOS).

The Case Management Team

The case management triad: the nurse case manager (RN-CM), the social worker case manager (MSW-CM), and the utilization reviewer (UR-CM).

The Setting/Population

Urban, diverse, and acutely ill populations; examples include patients with cardiac conditions, leukemia, and stroke.

Roles and Functions of the Case Management Team

The Case Management Team

- The team provides primary care and direct care on the assigned unit.
- The case manager and the physician (MD or DO) follow the same patient, if the patient is transferred to another unit.

The Case Manager

- Coordinates care for a group of patients. He or she may or may not be providing direct care. The care manager coordinates care over the course of the patient's entire hospitalization.
- Monitors the CPs and MAPs, and conducts variance analyses.
- Conducts case consultations.
- Designs the discharge plan.
- Is responsible for clinical and financial outcomes.
- Conducts limited follow-up after discharge.
- Educates the patient and family, and involves the family in goal setting, treatment planning, and discharge planning.

Outcomes

- Decreased LOS
- Decreased costs
- Adoption of the New England model for acute care settings as "the model" for other hospitals to imitate across the United States

In primary care case management, the case manager is responsible for care coordination as well as development and evaluation of the delivery of care and the quality of patient care on a 24/7 basis. Once assigned to a patient, the case manager follows that patient even if the patient is transferred to another unit. The case manager is assigned as a team member to a group practice (Huber, 2002; Woodall, 2005; Zander, 1988a, 1988b, 1991, 1992a, 1992b).

The Integrated Model for Acute Care

The integrated model for acute care was developed at St. Vincent's Catholic Medical Center in New York City. It weaves together three functions: clinical coordination/facilitation, utilization review, and discharge planning. All case managers are nurses and are unit based. The social workers are reassigned to counseling and social support; in this role, they deal with the end-of life issues, substance abuse, financial issues, and family support. The tool used to track outcomes is the MAP. The integration of the three roles reduces redundancy, duplication, and delays in obtaining ancillary services (Woodall, 2005).

The Goals

- Cost containment
- Decreased LOS
- Improved quality of care

The Case Management Team

The nursing team has three specific roles: coordination of care, utilization review, and/or discharge planning.

The Setting/Population

Urban, diverse, acutely ill patients.

Roles and Functions of the Case Management Team

- Coordination of care
- Facilitation of interdisciplinary interventions; attend daily rounds and team meetings
- Psychosocial assessments
- Facilitate access to ancillary services
- Monitor the utilization of resources
- Discharge planning
- Facilitate transitions to other services or settings
- Outcomes management

Outcomes

- Decreased LOS
- Decreased costs
- Improved quality of care
- Reduced duplication and fragmentation of resources, resulting in improved allocation of resources (Woodall, 2005)

In a 2004 article on evidence-based case management practice, McKendry and Van Horn stated that case management is continually challenged by the need to balance clinical and financial considerations. By integrating utilization review, case management, and discharge planning as part of the same model, case managers can achieve the following goals:

▪ Work more effectively when developing patient-specific care plans to meet complex care needs
▪ Identify more easily which patient-specific clinical outcomes need to be achieved
▪ Ensure that discharge planning needs are not only evaluated accurately, but also met

The Collaborative Model

The collaborative model (a transdisciplinary model) is commonly used today in acute care hospitals. Collaboration is a process of joint decision making among interdependent parties who are both accountable and responsible for the outcomes of their decisions. For example, at Moses Cone Behavioral Health in Greensboro, North Carolina, the case management team consists of a social worker, a nurse, and a licensed professional counselor.

The collaborative model was originally developed at Vanderbilt University Medical Center in Nashville, Tennessee. The Vanderbilt model recognized that a diverse skill mix is extremely effective and leads to the best outcomes (Koenig, 2005). The collaborative team includes the nurse case manager, who is the clinical coordinator; the social worker (MSW), who is the crisis interventionist and psychosocial assessor, and who provides brief therapy, when needed; and the utilization resource manager, who acts as the systems coordinator. The utilization resource manager is a specialist in DRGs and reimbursements. He or she examines precertifications, medical interventions, and recertification authorizations; conducts chart resource utilization reviews; monitors medical records; and collects quality and cost data.

The collaborative model is best described as a case management process that focuses on coordinating patient care across the hospital continuum of care to ensure optimal quality outcomes, patient satisfaction, and appropriate use of resources. All members of the team are accountable for realizing these goals (Koenig, 2005).

The Goals

▪ Quality, cost-effective care
▪ Improved allocation of resources
▪ Enhanced patient satisfaction
▪ Better discharge planning and improved continuity of care

The Case Management Team

The triad: the nurse case manager, the social worker case manager, and the utilization resource specialist. A nurse also serves as the utilization resource manager.

The Setting/Population

A large academic and urban medical center in a Southern city, serving a diverse population of acutely ill patients.

Roles and Functions of the Case Management Team

- Coordination of care (including discharge planning)
- Appropriate allocation of resources
- Crisis intervention with patients and families
- Certification, recertification, and authorizations
- Chart review/medical records
- Collection of outcomes data
- Responsibility for outcomes (shared by the case management team and the case management department)

Outcomes

- Quality, cost-effective care
- Improved patient satisfaction
- Better allocation of resources
- Improved continuity of care through better discharge planning

"BEYOND THE WALLS" MODELS: COMMUNITY-BASED CARE

The Broker Model

The traditional social work model matches patient and family needs with services. The social worker (MSW) links together a network of providers and services using assessment and referral strategies. At the same time, the social worker verifies the availability of needed services. This model is a generalist model that capitalizes on the social worker's knowledge of community resources (Herrick & Bartlett, 2004; Huber, 2002).

The Goals

Provide continuity of care.

The Setting/Population

Any community setting (rural or urban). Patients who have medical or social problems but do not have complex medical conditions.

The Case Management Team

A one-to-one relationship is forged between the social worker and the patient/family.

Roles and Functions of the Case Manager

Match patient needs with a network of services.

Outcomes

- Improved continuity of care
- Better access to health care and other resources

The Community Mental Health Model

The community mental health (CMH) model paved the way for many other case management models, such as the system of care model, the dyad model, and the collaborative model. The original CMH model was a broker model. When deinstitutionalization became the norm in the 1960s, however, it became clear that psychiatric patients had a multitude of needs. To meet these needs, the broker model was combined with a disease management model to form a psychosocial model, which included crisis intervention; supportive psychotherapy; family support; medication management, including home visitation and monitoring; and nonpsychiatric services, including access to food and housing, vocational training, rehabilitation, and other social services. The CMH model provided a lifeline to support independent living for severely mentally ill individuals. It was designed to provide 24-hour case management throughout the individual's life span.

Two specific models were developed to address these needs: the Program for Assertive Community Treatment (PACT) and Intensive Case Management (ICM). The latter model assigned smaller caseloads to case managers, thereby enabling them to provide more intensive case management. The goal of both programs is to keep people out of the hospital. If an individual is hospitalized, a safety net is activated upon patient discharge, allowing for a shorter LOS. With both PACT and ICM, outcomes research has demonstrated that these goals have been met (Herrick & Bartlett, 2004; Scott & Boyd, 2001).

The Goals

- Reduce recidivism and the "revolving door"
- Support mentally ill persons who live in the community, and improve their quality of life
- Reduce the LOS, if the patient needs hospitalization
- Improve medication compliance and compliance with other mental health regimens, including outpatient appointments

The Case Management Team

The nurse, social worker, rehabilitation counselor, and substance abuse counselor.

The Setting/Population

Chronically mentally ill persons who are living in the community. The Veterans Administration (VA) has established similar programs for mentally ill patients covered by this agency.

Roles and Functions of the Case Management Team

- Supportive individual, group, and family therapy
- Medication monitoring
- Home visitation
- Facilitation of access to community services, social services, health and mental health services
- Coordination of care across the healthcare continuum, thus enhancing the quality of care
- Assistance with access to housing and all other community services necessary to maintain the patient in the community
- Education of patients about self-maintenance (i.e., activities of daily living)

Outcomes

- Decreased recidivism (avoid the revolving door)
- Improved quality of life
- Reduced LOS
- Better medication compliance and compliance with other medical or mental health regimens, such as attending group therapy and keeping physician appointments

The Independent Practice Model

Case managers who work in private practice are entrepreneurs whose services are contracted for by individuals or families, or subcontracted for by groups, to coordinate health care and community services. These independent practitioners are case managers who want to chart their own careers (Miller, 2007). Some have established small independent firms. Others work for large, national case management companies (Huber, 2002).

The Goals

To facilitate continuity of care by assisting clients to access care across the healthcare continuum.

The Case Management Team

The case manager may have a solo practice or may work with a group of case managers.

The Setting/Population

Frail elderly individuals and other vulnerable populations who are living independently.

Roles and Functions of the Case Management Team

- Assist people to maintain a healthy life in their own homes
- Assist, educate, and empower the client toward achieving optimal health
- Provide support and counseling
- Coordinate healthcare and community resources

ve the case management team develop and implement care plans,
h the parents serving as integral members of the team.
power the family toward, and assist the family to reach, their
ximum potential (strengths based).

se Management Team

health counselors or nurses, social workers, teachers and principals,
and any other person designated by the child and/or family as signifi-
their stability and growth (for example, the minister or neighbor).
onal members of the team should not outnumber the patient/family
munity members. Power should be distributed equally among all team
rs. A team leader is selected by group consensus to be the care
ator.

tting/Population

y emotionally disturbed children and their parents, living in the
nity.

nd Functions of the Case Management Team

llaborate to provide comprehensive care and emotional support to
e child and family
ordinate care to include professional and community resources
ovide individual expertise (including the family's expert knowledge
out the child) to plan interventions
cilitate access to health care and other resources across the health-
re continuum
ild a network of professional and community services to sustain a
mily with complex needs in the community

nes

creased school dropout rates
creased hospitalizations
proved child and family functioning, including higher grades at
hool
creased trouble with the law
creased risk-taking behaviors (e.g., alcohol, drugs, and sexual
haviors)

Outcomes

- Coordinated care across the healthcare continu
- Clients who remain independent and conti
  community
- Improved access to health care and community
- Enhanced quality of life

The System of Care Model

The system of care is a community-based mental heal
oped core values and principles about the way service
severely emotionally disturbed children and their far
based model, the case manager assists family membe
sonal goals by helping them to access and maintain t
to provide an environment where parents can work and
attend school, and remain in their homes and commur
core values include care that is community based, cu
family centered.

Approximately 10 principles guide case manageme
model, only some of which are discussed here. One
principles is that services should be comprehensive and
management team. The "wrap-around" concept was d
fact that the continuum of care is not a straight line, bu
circle of services that are wrapped around the family. '
the family to provide a safety net for the child and fami
2002). In a system of care, care is holistic; that is, it (
healthcare continuum, including social services, menta
juvenile justice, educational, and other community ser
vices used are selected by the team to assist the fami
home, in school, and continuing to reside in the commun
him or her off to a residential program (Furman & Ja
Dosser, McCammon, & Powell, 1998; Herrick, 2006; He
Herrick, Bartlett, Pearson, Schmidt, & Cherry, 2006).

The Goals

- Keep the child at home and in school.
- Provide a seamless coordinated system of care tha
  and at the same time individualized to meet the nee
  family.

- Ha
  wi
- Er
  m.

The C

Mental
parents
cant to
Profess
and co
membe
coordi

The S

Severe
commu

Role a

- C
  th
- C
- P
  a
- F
  c
- P
  f

Outco

- I
- I
- I
  s
- I
- I
  l

- Improved family/community interactions, especially with educators, which result in better social support
- Improved quality of life
- Decreased family violence and abuse

CONTINUUM-OF-CARE MODELS: WITHIN THE WALLS AND BEYOND

Tucson–Carondelet, Arizona

The integrative collaborative care model developed in Tucson, Arizona, at Carondelet/St. Mary's Hospital integrates the services of nursing case management and home health, respite care, and home infusion therapy, while at the same time networking with the acute care hospital case managers and a community case manager (Lamb & Zazworsky, 2005). Carondelet/St. Mary's Hospital is an acute care medical center that delivers a full spectrum of nursing services, both in the hospital and in the community, including hospice, home health, long-term, and ambulatory care. The structure of the organization is a "nursing HMO"—that is, a system of care that is decentralized into nursing centers across the healthcare continuum (Ethridge, 1991). As part of this approach, nurse case managers are organized into nursing service networks. This patient/family-centered model combines nursing case management in acute care and community care, health promotion, and disease management. This model has been found to be especially effective with patients who have chronic diseases.

As part of the Tucson–Carondelet model, outcomes have been collected and documented over the years. Nurse administrators are constantly evaluating the nursing organization's performance and looking for innovative practices to meet the rapidly changing demands of health care. Tucson–Carondelet was among the first nursing case management programs to enter into contracts with managed care companies, including Medicare, Medicaid, and commercial contracts (Lamb & Zazworsky, 2005).

With this model, the case management team facilitates interdisciplinary collaborative care management for patients who have complex medical and psychosocial problems and are chronically ill. The purpose of case management is to decrease the excessive use of healthcare resources. The program encourages the development of long-term client–case manager partnerships in managing the patient's illness. Nurses are assigned to patients and follow them across the continuum of care (Cohen, 2005; Ethridge, 1991; Ethridge & Lamb, 1989; Lamb, 1992; Lamb & Zazworsky, 2005).

The Goals

- Provide quality care
- Deliver direct care nursing services
- Provide continuity of care across the healthcare continuum
- Empower patients for self-care to reach their maximum level of health and wellness
- Provide holistic care, to include the spiritual, psychosocial, and medical care
- Decrease the use of expensive resources, including the emergency department
- Decrease LOS through early case findings to facilitate hospital admissions before the patient is acutely ill

The Case Management Team

The nursing team: nursing roles have been redefined from care provider to case manager/healthcare coordinator.

- The *primary nurse* assesses, plans, and evaluates nursing care needs and provides direct and indirect care for the patient. This professional may delegate responsibilities to ancillary personnel, such as the LPN or NA. He or she follows the patient in the hospital from admission to discharge and works with the clinical nurse case manager at the time of admission and during discharge.
- The *clinical nurse case manager* manages the hospital stay for a caseload of patients, coordinating care with physicians, nursing staff, community nursing case managers, and other professionals to ensure patient outcomes are achieved within the established time frame.
- The *community nurse case manager* picks up the patient while he or she is in the hospital and follows the patient into the community, wherever the patient is transferred, to provide a smooth transition to community services. The community case manager also enrolls new patients and officially cancels agreements with patients when case management services are no longer needed.
- The *case managers* in the hospital and the community are collaborative partners, together and with the patient and family (Ethridge, 1991; Ethridge & Lamb, 1989; Lamb, 1992; Lamb & Zazworsky, 2005).

The Setting/Population

The nursing HMO where this model was developed is in the Southwestern United States. The population is diverse and urban, consisting of patients who are Hispanic, Native American, and Caucasian, and often elderly. The focus is on people who have chronic illnesses, who are considered high risk and problem prone. These patients are at increased risk for readmission to the hospital because of complex medical needs or lack of financial or social support systems. Many of the elderly are not covered for Medicare, home health services, or long-term care services.

Roles and Functions of the Case Management Team

- Through case finding, identifies high-risk patients or those with limited social and financial supports
- Educates patients for self-care activities
- Links patients to appropriate resources and coordinates the multidisciplinary relationships
- Provides direct care, if necessary, as well as emotional support, counseling, and referrals
- Serves as a liaison and advocate
- Follows the same patient along the continuum of care for a long time (until services are no longer needed)
- Conducts home visitations
- Monitors and evaluates care

Outcomes

- Reduced costs
- Fewer emergency room visits
- Reduced recidivism; decreased use of critical care services
- Increased coping
- Improved patient satisfaction
- Decreased LOS
- Timely admissions resulting in lower acuity levels for hospitalized patients
- Increased use of alternative healthcare services

The University of Colorado Hospitals Psychiatric Model

The Colorado Psychiatric Hospital/University of Colorado Health Sciences Center developed a psychiatric case management (PCM) model, which integrates concepts from brief solution focused therapy, assertive community treatment (ACT), and family preservation. System of care concepts are integrated into this model but not specifically mentioned.

Under the PCM model, case management spans the boundaries between inpatient and outpatient settings. The goal is to decrease LOS by rapidly reintegrating the patients back into the community. The program includes an intensive inpatient unit, a crisis intervention clinic that is open around the clock, and a day treatment program. Progression from inpatient to partial hospitalization is individualized, according to the needs of each patient. The patient, family, and community members all actively participate in treatment planning. Therapy focuses on strengths and available resources as well as addresses current concerns. The focus is on solutions to current problems rather than dealing with past problems. A case manager is assigned to the patient; this professional acts as an advocate and is the liaison between the acute care and the community settings, guiding the patient from the inpatient program to the community outpatient program, which offers a wide range of therapeutic and rehabilitation services.

Over time, the designers of the program found that nurses' and social workers' roles and responsibilities often overlapped, and they had many of the same skills. Recognizing this fact, rather than separating the two roles, they were combined into a single role, called the "psychiatric case manager." Both the nursing and social work disciplines provide leadership to the treatment teams on the unit and supervise the direct care staff (Herrick & Bartlett, 2004; Platter, Young, & Vaughn, 2005). In addition, both monitor the assigned patient's progress.

Initially, the nurse case manager's role included utilization management. Later, a utilization management specialist was hired, as it became clear that performing these functions detracted from the case manager's patient care responsibilities. Several positive outcomes were noted after the utilization manager was added as a separate role; namely, the success rate of authorizations increased, and there was better collaboration between the business and finance departments and the psychiatric units. The utilization manager role has several responsibilities: reviewing all cases, regardless of the patient's health coverage; using InterQual standards (see Definitions Chapter 1); reviewing all cases for which LOS exceeds two weeks or more; and serving as a financial counselor for patients and families.

The Goals

- Provide quality, cost-effective care
- Decrease the LOS; return the patient to the community as soon as possible
- Improve continuity of care through close clinical coordination

The Case Management Team

Originally, the nurses were the case managers; the social workers coordinated family work and discharge planning. Both worked with the physicians assigned to the patient. Each team was assigned five to eight patients. Later, the team evolved from a three-member team into a two-member team consisting of a physician and a psychiatric case manager (either a nurse or a social worker).

The Population/Setting

Diverse mentally ill population in an urban setting.

Roles and Functions of the Case Management Team

THE INPATIENT TEAM

The Case Manager

- Serves as the clinical coordinator, involving and coordinating ancillary providers
- Is responsible for driving the treatment forward
- Develops treatment plans and supervises the implementation of the care plan by the inpatient staff
- Maintains a solution-focused approach
- Documents the treatment plans and the patient's progress
- Serves as the liaison between the inpatient program and the outpatient program
- Guides the patient and family through the care continuum
- Coordinates follow-up appointments

The Utilization Manager

- Works with third-party payers and the organization's business and finance departments
- Is a financial specialist with knowledge of third-party reimbursements
- Acts as a financial counselor for patients and families

THE OUTPATIENT TEAM

- Provides family-centered care
- Conducts home visitations and monitors medications
- Provides supportive psychotherapy and group therapy
- Conducts parenting classes and provides patient education

Outcomes

- Improved teamwork
- Improved patient and family satisfaction
- Improved care coordination between inpatient and outpatient services to accomplish a well-developed and functional continuum of care
- Decreased recidivism and avoidance of the "revolving door"
- Decreased LOS

The Catastrophic Case Management Model

Acquired immune deficiency syndrome (AIDS)/human immunodeficiency virus (HIV) infection is one of many diseases that require catastrophic case management. The catastrophic model is also used with worker's compensation cases in which individuals experience severe injuries leading to chronic disability. This integrated and collaborative model usually requires life care planning. According to Sonnwald (2007), who wrote about brain and spinal cord injuries, the case manager can ensure early intervention and rehabilitation for patients with potentially catastrophic conditions by facilitating a cooperative relationship between patients, families, rehabilitation providers, and payers.

Under this model, a life care plan is developed to identify the needs and services required to care for the patient over his or her lifetime. The purpose of the life care plan is not only to plan care, but also to control the use of available resources and costs, thereby making the case manager accountable for the use of these resources (McCollom, 2006). The goal is to economize—and at the same time optimize—use of resources. The developer of the life care document may be asked to present it in court (J. Perkins, personal communication, class presentation, NUR 541, Greensboro, NC: University of North Carolina–Greensboro, 2008). Because of the complexity of catastrophic illnesses and injuries, not only is an integrated case management model necessary, but the approach must also take the form of a collaborative–interdisciplinary model (Huber, 2002). One such model is AIDS Atlanta.

AIDS Atlanta was established during the height of the AIDS/HIV epidemic, prior to the introduction of the drugs that now make it possible to live a symptom-free life for a relatively long period time. This organization utilizes a four-phase continuum of care model to meet the long-term needs of its patients. Each of its interdisciplinary teams takes advantage of the varied expertise of nurses, social workers, family nurse practitioners, pastoral care counselors, psychotherapists, and physicians to deliver holistic and comprehensive care.

The outpatient intake clinic is where a first brief contact is initiated and anonymous testing is performed. Hospital and outpatient services are available once a diagnosis has been made. Walk-in clinics are available 24 hours per day, 7 days per week, to handle crises. Shelters have been established for homeless individuals with HIV/AIDS. Services are provided along the healthcare continuum to meet each patient's current and future needs. The continuum of care goes from outpatient facilities, which maintain patients' stability, to hospice care when end-of-life issues are imminent (Sowell & Meadows, 1994).

The Goals

- Provide access to HIV/AIDS-related services
- Respond to complex needs across the continuum of care
- Link diagnostic and early intervention services to other services, including community, hospital, and hospice care, thereby providing a seamless continuum of holistic care (i.e., includes the mind, body, and spirit)

The Case Management Team

Team members include nurses, family nurse practitioners, pastoral care counselors, case managers, social workers, psychotherapists, physicians, and any other professionals needed to provide holistic care to the patient to meet his or her needs, such as dieticians, phlebotomists, and respiratory therapists. Many of the professionals are volunteers.

The Setting/Population

Clients residing in the metropolitan area of Atlanta with the diagnosis of AIDS/HIV infection in various stages of the disease. The setting consists of the entire continuum of care.

Roles and Functions of the Case Management Team

A four-phase system of care was developed:

1. Brief Contact
Diagnostic services, counseling, education and information. An informative newsletter is sent to all patients.

2. **Medical Intake**
   Services that are needed are identified and matched with the client's
   need for an array of services.
3. **Low-Need Case Management**
   - Ongoing education and information
   - Negotiation for needed services
   - Crisis intervention
   - Tele-links, contacting patients on a monthly schedule
   - Coordination of volunteer support services
4. **High-Need Case Management**
   - Identification of clients who are at high risk for emotional, medical,
     or financial crises
   - Ongoing assessments, reassessments, and evaluations
   - Broker services along the continuum of care

The Chronic Care Model

The chronic care model of case management is a departure from traditional
patient care. This empowerment model (Anderson & Knickman, 2008) serves
people with chronic conditions who are being cared for in their communities.
Continuum-of-care/community-based healthcare programs are important to
people with chronic conditions, especially those programs that stress prevention. Self-care and self-management are the focus of the chronic care model.
Such a model integrates guidelines for the care of the chronically ill into a
community-based healthcare delivery system using reminders, feedback, and
standing orders, with an emphasis on prevention and primary care. The reminders may take the form of emails, phone calls, or drop in-clinics; such reminders
of needed services assist patients in maintaining their highest level of wellness.
In a chronic care model, clinical information systems allow easy access to
information. Telephone case management, group visits, and emails are then
used to keep people attending to their own healthcare needs on an ongoing
basis.

   With this model, prevention is the focus of care, rather than expensive
emergency room and hospital visits. If hospitalization is necessary, a designated person from the community case management team works with the
hospital case manager to prepare the patient and family for a timely discharge.
By working closely with the hospital, the case management team provides
continuity of care, which improves the overall quality of care. The chronic care
model offers the chronically ill patient ongoing support across the continuum
of care.

The Goals

- Maintain the highest level of wellness
- Reduce the number of emergency room visits
- Limit hospital recidivism
- Prevent complications
- Improve the quality of care
- Enhance the patient's quality of life
- Facilitate continuity of care across the healthcare continuum

The Case Management Team

Consists of the primary care provider, the nurse case manager, the social worker, the health educator/coach, and the exercise specialist.

The Population/Setting

- Chronically ill individuals who are living in the community
- Elderly persons who are living independently in the community
- Visitors to senior community centers and other outpatient facilities that provide the opportunity to deliver messages related to prevention and health maintenance

Roles and Functions of the Case Management Team

- Health education
- Monitoring (i.e., sending reminders about needed services)
- Coordinating and facilitating services
- Improving access to care
- Providing information about disease management
- Providing support for self-care

Outcomes

- The patient is able to maintain the highest level of wellness possible by participating in prevention and early intervention programs.
- The patient has a better understanding of the chronic condition and needs related to self-care, and this education leads to fewer emergency room visits and less frequent hospitalizations.
- The patient's quality of life with the family and in the community is improved.

- Access to information and care across the healthcare continuum improves the quality of care and contains costs.

The chronic care model emphasizes health coaching and education, monitoring people with chronic conditions, and providing support for healthy behaviors and activities that involve prevention, such as exercise classes in senior centers, nutrition-related education, and other preventive activities. Because this community model takes advantage of services from a variety of community agencies, the case management team must select one of the providers to be responsible for oversight of the patient's condition. Any one of the team members could fill this role, although the most likely candidate is the social worker or a community health nurse. The case management team or the designated first responder supervises the patient's care in both the acute care and community settings. Given this arrangement, the chronic care model can be considered a continuum-of-care model even though it is primarily a community-based model.

■ SUMMARY

A variety of models have been developed in a number of settings, both inpatient and outpatient, that are designed to meet the needs of specific populations of patients with different conditions. The core interventions used in the various models and the roles of the nurse case managers are similar, as are the goals and resulting outcomes in many instances. All of these models were designed to facilitate access to care, coordinate care so as to overcome the challenges of fragmentation of the healthcare system and the duplication of resources, and reduce costs, while continuing to provide high-quality care. The precise structure of each model depends on the institution that uses it and the target population. Each model provides guidelines for nurse case manager practice and the practice of the interdisciplinary case management team.

■ CASE STUDIES

Mrs. B. is 56 years old, is married, and works at a full-time job. She has been recently diagnosed with chronic obstructive pulmonary disease. Mrs. B. has smoked two packs of cigarettes per day for more than 30 years and has no intention of quitting, regardless of her diagnosis. Recently, she was admitted to the hospital with shortness of breath and hypoxia. Her husband has been laid off from his job and is currently collecting unemployment. He smokes as well, but does not feel that he can quit given his current stress level. Mrs. B. will be discharged from the acute care setting with supplemental oxygen and bronchodilator therapy.

Compare and contrast two case management models that might be used with Mrs. B. and her husband—one from an acute care setting and another from a community-based or continuum-of-care setting. Describe the following aspects of each model:

1. The setting
2. The goals of case management
3. The target population
4. The roles and functions of the case manager or the case management team
5. Outcomes from the model

■ DISCUSSION QUESTIONS

1. Why are there variations in the role of the case manager in different case management models?
2. Which factors contribute to these variations?
3. Which factors influence the roles and activities of the case manager and the process of case management?
4. Why do you think so many models have been developed to guide case management practice?
5. Describe acute care case management.
6. Describe community-based case management.

■ CLASSROOM EXERCISES

Discuss a complex case from either your personal or professional experience. Discuss both the collaborative model and the independent practice model, comparing and contrasting them on the following points in relationship to your case:

1. Setting
2. Goals of case management in this setting
3. Target population
4. Roles and functions of the case manager or case management team
5. Outcomes based on each of the models
6. Rationale

■ RECOMMENDED READINGS

Huber, D. L. (2002). The diversity of case management models. *Lippincott's Case Management, 7*(6), 212–220.

McCollom, P. (2006, September/October). Applying life care planning: Principles in acute situations. *Case Manager, 17*(5), 66–68.

McKendry, M. J., & Van Horn, J. (2004). Tips, tools and techniques: Today's hospital-based case manager. How one hospital integrated and adopted evidence-based medicine using InterQual criteria. *Lippincott's Case Management, 9*(2), 61–71.

Terra, S. M. (2007). An evidence-based approach to case management model selection for an acute care facility: Is there really a preferred model? *Professional Case Management, 12*(3), 147–157.

Thomas, M. E. (2008). The providers' coordination of care: A model for collaboration across the continuum of care. *Professional Case Management, 13,* 220–227.

■ REFERENCES

Anderson, F., & Knickman, J. R. (2008) Chronic care. In A. R Kovner & J. R. Knickman (Eds.), *Health care delivery in the United States* (9th ed., pp. 232–234). New York: Springer.

Cohen, E. L. (2005). Beyond-the-walls case management. In E. L. Cohen & T. G. Cesta (Eds.), *Nursing case management: From essentials to advanced practice* (4th ed., pp. 125–128). St. Louis, MO: Elsevier/Mosby.

Cohen, E. L., & Cesta, T. G. (2005a). Contemporary models of case management: Beyond the walls. In *Nursing case management: From essentials to advanced practice* (4th ed., pp. 125–177). St. Louis, MO: Elsevier/Mosby.

Cohen, E. L., & Cesta, T. G. (2005b). Contemporary models of case management: Within-the-walls case management. In *Nursing case management: From essentials to advanced practice* (4th ed., pp. 4–122). St. Louis, MO: Elsevier/Mosby.

Daniels, S., & Ramey, M. (2005). Hospital case management models. In *The leader's guide to hospital case management* (pp. 94–97). Sudbury, MA: Jones and Bartlett.

Ethridge, P. (1991) A nursing HMO: Carondelet St. Mary's experience. *Nursing Management, 22*(7), 22–27.

Ethridge, P., & Lamb, G. S. (1989). Professional nursing case management improves quality, access, and costs. *Nursing Management, 20*(3), 30–35.

Furman, R., & Jackson, R. (2002). Wraparound services: An analysis of community-based mental health services for children. *Journal of Child and Adolescent Psychiatric Nursing, 15*(3), 124–130.

Handron, D. S., Dosser, D. A. Jr., McCammon, S. L., & Powell, J. Y. (1998)."Wraparound" the wave of the future: Theoretical and professional practice: Implications for children and families with complex needs. *Journal of Family Nursing*, *4*(1), 65–86.

Herrick, C. A. (2006). Building collaborative relationships: A paradigm shift to family-centered, interprofessional partnerships. In M. Arbuckle & C. Herrick (Eds.), *Child and adolescent mental health: Interdisciplinary system of care* (pp. 31–56). Sudbury, MA: Jones and Bartlett.

Herrick, C. A., & Bartlett, R. (2004). Psychiatric nursing case management: Past, present and future. *Issues in Mental Health Nursing*, *25*(6), 589–602.

Herrick, C. A., Bartlett, T. R., Pearson, G. S., Schmidt, C., & Cherry, J. (2006). System of care in nursing: Across the life span and across settings. In M. Arbuckle & C. Herrick (Eds.), *Child and adolescent mental health: System of care interdisciplinary practice* (pp. 129–157). Sudbury, MA: Jones and Bartlett.

Huber, D. L. (2002). The diversity of case management models. *Lippincott's Case Management*, *7*(6), 212–220.

Koenig, E. (2005). Collaborative models of case management. In E. L. Cohen & T. G. Cesta (Eds.), *Nursing case management: From essentials to advanced practice applications* (4th ed., pp. 79–86). St. Louis, MO: Elsevier/Mosby.

Lamb, G. S. (1992). Conceptual and methodological issues in nurse case management research. *Advances in Nursing Science*, *15*(2), 16–24.

Lamb, G. S., & Zazworsky, D. (2005). Carondelet community-based nurse case management program: Yesterday, today, and tomorrow. In E. L. Cohen & T. G. Cesta (Eds.), *Nursing case management: From essentials to advanced practice applications* (4th ed., pp. 580–589). St. Louis, MO: Elsevier/Mosby.

McCollom, P. (2006, September/October). Applying life care planning: Principles in acute situations. *Case Manager*, *17*(5), 66–68.

McKendry, M. J., & Van Horn, J. (2004). Tips, tools and techniques: Today's hospital-based case manager. How one hospital integrated and adopted evidence-based medicine using InterQual criteria. *Lippincott's Case Management*, *9*(2), 61–71.

Miller, D. (2007, February/March). Do you have what it takes to be an independent case manager? *Case in Point*, 10–11.

Platter, B. K., Young, R. C., & Vaughn, K. (2005) The University of Colorado hospital psychiatric services health case management model: An innovative approach to client-centered care. In E. L. Cohen & T. G. Cesta (Eds.), *Nursing case management: From essentials to advanced practice applications* (4th ed., pp. 97–122). St. Louis, MO: Elsevier/Mosby.

Scott, J., & Boyd, M. (2001). Outcomes of community-based nurse case management programs. In E. L. Cohen & T. G. Cesta, *Nursing case management: From essentials to advanced practice applications* (3rd ed., pp. 127–138). St. Louis, MO: C.V. Mosby.

Scott, R. (2007, February/March). The essence of hospital case management. *Case in Point*, 10–11.

Sonnwald, K. (2007, February/March). Catastrophic case management: Focus on brain and spinal cord injuries. *Case in Point*, 26–29.

Sowell, R. L., & Meadows, T. M. (1994). An integrated case management model: Developing standards, evaluation and outcomes criteria. *Nursing Administration Quarterly, 18*(2), 53–64.

Woodall, J. (2005). Case management. In E. L. Cohen & T. G. Cesta (Eds.), *Nursing case management: From essentials to advanced practice applications* (4th ed., pp. 55–67). St. Louis, MO: Elsevier/Mosby.

Zander, K. (1988a). Managed care within acute care settings: Designing and implementation via nursing case management. *Health Care Supervisor, 6*(2), 24–43.

Zander, K. (1988b). Nursing case management: Strategic management of cost and quality outcomes. *Journal of Nursing Administration, 18*(5), 23–30

Zander, K. (1991, Fall). Care maps TM: The core of the cost/quality care. *New Definition, 6*(3), 1–3.

Zander, K. (1992a). Physicians, care maps and collaboration. *New Definition, 7*(1), 1–3.

Zander, K. (1992b). Quantifying, managing and improving quality: How care maps link CQI to the patient. *New Definition, 7*(1) 1–4.

Nursing Case Management: Building Collaborative Relationships with Patients

Laura J. Fero
Charlotte A. Herrick

6

■ **OUTLINE**

Introduction
Collaboration: An Essential Ingredient
Building an Interdisciplinary Team
The Social Work–Nurse Dyad: A Collaborative Case Management Team

■ **OBJECTIVES**

1. Discuss collaborative relationships, the characteristics of collaboration, and the steps and strategies necessary to build a collaborative relationship, including the benefits and barriers.

2. Identify the roles and skills of the team leader on an interdisciplinary team, the phases of group development, and the characteristics of an effective team.

3. Discuss conflict resolution.

4. Describe the nurse–social worker collaborative dyad.

5. Describe the collaborative process in partnering with families, family-centered care, and empowering patients and families for self-care.

INTRODUCTION

Case managers work with many different people, including professionals from other disciplines, patients and families, third-party payers, vendors, and personnel at many different agencies. The art of collaboration is exceedingly important in this field. By mastering the ability to work with others well, the case manager can successfully maneuver the patient and family through the maze of the current complex healthcare delivery system. Care management or nursing case management (NCM) represents a shift from the traditional discipline, in which an episodic approach is used, to a continuing approach as part of an integrated interdisciplinary model of healthcare delivery, across time and across the continuum of care. Nurse case managers work with many community agencies, including organizations that are the natural resources in the community, such as the Boys and Girls Clubs and the YMCA. Their goal is to build a supportive network for the patient and family, so that the patients can remain in the least restrictive and most therapeutic environment—namely, in their own homes and communities (Herrick, 2006; Herrick & Bartlett, 2004). NCMs strive to ensure that all patients receive quality, cost-effective care that meets the standards of care.

COLLABORATION: AN ESSENTIAL INGREDIENT

Sullivan and Decker (2009) defined *collaboration* as mutual attention to a problem, using the expertise of the collaborators from different agencies and/ or disciplines to contribute to finding a solution. In collaborative efforts in health care, the focus is on cooperation. The goal is to develop a plan where everyone is satisfied, including the patient and family. Compromise may be necessary to reach a solution. Among the partners, equality, mutual respect, and trust are required (Hogan & Nickitas, 2009). Table 6-1 gives some other definitions of collaboration that are found in the literature.

Collaboration is an essential ingredient for case management because the nurse case managers must work with all professionals who are providing services to benefit the patient and the family. As part of their duties, nurse case managers work with other professionals to establish partnerships with the patient and family. The partners are equal participants in the decision-making process, during the course of the patient's treatment and rehabilitation. All disciplines act as change agents, so that patients and families can reach their fullest potential for health. The end result is a better understanding of each provider's capabilities. Along the way, a network of comprehensive services is developed that takes advantage of every professional's capabilities (Herrick, 2006). The key elements of collaboration are good communication and teamwork.

Characteristics of Collaboration

The characteristics of collaboration include the necessary steps to building collaborative relationships. Naturally, there are both benefits and barriers to building these relationships. The three steps in building collaborative relationships are identified here:

1. *Coordination*: The first step is to coordinate activities so that there are no duplications or fragmentation of services.
2. *Cooperation*: The partners agree to help one another while providing services across the healthcare continuum.

TABLE 6-1 Collaboration: Key Terms and Definitions

Collaboration is a partnership where there is joint decision making, involving joint ownership of the decisions and collective responsibility for the outcomes (Koenig, 2005).

Collaboration is a relationship, where power, knowledge, and resources are shared so that all parties can work together to reach a common goal. The roots of the word are "co-", meaning together, and "labor" meaning work; thus collaboration means working together (Herrick, 2008).

Collaboration consists of two or more people working together toward a common goal by sharing a vision, information, resources, successes, and failures. Each partner is committed to the team and is responsible and accountable for the outcomes and the effectiveness of the collaborative whole. Collaboration is a cooperative effort that focuses on a "win-win" strategy. Diverse values are respected (Herrick, 2008).

Collaboration is "two or more consenting adults engaging in unnatural behaviors." Consensus is the goal (personal communication with Laura Weber, 2002, UNCG doctoral student in Education Leadership and instructor at the UNCG School of Public Health).

Collaboration involves joint planning, pooling resources, and evaluating outcomes together. When working individually, the healthcare provider operates separately to care for the patient, according to his or her own standards and expertise. Changes must be made by all partners, including (1) opening channels of communication; (2) making a commitment to work together; (3) sharing information, expertise, and resources; and (4) being willing to spend time with one another to collaborate. The partners take equal responsibility for the outcomes. Flexibility is the key to being able to share responsibilities; delivery of care can no longer be regarded as "business as usual" (Herrick, 2008).

A **collaborative relationship** involves pooling resources and having all parties work together to evaluate the results of their efforts. The talents and expertise of all parties are considered when planning strategies to reach mutually agreed-upon goals. Individual talents contribute to the plan (Herrick, 2008).

Interagency collaboration develops when members of different agencies participate in community projects as equal partners. In the "system of care" case management model and other continuum-of-care models, services are coordinated to provide a network of services around families so that families and patients do not get lost while going from one service delivery system to the next one (Herrick, 2006). One of the goals of care management is to facilitate transitions from one care system to another in such a way that the quality of care is maintained (Tahan, 2007). Commitment to interagency partnerships means that people work through the barriers and stereotypes that exist between agencies to sustain collaborative partnerships. Boundaries between agencies become more porous and professionals become more flexible and inclusive, so as to provide comprehensive quality care to families who require multisystem interventions.

3. *Collaboration*: The partners make a commitment to providing information and resources to reach the identified goal(s). They share power and are accountable for the outcomes.

Benefits of and Barriers to Building Collaborative Relationships

Although building collaborative relationships bring some distinct benefits, a series of barriers must be overcome before those benefits become reality (Table 6-2). Unfortunately, in some institutions, their historical legacy may place constraints on any chances of developing collaborative relationships among the disciplines to work in teams (Daniels & Ramey, 2005).

Strategies for Forming Collaborative Partnerships

Table 6-3 lists the actions that must be accomplished to successfully build a collaborative team. One of the most essential strategies for effective collaboration is good communication. Good communication is the "oil" that keeps the collaborative partnership humming along smoothly. It is the "glue" that holds all of the disparate personalities together so that they function as a whole. Each team member adds a new perspective to the patient's plan of care. Pursuit of a broader approach to the patient's care enhances the quality of care (Daniels & Ramey, 2005).

BUILDING AN INTERDISCIPLINARY TEAM

Manion and Huber (2006) defined "team building" as the process of unifying a group of people into a functioning unit so that specific goals are accomplished (Table 6-4). According to Hogan and Nickitas (2009), team building supports the efforts of a group of people who are working together on specific tasks. To build a team, the leader must motivate, persuade, coach, and mentor the team members so that they develop "team spirit." It is important to select the right team members so that there will be a "goodness of fit" of personalities, beliefs, values, and interests, which is crucial to developing cooperation. The leader is a cheerleader, celebrating "togetherness" (Brooks, 1990, cited in Herrick, 2008). Although individuality is honored within the team, at the same time the group as a whole is valued. Ideally, the team will strike a healthy balance between the needs of the individual and the needs of the group.

Understanding Group Concepts = Understanding Group Dynamics

Both the team leader and team members must understand group dynamics so that the team can function smoothly. The team leader should understand the

TABLE 6-2 Collaboration: Benefits and Barriers

Benefits	Barriers
• An increased likelihood of obtaining funds where there is cooperation rather than competition.	• Time to attend collaborative meetings.
• Decreased fragmentation and duplication of services, which improves the quality of care and decreases costs.	• Lack of clarity about the leadership. • Leaving out important stakeholders. • Lack of a common vision.
• The creation of a network of complementary services to provide holistic and comprehensive health care, mental health care, and social services, thereby ensuring continuity of care.	• Poor communication that leads to misunderstandings. • Poor negotiating skills. • Poorly established ground rules. • Lack of incentives to collaborate.
• The political strength of a broad-based advocacy group, which often leaves a greater impression on the officials and/or legislators who develop policies and hold the purse strings.	• Lack of resources to contribute equally to the collaborative effort. • Inadequate knowledge about the necessary requirements to contribute to the joint effort. • Lack of administrative support.
• Opportunities provided for group support, enabling multiple parties to share their problems and brainstorm solutions. Support from other professionals can lessen feelings of helplessness and prevent burnout, especially when working with complex patients and families. Professionals' job satisfaction is often improved.	• Most Americans have been schooled in a competitive environment rather than a cooperative one. Consequently, many Americans are more comfortable competing rather than cooperating (Herrick, 2006).
• Improved patient satisfaction because of better access to care and the continuing support of the case manager and other healthcare providers.	
• Cost-effective, evidence-based nursing interventions (Grossman & Batista, 2002).	

phases of group development, so that he or she can match the appropriate leadership style to each phase of group development. Table 6-5 identifies important group concepts—namely, norms, conformity, and trust—that are essential to effective team building.

Group/Team Leadership Skills

The group leader must have good interpersonal skills, including active listening skills. He or she must be a visionary who is able to clearly convey to the group

TABLE 6-3 Strategies for Collaboration

1. Establish a dialogue. Build trust. Share information. Motivate others to coordinate their activities.

2. Identify and establish common goals and reasons for collaborating.

3. Define the mission.

4. Establish priorities.

5. Identify the shared resources to accomplish goals.

6. Develop a plan and distribute it to all of the team members and other stakeholders, such as individual agency administrators.

7. Seek administrative support from the participating agencies.

8. Clarify the roles and tasks of each contributor/partner.

9. Apply the interventions identified in the plan by the assigned participants.

10. Evaluate the outcomes and modify as needed. Celebrate accomplishments.

Source: Herrick, 2006.

TABLE 6-4 Building an Interdisciplinary Team

Definitions of Teams

A group of people on the same side. A group of individuals organized to work together (Brooks, 1990, cited in Herrick, 2008).

People with complementary skills, working together toward a common purpose, who are all accountable for the outcomes (Manion & Huber, 2006, p. 563).

Teams can vary in size or purpose, ranging from a small number who are together for a specific purpose, to large groups. Groups are expected to produce results, such as a winning record, making a new product or completing a project or providing a service. Frequently, the nurse case manager is the team leader because he or she is the "linchpin" for coordinating care among all of the disciplines (Winters & Terrell, 2003, cited in Herrick et al., 2006, p. 139).

how the future should ideally evolve. In addition, the leader must be able to facilitate the members' cooperation to establish agreed-upon goals and to determine how the group will be structured and operate to meet those goals. He or she must also have the skills necessary to delegate responsibilities, assigning functions fairly and according to each member's strengths and abilities. Working together, the leader and the team members make decisions. The leader empowers the members to be self-directed, which in turn motivates the members to succeed.

TABLE 6-5 Group Concepts

Group Norms
Norms are rules that are spoken or unspoken, but that govern behavior and provide predictability.
Norms change over time.
Norms protect the group from conflict.
The expectation of the team members is that each will respect the others.

Conformity
Similar values and behaviors result from peer influences.

Trust
Shared expectations and resources result from open and honest communication.

Inevitably, groups will experience some conflict, so the group leader will need to be skilled in conflict resolution (Manion & Huber, 2006). Managing conflict is a top priority for all groups. Conflict can be both negative and positive. It can be beneficial, for example, when it serves as the forerunner of constructive change (Sullivan & Decker, 2009).

Table 6-6 examines group dynamics and the leadership styles that are appropriate for each phase of the group's development.

Termination of the Group

Termination occurs when one member leaves the group or when all of the members disband. If one member leaves and another individual replaces that person, then the group dynamics will change. The group should then be restructured into a "new" group to take advantage of the new member's expertise. Both the member who is leaving and the new member should participate in the termination meeting as a way of saying "hello" and "goodbye." The group leader provides a more directive approach during this phase. He or she facilitates the transformation of the new group from the former group using the following strategies listed in Table 6-7.

Conflict Resolution

Conflict occurs when perceived threats or differences exist in the desires, thoughts, attitudes, feelings, or behaviors of two or more parties (Cox, 2006).

TABLE 6-6 Group Dynamics

Phase	Team	Leadership Styles
Orientation Phase		
Forming	• Group of individuals: initial meeting	• Directive • Authoritarian
Storming	• Struggles for power • Conflicts • Resistance	• Directive • Authoritative • Supportive
Conforming	• Cooperative members	• Nondirective • Facilitative
Working Phase		
Performing	• Cohesion • Interdependence • Productive • Self-directive	• Nondirective • Delegative • Laissez-faire • Consultative

Source: Tuckman & Jensen, 1977, cited in Amos, Hu, & Herrick, 2005.

TABLE 6-7 Leadership Strategies During the Group Termination Phase

The leader:
• Provides positive affirmations about the previous group
• Reviews what members have learned from one another and highlights the group's accomplishments
• Acknowledges the loss of the departing member and describes the person's contributions to the group's success
• Encourages all members of the group to express their good wishes to the departing member(s)
• Introduces the new member, encouraging the new member to share his or her interests and talents that he or she envisions will contribute to the group

Conflict resolution is an ongoing strategy that case managers and team leaders must use to resolve the inevitable differences that arise among group members (Table 6-8). In fact, conflict resolution skills are among the most essential skills necessary for leaders to acquire, because interpersonal conflicts may be the biggest challenge that leaders, managers, and case managers must face. The ability to resolve conflict hinges on the leader's skill in moving the parties engaged in the dispute through the following progression:

Mediate → Explain → Feedback → Agree → Explore → Review

TABLE 6-8 Leadership Strategies to Resolve Conflicts

The leader should:
- Be aware of antecedent conditions, such as differences in beliefs and values, incompatible goals, role conflicts, and/or competition for scarce resources
- Monitor tensions among members
- Be the *mediator or arbitrator*; do not take sides
- Protect minority opinions
- Clarify a common purpose
- Define the problem and identify the reasons for the problem to be resolved
- Provide feedback and reflect the various points of view from all sides
- Facilitate problem solving so that each person can contribute to the resolution
- Explore acceptable options or alternatives and select the best alternative(s)
- Focus on outcomes
- Promote full participation by all group members
- Review the solutions that everyone has agreed to and set a date for follow-up

Sources: Herrick, 2008; Hogan & Nickitas, 2009; Sullivan & Decker, 2009.

Frequently, when a conflict arises, each party sees only his or her own point of view rather than viewing the problem as one that everyone needs to work on to find a solution. Over time, the conflict may come to be seen as a personal affront to each party's self-esteem. To overcome this difficulty, the leader must focus on helping each party view the conflict as an opportunity to learn objectivity and to see another perspective. Table 6-9 lists some conflict resolution strategies developed by Filley in 1975 (cited in Sullivan & Decker, 2009).

The group leader should take conflicts in stride, and should ensure that disagreements are managed in a timely manner. The leader should not let anger and hostility in others cause him or her to lose sight of the mission. Leaders with excellent critical thinking skills bring to potential conflicts many of the abilities needed to provide win-win resolutions to conflicts (Cox, 2006; Sullivan & Decker, 2009). As part of the conflict resolution process, for example, the leader should demand that team members respect one another and actively listen to others' opinions. Table 6-10 highlights some specific skills that leaders may use to resolve group conflict.

Characteristics of an Effective and Successful Interdisciplinary Team

The literature describes a number of characteristics that are key to successful team building. Table 6-11 lists the characteristics of an effective team. In addition, Blanchard (2000, cited in Herrick, 2006), who has written several books on leadership, has developed an easy-to-remember formula (mnemonic) describing the characteristics of a high-performing team.

TABLE 6-9 Potential Solutions to Conflicts

Win-Lose: An all-out effort to win. Competition is the main strategy. The goal is to gain power over someone else.

Lose-Lose/Win-Win: Compromise occurs—splitting the difference and making concessions, dividing the rewards and the liabilities.

Lose-Lose: Neither side wins. Not confronting the conflict and avoiding it means that the conflict goes underground, unresolved, only to emerge later.

Win/Lose-lose: Winning is temporary. Accommodating in favor of others and neglect of one's own concerns leads to groupthink, meaning all participants must think alike and agree, whether right or wrong.

Win-Win: All parties collaborate to negotiate differences. Conflicts are resolved by building consensus. Participants become a cohesive team.

Sources: Cox, 2006; Sullivan & Decker, 2009.

TABLE 6-10 Leadership Skills for Conflict Resolution

- The ability to listen actively and reflect on what was said
- The ability to confront problems
- Flexibility and an open mind
- The ability to mediate and negotiate
- The knowledge and skills to teach critical-thinking and problem-solving skills to followers
- The ability to create a culture where errors are seen as opportunities for learning

Source: Lachman, 1999, cited in Herrick, 2008.

TABLE 6-11 Other Important Characteristics of Successful Teams

- **Trust** established among group members
- Ongoing, honest, and **open communication**
- **Shared values**, purpose, mission, responsibilities, and accountability
- Adherence to **group norms**
- **Commitment** to the group's goals and measurable outcomes
- **Genuine reason** for each member to be a participant
- **Individual competence** in a variety of skills with a focus on strengths that enhance group competence
- **Participative leadership** and decision making
- **Empowered group members** who are encouraged to make joint decisions
- **Rewards** for team accomplishments
- **Cohesiveness** "togetherness"
- Ability of the team to **objectively review, evaluate, and modify the group's processes and functions** as needed
- **Teamwork** = cooperation and collaboration
- **Excellent teamwork** = optimal patient care

Sources: Bronstein, 2003; Herrick et al., 2006; Herrick 2008.

PERFORM:

P = Purpose and shared values
E = Empowerment
R = Relationships that are respectful and characterized by open communication
F = Flexibility
O = Optimal performance
R = Recognition and appreciation
M = Morale
Source: Blanchard, 2000, cited in Herrick, 2006.

Collaboration requires a commitment to working together as a team. The leader recognizes each member's contributions to the group's success and celebrates everyone's accomplishments. The result is a healthy atmosphere where morale is high and all team members feel valued. Although conflicts may arise, a good leader and motivated followers, who have a sense of belonging, can resolve conflicts to the benefit of the entire team.

THE SOCIAL WORK–NURSE DYAD: A COLLABORATIVE CASE MANAGEMENT TEAM

Case management and disease management are transdisciplinary healthcare strategies. In fact, case management is not a profession in itself, but rather an area of practice within one's profession (CCMC, 2001, cited in Schuetzee, 2005). It is a service delivery system, coordinated by either a partnership or a group of different disciplines that make up a team, to provide health care to patients. The partnership or the team is made up of nurses and social workers and/or other healthcare professionals, such as rehabilitation specialists, who act as patient advocates. The case management partnership or team identifies and coordinates the necessary resources to provide holistic care (Schuetzee, 2005).

The concept of the dyad of a nurse and a social worker collaborating to provide continuity of care dates back to the late 1900s, according to Robbins and Birmingham (2005). With the advent of managed care during the 1980s medical care became more community based. Once patient care moved out of the hospital, a more holistic approach to patient care by nurses and other disciplines was required. The nurse and the social worker dyad became the most common partnership both in acute care hospitals and in community settings. Case management serves as the bridge between the two professions.

The Dyad Model

The dyad model is currently used in many healthcare institutions, which have found that together the two professions can provide more holistic and com-

TABLE 6-12 The Dyad Model in an Emergency Department

Social Worker (MSW)	Nurse (RN)
• Makes psychosocial and strength-based assessments.	• Monitors the medical necessity of hospital admissions.
• Conducts patient/family assessments, including evaluating the resources to care for the patient in the home.	• Conducts physical assessments. Contributes to the nursing care plan.
• Develops a service plan based on the patient's and family's strengths.	• Is a resource for the medical team and the interdisciplinary team to develop a care plan.
• Conducts substance abuse counseling.	• Understands emergency care, disease processes, and utilization management, plus payers' requirements within the prospective payment system.
• Provides family counseling.	• Negotiates with third-party payers within the managed care contract.
• Does crisis intervention.	• Coordinates follow-up care with the primary care provider and community agencies.
• Provides bereavement counseling.	• Ensures continuity of care, acting as a liaison with community healthcare agencies.
• Arranges community referrals. Provides follow-up to ensure that the family can care for the patient.	• Makes follow-up medical appointments, arranges home health care, and orders durable medical equipment. Provides follow-up to ensure that the medical equipment has arrived and the family knows how to use it. Reviews the teaching that was done prior to discharge.

prehensive care. One example is the nurse–social worker dyad found in the emergency department in a large teaching hospital in the Southeast (Bristow & Herrick, 2002; Bristow & Herrick-Hicks, personal communication, class presentation in Nursing Case Management, NUR 541, Greensboro, NC: University of North Carolina at Greensboro, August 2006; Kiernan-Stern, 2005). Table 6-12 lists the contributions of each of the professions, the social worker (MSW) and the nurse (RN), in this partnership.

TABLE 6-13 Shared Roles

Collaborator	Consultant	Listener
Partner	Facilitator	Allocator of resources/utilization specialist
Advocate	Educator	Discharge planner
Negotiator	Assessor	Monitor/coordinator

Overlapping Roles Within the Dyad

The RN/MSW partners work together to provide cost-effective quality patient care. They educate the patients and families to manage their own care. Lastly, they inform patients and their families about the various healthcare options and encourage them to select the options that they think are best for them. The dyad acts as advisors, advocates, collaborators, negotiators, consultants, discharge planners, facilitators, risk managers, and teachers or educators (Table 6-13). Over the duration of the patient's care, the partners monitor the patient's progress and coordinate care across the healthcare continuum. They divide the responsibilities according to their individual expertise (Bristow & Herrick, 2002; Bristow & Herrick-Hicks, personal communication, August 2006).

In a 1997 study by Brewer (cited in Herrick, 2008), the roles of the two disciplines were divided into two foci. The social worker's roles included crisis management and discharge planning. The nurse case manager's roles included the following responsibilities:

- Emergency care
- Nursing care related to the disease
- Utilization management
- Negotiating with third-party payers

Both roles overlapped in terms of discharge planning and communicating with the interdisciplinary team, the patient and family, and administrators. The outcomes in the studies conducted by Bristow and Herrick (2002) and Brewer (1997, cited in Herrick, 2008) demonstrated that use of the nurse–social worker dyad provided the following benefits:

- Improved discharge planning
- Decreased inappropriate admissions
- Cost savings
- Improved patient and staff satisfaction
- Improved clinical management of patients
- Better quality of care
- Improved continuity of care

Bristow and Herrick (2002) found that there was a decrease in the use of emergency department (ED) services by high utilizers as the result of better patient education, thus decreasing not only costs but also the wait times for other patients in the ED.

Other Studies on the Nurse–Social Worker Dyad Model

In a study conducted by Holliman, Dziegielewski, and Teare (2003), these social workers found that members of both the nurse and social worker professions were effective discharge planners, with no significant differences being discerned between the two professions regarding discharge planning. The tasks done by both social work and nursing included coordination of services, assessments, supportive counseling, documentation, treatment team participation, and quality assurance. The major differences between the two related to their work settings: Social workers worked in larger hospitals and nurses in smaller hospitals. Social workers tended to provide case management services to individuals with AIDS, psychiatric patients, and homeless persons. Nurse case managers tended to work more with people who were medically ill. Social workers provided more comprehensive mental health assessments, helped patients complete advanced directives, and assessed children and the elderly for abuse, whereas nurses provided more physical assessments. Nurses' knowledge of medicine, diagnosis, treatment, statistics, and research provided a background for more comprehensive medically oriented discharge planning.

The authors of this study concluded that both types of professionals provided quality discharge planning. The social worker's perspective focused more on the patient's and family's strengths, while the nurse was more problem oriented. Both were equally competent as discharge planners, albeit while taking slightly different perspectives. The social workers were better able to address the needs of the mentally ill, patients with substance abuse, or the homeless, while the nurses were better able to address the needs of people with complex medical problems.

Dyzacky (1998, cited in Herrick, 2008) described the process of building a case management team with a social worker and a nurse. Their roles were redesigned to take advantage of the respective strengths of both professions. One of the important outcomes was that families appreciated the time given to them by the dyad team. Another positive outcome of the collaborative relationship was better communication between the two disciplines.

Carr (2009) described the benefits of a RN case manager/social work dyad in critical care. One especially important benefit was that the dyad team enhanced the functioning of the ICU multidisciplinary team. The team of social worker and nurse case manager could integrate their respective strengths to promote continuity of care, especially during transitions of patients from the ICU to other forms of care, such as the step-down unit or home care. The social worker's attention to the psychosocial and behavioral health issues complemented the clinical approach, which is the focus of the nurse case manager and the interdisciplinary ICU team. Consequently, both the patient and the family received emotional support throughout the course of the illness. According to Carr (2009), the MSW/RN dyad shares a commitment to "the delivery of patient-centered, quality-focused, efficacious care" (p. 127). Such a team can facilitate smoother transitions between one care delivery system and the next, all the while ensuring that quality is not compromised. According to Powell and Zander (2005, cited in Carr, 2009), the dyad structure can better meet the goal of patient-centered care.

Robbins and Birmingham (2005) have noted that a number of turf issues between the two professions need to be confronted to build effective collaborative relationships. The differences between the two professions that may interfere with building a good collaborative relationship include the following:

- Lack of understanding about what each profession does
- Educational differences: RNs have 2, 3, or 4 years of schooling, whereas MSWs have 4, 5, or 6 years of education
- Salary differentials: Salaries for MSWs are lower than salaries for RNs

The differences in their educational backgrounds and salaries may sometimes result in resentment by the social worker and hostility between members of the two professions. Robbins and Birmingham suggest that these issues should be confronted during the initial phase of establishing the dyad, and recommend implementing the three R's—reciprocity, responsibility, and respect for each other's expertise—as a means to ensure a good working relationship.

Building collaborative relationships takes time, effort, patience, and a commitment on the part of both partners. Many authors, including those working for the Institute of Medicine, have suggested that both the social work and nursing disciplines should be taught together during a portion of the preprofessional education by co-teachers from both disciplines, who can serve as role models of collaborative behaviors while teaching interdisciplinary collaboration (Crow & Smith, 2003; Finkelman & Kenner, 2007; Greiner & Knebel, 2003; Herrick & Arbuckle, 2006; Herrick, Arbuckle, & Claes, 2002). In today's complex healthcare environment, the expertise of each profession is clearly necessary to provide quality comprehensive case management services. The healthcare system needs professionals who are caring, competent, and compassionate, and who understand the importance of collaboration (Robbins & Birmingham,

2005). Schuetzee (2006), a social worker, has expressed the opinion that the diversity among case managers adds to the richness of the field and contributes to the depth of case management knowledge. Case managers should value their diversity.

Patient- and Family-Centered Care

Nursing has a history of being patient centered, but acute care nurses often have ignored families as part of patient care. In the past, children were isolated from their parents and siblings during hospitalizations because of the threat of infection. Now we know that isolating children from their parents has terrible psychological effects (Herrick & Bartlett, 2004; Herrick et al., 2006). Studies have shown that patients recover more rapidly when they are surrounded by loved ones. For this reason, the focus of nursing case management should be on the family as the unit of care (Reagan, 2006).

The one thing that families want from their caregivers is a sense of hope (Washington, 2001). In a qualitative study conducted by Goodwin and Happell (2007), the researchers examined the opinions of family members and significant others in Australia who shared caregiving responsibilities with healthcare providers. They found that family members and significant others wanted nurses to respect and communicate with them, and to provide them with education and information; they also wanted to be active participants with the nurses as caregivers.

In today's healthcare environment, patients are typically discharged from the hospital early in the course of the illness. The family then provides most of the care for the patient after hospitalization. Consequently, the whole family, as well as the patient, must be the focus of the case management process.

The case manager's assessment should include an assessment of the family's strengths and resources, thereby allowing the case manager to build on what they currently know or have. Once their strengths are identified, the case manager can teach new skills that the family needs to care for the patient. Educational support and supervision, as well as providing an empowering environment, are essential for the family to be able to provide adequate home care. Building a network of services to "wrap around" the family will support the family's ability to provide adequate patient care (Handron et al., 1998; Herrick et al., 2006). After the family masters the new skills, their perspective will change from helplessness to a positive "can do" attitude. Family-centered care involves a paradigm shift, making the focus of care broader in order to include the family and the community (Table 6-14).

TABLE 6-14 The Principles of Family-Centered Care

- Providers establish a caring atmosphere that fosters collaboration.
- Communication between the case manager and the family is bidirectional.
- Trust and mutual respect are conveyed from the family to the professional, and vice versa.
- The family's cultural, ethnic, religious, and socioeconomic values are honored.
- The diverse needs of family members are considered when planning care.
- The family's strengths and individuality are respected. By focusing on their assets rather than their problems, the family will feel empowered.
- Unbiased information is provided, including all available options for treatment, risks, and potential outcomes.
- All decisions rest with the family. Nurse case managers respect the patient's and family's decisions, and they set aside their own biases.
- Case managers provide emotional support to family members so that they can nurture one another, flourish, and survive crises.
- Family perceptions and opinions are solicited.
- The case manager ensures that the patient's and family's goals are identified and addressed.
- The nurse case manager assists families to care for themselves.
- Institutional policies are flexible to meet the individual needs of patients and families (e.g., visiting hours).

Sources: Herrick, 2008; Herrick et al., 2006.

Roles of the Nurse Case Manager and the Family as Collaborative Partners

The nurse case manager shares with the family a conceptual framework for his or her practice, knowledge, and education, and provides them with emotional support. This professional teaches the family self-help skills, including skills to cope with stress, and educates them about the patient's illness. He or she also facilitates access to healthcare resources, and helps the family negotiate the healthcare system. The case manager explains the healthcare system, including both its assets and its liabilities. He or she monitors the patient's progress and the family's ability to care for the patient. The case manager is the advocate, the family counselor, the educator, and the coordinator of home services (Herrick et al., 2006).

In turn, the family provides the direct home health care. The family provides the historical information to the healthcare providers, prior to and at the onset of the illness, describing the manifestations of the illness, both signs and symptoms, and the patient's idiosyncrasies and personal preferences. When caring for the patient in the home, the family monitors the patient's progress and reports it to the case manager (either the social worker or the nurse). The family participates in planning care, identifies for the case manager those resources that they have currently at their disposal, and indicates the additional resources that they will need to care for the patient at home (Herrick et al., 2006).

Barriers to Providing Family-Centered Care

Sometimes there may be a resistance on the part of the nurse or the social worker to change from the traditional problem-oriented model of care and instead focus on the individual patient through a new paradigm—namely, a family/strength-based orientation (Kiernan-Stern, 2005). Other barriers may also be encountered, including a lack of administrative support to establish collaborative relationships with other disciplines for the sake of the patient. In addition, family attitudes can be problematic if families believe that health professionals should "fix the problem" and that, once they present the patient to the healthcare system, the patient is no longer their responsibility but rather the responsibility of the healthcare providers. At times, families may exhibit anger at the case manager for not immediately "fixing the problem" (Griffin, 2003; Herrick et al., 2006).

Empowered Families

Empowerment: Patient and Family Education

The purpose of education is to empower the patient and family for self-care. Thus these two concepts—education and empowerment—are inevitably intertwined. As part of his or her duties, the nurse case manager conveys information and teaches specific nursing care skills necessary to care for the patient. The case manager should assess the capabilities of each family member, so as to determine the best caregiving roles for each person. In fact, coordinating the family members is as important as coordinating services for them. When the patient and family are educated appropriately, however, they are empowered to take responsibility for themselves. There is power in knowledge.

Empowerment entails giving people the authority, responsibility, and freedom to act on what they know and think is best (Huber, 2006). It is a process in which individuals feel in control and have some degree of power over their own destinies (Grossman & Valiga, 2000). Empowerment occurs when a person feels strengthened by an experience or finds inner strength within a relationship, such as the nurse case manager–patient relationship. In family-centered care, power is shared by an agreement forged between the case manager and the patient/family. Empowerment is a dynamic, ongoing

TABLE 6-15 Essentials for Patients to Be Self-Advocates

Families must:
- Have complete knowledge about both their medical and social histories, and their family's background.
- Make choices. Patients cannot make decisions without complete information, requiring the nurse case manager to be an educator.
- Understand their health insurance contract. Patients need to understand the implications financially for their choices.

Source: Busch, 2003.

process through which families identify their own goals and strive to reach them. Empowered families believe in themselves and their own competence. They recognize their own abilities (Hogan & Nickitas, 2009).

To provide an empowering environment, the case manager develops an atmosphere where people are motivated to succeed and act on their own behalf (Table 6-15). The case manager mentors the family, providing them with supervision and support as they try out new skills. Sharing power and providing an empowering environment, where people can grow and develop to their maximum potential, means that the leader/case manager recognizes the inherent power in each individual. Professionals who are empowered themselves can provide patients with an empowering environment and, therefore, are effective case managers. Empowerment means that case managers do "not do" for the patient" but rather "work with" the patient. The result of empowerment means that the patient and family have acquired a new and/or renewed sense of self.

Building on Strengths

Because family members are typically adult learners, adult learning principles should guide the teaching plan used to educate them. The family knows their loved one better than the healthcare providers do. These individuals should be considered the experts about the patient. Prior to developing a teaching plan, an assessment of the family's knowledge and skills and the information that they consider important to learn should be conducted. By building on strengths, the case manager can help the patient and family to improve their quality of life (Huber, 2002). Emphasizing what people can do, rather than what they cannot do, instills confidence, which in turn gives them a sense of self-worth: It makes them feel that they are in control and self-directed and, therefore, empowered. Good self-esteem promotes a positive vision for the future (Brun & Rapp, 2001).

■ SUMMARY

Collaboration is the key to the future in health care, as it is essential to create exceptional outcomes for patients, families, nurses, and healthcare organizations alike (Esposito-Herr et al., 2009). According to Michaels and Cohen (2005), a seamless case management system must adhere to the following principles:

- Case management is a community effort that goes across the healthcare continuum.
- Patients are grouped by similar health and functional problems, making early identification and interventions more timely.
- A system of care is built to support the therapeutic relationship between the provider(s) and patients.

Organizing case management into a seamless system, using an interdisciplinary team of healthcare professionals and interagency connections, will effectively serve patients, caregivers, and the healthcare system. Partnering with other disciplines, families, and others, including community leaders, will be necessary to lobby for healthcare funding, especially as more Americans remain or become uninsured. Partnerships are especially essential in the current system of care so that people working together can improve healthcare services for vulnerable populations with complex medical and social needs (Herrick et al., 2006). According to Finkelman and Kenner (2007), the top two most recommended core competencies for all healthcare providers, as identified by the Institute of Medicine, include patient-centered care and working in interdisciplinary teams. Manion and Huber (2006) conclude that a group of people who have complementary skills and a common purpose, working together collaboratively, can achieve better and more reliable outcomes than one discipline can achieve alone.

■ CASE STUDIES

Mr. B. is a 76-year-old male who lives alone on a family farm. He has two sons and one daughter, all of whom live within 5 miles of his home. Mr. B. has been diagnosed with high blood pressure, type 2 diabetes, early-stage dementia, peripheral vascular disease, and neuropathy. He has been admitted to the acute care facility with uncontrolled hypertension, and the physicians believe that he has had a small stroke based on his presenting symptoms and recent confusion. Mr. B. insists that he will be going home independently at discharge; however, his children have expressed that they feel he is failing at home and at risk for falling and noncompliance with his medication regimen. The children cannot take him into their homes due to strained family relationships.

1. Discuss both the inpatient and community collaboration opportunities to manage Mr. B.
2. What are the potential benefits and barriers to his care?
3. How could an inpatient and community case manager influence Mr. B.'s care?
4. Which communications strategies could be used with both Mr. B. and his family?
5. How could both the patient and family be empowered?

■ DISCUSSION QUESTIONS

1. What is the role(s) of the case manager on an interdisciplinary team?
2. Why is communication so important to building effective partnerships?
3. What are the barriers to collaborative team management?
4. Which strategies are useful in building collaborative relationships?

■ CLASSROOM EXERCISES

Share with your peers your experiences and comment on their experiences:

1. As a manager or case manager, which strategies would you use to empower your staff and/or patients so as to enhance their welfare? Give specific examples of what you may have done or may want to do in the future.
2. Which experiences have you had, as a staff nurse (or patient), whereby another professional empowered you in terms of your own professional or personal growth and development? Describe the experience.

Discuss your experiences in collaborating with other disciplines or any experiences that you may have had as a member of an interdisciplinary team.

■ RECOMMENDED READINGS

Family-Centered Care/Wrap-around Care

Furman, R., & Jackson, R. (2002). Integrating nursing care into systems of care for children with emotional and behavior disorders. *Journal of Child and Adolescent Psychiatric Nursing, 15*(3), 124–130.

Holistic Care: Integrating Medical and Mental Health Care
Aliotta, S. L. (2004). Integrating medical and mental health care. *Case Manager,*
    15(1), 56–60.

▪ REFERENCES

Amos, M. A., Hu, J., & Herrick, C. A. (2005). The impact of team building on
    communication, job satisfaction of nursing staff. *Journal of Staff Development,*
    2(1), 1–7.

Bristow, D. P., & Herrick, C. A. (2002). Emergency department case management: The
    dyad team of nurse case manager and social worker. *Lippincott's Case
    Management, 7*(3), 121–128.

Bronstein, L. R. (2003). A model for interdisciplinary collaboration. *Social Work, 48,*
    297–306.

Brun, C., & Rapp, R. C. (2001). Strength-based case management: Individual's
    perspectives on strengths and case manager relationships. *Social Work, 46*(3),
    278–289.

Busch, R. (2003). Empowering patients to direct their health care. *Case Manager,*
    14(6), 62–65.

Carr, D. D. (2009). Building collaborative partnerships in critical care: The RN case
    manager/social work dyad in critical care. *Professional Case Management, 14*(3),
    121–132.

Cox, K. S. (2006). Power and conflict. In D. L. Huber (Ed.), *Leadership and nursing
    care management* (3rd ed., pp. 501–542). Philadelphia: Saunders/Elsevier.

Crow, J., & Smith, L. (2003). Using co-teaching as a means of facilitating
    interpersonal collaboration in health care and social care. *Journal of
    Interprofessional Care, 17*(1), 45–55.

Daniels, S., & Ramey, M. (2005). *The leader's guide to hospital case management.*
    Sudbury, MA: Jones and Bartlett.

Esposito-Herr, M. B., Persinger, K. D., Regier, A., & Hunt, S. S. (2009). Partnering
    for better performance: The nursing–finance alliance. *American Nurse, 4*(4),
    29–31.

Finkelman, A., & Kenner, C. (2007). *Teaching IOM: Implications of the Institute of
    Medicine report for nursing education.* Silver Spring, MD: American Nurses
    Association.

Forest, C. (2003). *Empowerment skills for family workers: A Worker Handbook.*
    Ithaca, NY: Family Development Press/Cornell University.

Goodwin, V., & Happell, B. (2007, June). Consumer and carer participation in mental
    health care: The carer's perspective. Part I: The importance of respect and
    collaboration. *Issues in Mental Health Nursing, 28*(6), 607–623.

Greiner, A. C., & Knebel, E. (2003). Executive summary. In Commission on Health Professions Education Summit Board on Health Services, Institute of Medicine of the National Academies, *Health professions education: A bridge to quality.* Washington, DC: National Academies Press. www.nap.edu.

Griffin, T. (2003). Facing challenges to family-centered care. II: Anger in the clinical setting. *Pediatric Nursing, 29*(3), 212–214.

Grossman, S., & Batista, C. (2002). Collaboration yields cost-effective, evidence-based nursing protocols. *Orthopedic Nursing, 21*(3), 30–36.

Grossman, S., & Valiga, T. M (2000). *The new leadership challenge.* Philadelphia: F. A. Davis.

Handron, D. S., Dosser, D. A., McCammon, S. L., & Powell, J. Y. (1998). "Wraparound": The wave of the future: Theoretical and professional practice. Implications for children and families with complex needs. *Journal of Family Nursing, 4*(11), 65–68.

Herrick, C. A. (2006). Building collaborative relationships: A paradigm shift to family-centered interprofessional partnerships. In M. Arbuckle & C. Herrick (Eds.), *Child and adolescent mental health: Interdisciplinary system of care* (pp. 31–56). Sudbury, MA: Jones and Bartlett.

Herrick, C. A. (2008). *Learning module: Nursing case management* (NUR 541) [unpublished document]. Greensboro, NC: University of North Carolina at Greensboro School of Nursing.

Herrick, C. A., & Arbuckle, M. B. (2006). Where are we going? In M. Arbuckle & C. Herrick (Eds.), *Child and adolescent mental health* (pp. 367–393). Sudbury, MA: Jones and Bartlett.

Herrick, C. A., Arbuckle, M. B., & Claes, J. A. (2002). Teaching interdisciplinary practice: A course in system of care for severely emotionally disturbed children and their families. *Journal of Family Nursing, 8*(3), 264–281.

Herrick, C. A., & Bartlett, T. R. (2004). Psychiatric nursing case management: Past, present and future. *Issues in Mental Health Nursing, 6*, 589–602.

Herrick, C. A., Bartlett, T. R., Pearson, G., Schmidt, C., & Cherry, J. (2006). System of care in nursing across the life span and across practice settings. In M. Arbuckle & C. Herrick (Eds.), *Child and adolescent mental health: Interdisciplinary systems of care* (pp. 129–157). Sudbury, MA: Jones and Bartlett.

Hogan, M. A., & Nickitas, D. M. (2009). *Nursing leadership and management: Reviews and rationales.* Upper Saddle River, NJ: Pearson/Prentice Hall.

Holliman, D., Dziegielewski, S. F., & Teare, R. (2003). Differences and similarities between social work and nurse discharge planners. *Health & Social Work, 28*(3), 224–231.

Huber, D. L. (2002). The diversity of case management models. *Lippincott's Case Management, 5*(6), 248–255.

Huber, D. L. (Ed.). (2006). Leadership principles. In *Leadership and nursing care management* (3rd ed., pp. 1–30). Philadelphia: Saunders/Elsevier.

Kiernan-Stern, M. (2005, September/October). Managing resistance to change: The social worker's role in case management. *Case Manager, 16*(5), 48–51.

Koenig, E. (2005). Collaborative models of case management. In E. L. Cohen & T. G. Cesta (Eds.), *Nursing case management: From essentials to advanced practice applications* (4th ed., pp. 79–86). St. Louis, MO: Elsevier/Mosby.

Manion, J., & Huber, D. L. (2006). Team building and working with effective groups. In D. L. Huber (Ed.), *Leadership and nursing care management* (3rd ed., pp. 561–586). Philadelphia: Saunders/Elsevier.

Michaels, C., & Cohen, E. L. (2005). Two strategies for managing care. In E. L. Cohen & T. G. Cesta (Eds.), *Nursing case management* (4th ed., pp. 33–37). St. Louis, MO: Elsevier/Mosby.

Reagan, K. M. (2006). Paradigm shifts in inpatient psychiatric care of children: Approaching child and family-centered care. *Journal of Child and Adolescent Psychiatric Nursing, 10*(1), 29–40.

Robbins, C. L., & Birmingham, J. (2005). The social worker and nurse roles in case management: Applying the three R's. *Lippincott's Case Management, 10*(3), 120–127.

Schuetzee, K. (2005). Social work and nursing. In D. L. Huber (Ed.), *Disease management*. St. Louis, MO: Elsevier/Saunders.

Schuetzee, K. (2006). Professional diversity adds richness to the case management field. *Lippincott's Case Management, 11*(5), 238–239.

Sullivan, E. J., & Decker, P. J. (Eds.). (2009). Handling conflict. In *Effective leadership & management in nursing* (7th ed., pp. 163–171). Upper Saddle River, NJ: Pearson//Prentice Hall.

Tahan, H. A. (2007). One patient, numerous healthcare providers and multiple care settings: Addressing the concerns of care transitions through case management. *Professional Case Management, 12*(1), 37–46.

Washington, G. T. (2001). Families in crisis. *Nursing Management, 32*(5), 28–33.

The Case Manager in Private Practice

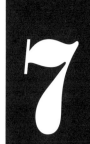

Laura J. Fero
Charlotte A. Herrick

■ OUTLINE

Introduction
Definitions: What Is an Entrepreneur?
Intrapreneurship
Challenges Faced by Entrepreneurs
Important Considerations for Nurse Entrepreneurs

■ OBJECTIVES

1. Define *entrepreneurship.*

2. Identify the benefits and challenges of working in private practice.

3. Describe the characteristics needed to be a successful entrepreneur.

4. List the guidelines and resources available to entrepreneurs.

5. Discuss important considerations when contemplating starting your own business.

6. Identify the mistakes that frequently are made during a business start-up.

INTRODUCTION

As nurses become better educated and more community oriented, many are looking at the private practice model in conjunction with their work as case managers and as advanced practice nurses. Boling (2009) labeled the private practitioner in case management as the "direct to the patient or consumer" case manager, who practices alone or with a physician's group, a law firm, or a business. The focus of this practitioner is on the patient's care as an advocate. Numerous opportunities are available for nurses to form their own small businesses with the support of governmental and nongovernmental agencies (Danna, 2006).

The authors of this book have known several nurses and case managers who started their own businesses. Examples include a nurse who established her own business as a consultant to nursing organizations, such as the American Nurses Association; a psychiatric nurse who started a group home for chronically mentally ill individuals; and a geriatric nurse who has a case management practice for the elderly. This geriatric nurse has recently hired a couple of other case managers with gerontological expertise. The author of *The Case Manager's Handbook*, Catherine Mullahy (2004, 2009) is also the owner of a small business known as "Options Unlimited," which provides services to injured workers.

You, too, can be a nurse entrepreneur. This chapter introduces nurses and nurse case managers to the possibilities of becoming entrepreneurs, including the benefits and challenges inherent in following that path.

DEFINITIONS: WHAT IS AN ENTREPRENEUR?

What is an entrepreneur? Table 7-1 offers some definitions to help clarify the scope of entrepreneurship.

Other examples of nurse entrepreneurs come from a lifetime of observations across many states. A family nurse practitioner has gone into the home health business with a nurse, whose master's degree is in community mental health nursing, serving the poor of New Orleans. A Houston pediatric nurse designed and marketed a pacifier that parents and their babies liked better than those that were on the market. A psychiatric nurse in North Carolina is in private practice, counseling the mentally ill. A nurse who has expertise in item writing for the National Council Licensure Examination (NCLEX) testing consults with faculty in schools of nursing about item writing for developing tests for nursing students. A nurse who is a family nurse practitioner developed her own private practice in rural Alabama. Another nurse practitioner in rural Alabama joined a physician's practice in family medicine as a partner. Because of her past experience in psychiatric nursing and her finely honed assessment skills, she proved an invaluable member of the family practice team. Many nurse case managers work independently for insurance companies caring for patients on worker's compensation. Nurse practitioners in New York City are serving families in Harlem in local clinics and small community agencies, as independent practitioners. Targeting the medically underserved lies in the future for many advanced practice nurses and nurse case managers. Table 7-2 provides other examples of case managers who have ventured out on their own.

Today, business does not necessarily take place in an office, but rather is frequently conducted at a temporary station on a portable electronic terminal. Many nurses work out of their homes. Such a home office or temporary station may be equipped with a phone, a computer, a fax machine, a television, a copy machine, or other necessary items. Many employees who work for community

TABLE 7-1 Definitions of Entrepreneurship

- An entrepreneur is someone who starts a business and is willing to assume all of the risks and rewards (Herrick, 1990–1995, 2008; Schrull, 1997–2006).
- The entrepreneur organizes and manages a new enterprise, taking the risk of not making a profit and getting the profit when there is one (Schrull, 1997–2006).
- One who undertakes an enterprise and especially one involving risk (*Webster's New Dictionary*, 1990, p. 111).
- An entrepreneur is a person who plans, organizes, finances, and operates his or her own business (Herrick, 2008).
- An entrepreneur is a person with an innovative spirit who is receptive to new opportunities (Herrick, 2008).
- The entrepreneur creates an idea and follows it to fruition, developing the idea, inventing a product, or establishing a business, and then marketing it (Vollman, 2004).
- An entrepreneur is a person who organizes, operates, and assumes the risk of a business enterprise (Mericle, 2009).
- An entrepreneur is a person who searches for a challenge, responds to it, and explores it as a new opportunity (Schrull, 1997–2006).
- Entrepreneurs are part of the economic forces that generate new markets.
- Entrepreneurs are the nurses who organize, manage, and assume the risk of a business with the goal of making nursing more accessible to the public.
- The entrepreneur assumes total responsibility and risk for discovering and creating unique opportunities to use his or her personal talent, skills, and energy, and employs a strategic planning process to transform an opportunity into a marketable service or product (Schrull, 1997–2006).
- The entrepreneur is a person who launches and manages a business venture and takes the responsibility for its success or failure (Mericle, 2009).

TABLE 7-2 More Real-Life Examples of Nurse Entrepreneurship

- Selling healthcare products or surgical and medical supplies or equipment
- Consultation to educational services in hospitals or healthcare agencies
- Developing a tool for public consumption or one that a nurse might use
- Consultation to hospitals regarding developing discharge plans to ensure smooth transitions from one healthcare agency to another
- A nurse-owned agency providing hospitals with travel nurses
- Establishing a retail business that sells diabetic books and products

agencies, including nurses, go to the office just two or three times each week or month; they spend the rest of their time seeing customers or patients, researching materials, or working in a home office. In the past, nurses often assumed that they had to work for someone else. Today, however, more nurses are becoming independent contractors as they pursue new horizons in nursing (Mericle, 2009). Today, the independent practitioner or contractor is among a growing number of nurses who are in the midst of dramatic changes in how nurses perceive their destinies.

TABLE 7-3 The Benefits and Challenges of Entrepreneurship

Positive Benefits	Negative Challenges
Work for yourself (autonomy)	Work more hours, and harder
Work on what you want and like to work on	No administrative support
Unlimited income	Income fluctuates; you are the last to get paid
Experience a great sense of accomplishment	Uncertainty
A great feeling of control and ownership	Ultimately responsible
Manage your own time	More to worry about
Ego boost	Ego deflating
Flexibility	High failure rate within the first year

Sources: Elango, Hunter, & Winchell, 2007; Herrick 2008; Schrull, 1997–2006.

As in most things in life, there are both benefits and liabilities involved in being an entrepreneur (Elango, Hunter, & Winchell, 2007). Table 7-3 describes the positive and negative aspects of entrepreneurship.

It takes a special type of person to be an entrepreneur. To be an entrepreneur, you must be self-directed and like not having a boss. You must be achievement oriented, optimistic about the future, and passionate about what you plan to do. If you are a member of a family who owns a small business, you will probably be more likely to consider being an entrepreneur rather than working for someone else. Bergman (1998) interviewed nurse entrepreneurs in different states and concluded that a master's degree in nursing administration is helpful for a future entrepreneur because it enables that individual to understand the financial aspects of health care. The master's degree in nursing administration frequently includes some business courses (Herrick, 2008). If you have a clinical degree, as a potential entrepreneur you should take some business courses.

Table 7-4 contains words that describe an entrepreneur, and Table 7-5 compares the characteristics of a nurse manager with a nurse entrepreneur. Table 7-6 provides a self-assessment tool for determining whether entrepreneurship might be right for you. As part of the preparation to be an entrepreneur, a careful self-examination is important.

Boling (2009) has suggested that the aspiring entrepreneur should have experience in multiple clinical settings. This individual should also be knowl-

TABLE 7-4 Personal Characteristics Necessary to Be an Entrepreneur

Innovator	Likes challenges	Self-starter
Persistent	Reliable	Self-disciplined
Creative	Has foresight	Is a visionary
Driven to succeed	Likes to work alone	Independent
Has stamina and lots of energy	Doesn't like to work for others	Manages time, money, and resources well
Strong ego	Not shaken by rejection	Understands the scope of practice
Professional	People oriented	
Opportunity seeker	Resilient	Committed to excellence
Realistic	Assertive	Future oriented
Resourceful	Adaptable and flexible	Keen negotiator
Confident	Has high self-esteem	Ambitious
		Builder rather than a maintainer

Sources: Finkelman, 2006; Harper, 2003; Herrick, 1990–1995, 2008; Schrull, 1997–2006.

TABLE 7-5 Differences Between a Nurse Manager and a Nurse Entrepreneur

Manager	Entrepreneur
Likes to maintain the status quo	Change agent
Efficient	Visionary
Social	Independent
Security oriented	Risk taker
Data oriented	Intuitive

TABLE 7-6 Self-Assessment for Aspiring Entrepreneurs

Which Entrepreneurial Characteristics Do I Have?

- Can I make my own decisions?
- Do I enjoy being challenged?
- Do I thrive on competition?
- Do I believe in myself?
- Am I creative?
- Do I enjoy working alone?
- Can I accept criticism?
- Am I assertive?
- Am I patient and persistent?
- Do I plan well and manage my time well?
- Can I delegate?
- Do I seek out and listen to advice from other professionals?
- Am I willing to work long hours?
- Do I understand the financial and business side of health care?

edgeable about starting a new business, including the need for liability insurance, personal health insurance, accounting services, financial and banking matters, and other expertise necessary to start a new business and sustain it. Most of all, the would-be entrepreneur should be passionate about the venture, and resilient enough to withstand the challenges ahead. The advantages of being a private practitioner, who is hired by a patient and his or her family, is that the entrepreneur does not have divided loyalties but can advocate fully for the patient and family.

Before embarking on a new enterprise, ask yourself the following questions: What events are happening that make you want to become an entrepreneur? Do you know yourself well—including both your attributes and your faults? Do you have what it takes to be an entrepreneur? Be sure to conduct a self-assessment.

INTRAPRENEURSHIP

An *intrapeneur* is someone who organizes, manages, and assumes a portion of the risk of a business that is part of another business or organization. A nurse does not necessarily have to leave the hospital to be a creative intrapreneur, but he or she does need to think like an entrepreneur (Dayhoff & Moore, 2003, 2005). With this business model, the larger entity provides administrative support and assumes the major part of the risk. For example, intrapreneurship might be required for starting a new unit in a hospital.

According to Finkelman (2006), there are probably more intrapreneurs in nursing than there are entrepreneurs. Consider the following examples:

- Acting as an internal consultant—for example, as a psychiatric liaison nurse or wound specialist in an acute care hospital.
- Developing a new program for an institution—for example, a palliative care unit in an acute care hospital.
- Developing a new role in an institution—for example, a case manager in an emergency department.
- Developing and managing an Alzheimer's disease unit in a long-term care facility.
- Being a nurse case manager in a child welfare department in the foster care division as a liaison from the Public Health Department. Traditionally child welfare departments employ only social workers.

Both the intrapreneur and the entrepreneur roles have both advantages and disadvantages. Table 7-7 addresses the advantages and the disadvantages of each of these roles.

TABLE 7-7 Advantages and Disadvantages of the Intrapreneur and Entrepreneur Roles

Intrapreneur	Entrepreneur
It is an advantage to know the institution and its culture and to have institutional support.	The entrepreneur has no support except what he or she seeks out from other professionals, the community, and his or her own family.
The status as an insider is an asset. However, the intrapreneur's reputation may include mixed reviews.	The status of an entrepreneur has to be earned from the community, other professionals, and the people whom the entrepreneur serves. A reputation takes time to build.
The insider's perspective is limited to knowledge about one institution.	The entrepreneur must have a broader perspective, including knowledge of the community and its many institutions.
The risk is shared between the intrapreneur and the institution.	All of the risk resides in the entrepreneur.

CHALLENGES FACED BY ENTREPRENEURS

An independent entrepreneur works longer and harder than the intrapreneur, who has administrative support. The only security for an entrepreneur comes from within. At first, there will be no steady paycheck and the entrepreneur will be the last to get paid, paying the office personnel and the bills first. It takes time to reach the break-even point, when the private practitioners can start paying himself or herself. And there is always the risk of losing the business: High rates of failures occur during the first year of a new venture. According to Schrull (1997–2006), two-thirds of all new businesses fail during the first year. The entrepreneur is ultimately responsible for the business and welfare of the people who are hired. There is a great deal of uncertainty until the enterprise is fully established and well known in the community and the entrepreneur has developed a good reputation among other healthcare professionals.

The entrepreneur (and intrapreneur) should seek guidance from a number of different experts to assist him or her in setting up and running the business. Table 7-8 lists some of the many resources that are recommended when planning, developing, and maintaining a new enterprise.

Use all of the resources that are available. The entrepreneur may have to pay some of the consultants, but it is well worth the expense. Find a mentor—

TABLE 7-8 Resources for Entrepreneurs

Advisors	Consultants	Assistants	Organizations
Librarian	Marketing/Advertising consultant Business manager as a consultant and/or assistant	Secretary	Professional organizations (e.g., American Nurses Association [ANA], Case Management Society of America [CMSA], American Case Management Association [ACMA])
Community leaders and professional leaders	Members and leaders of the National Nurses in Business Association, Inc.	Insurance agent	Local small business association such as the Rotary Club
Accountant	Consultants from the U.S. Small Business Administration	Bookkeeper	Consumer organizations (e.g., American Cancer Society [ACS])
Attorney	Consultants from the National Association of Small Business Investment Companies (NASBIC)	Banker	American Organization of Nurse Executives (AONE)

someone who is in your field of nursing. Seek out a nurse expert—someone who has become an intrapreneur or entrepreneur (Royal College of Nursing, 2007). And be aware that you may need more than one mentor, given the many different aspects of the business to be considered.

IMPORTANT CONSIDERATIONS FOR NURSE ENTREPRENEURS

Determine Which Business to Start

- Develop a business that focuses on what you enjoy doing.
- Analyze the market and develop a marketing plan (Chapter 8).
- Determine what unmet need exists in the community that you can fulfill.
- What do you see in the future that others do not see?

Raise Capital

How much money will be needed to start and support the business, especially over the first year when profits are unlikely? Where will that money come from?

Develop a Business Plan

The wise nurse entrepreneur will formalize his or her business strategy and *write it down*. To translate an idea into a business that is sustainable, a great deal of preplanning is necessary. The business plan outlines your dream and specifically addresses why and how that dream will become a reality and a profitable venture (Mericle, 2009). The words and numbers in the business plan document should specifically detail your plans for the new enterprise. It must be a complete package, without ambiguity.

You may learn to write a business plan in a course in nursing administration. If not, take a course on developing your own business at a community college.

The business plan must be a realistic presentation of the enterprise and the foundation of your operating strategy. Table 7-9 offers a guideline for developing a business plan.

Mistakes are common when first establishing a new enterprise (Table 7-10). Learn from your own mistakes and from the mistakes made by others. Every entrepreneur experiences a few setbacks along the journey. Heed the warnings in Table 7-11; they are not meant to discourage you, but to help you look at the venture realistically and prepare you for the potential troubles that may be encountered.

TABLE 7-9 Suggested Organization of a Business Plan

- Title page
- Table of contents
- Nondisclosure agreement
- Niche in the market for the potential product or services

Overview of the Basics
- What is the business?
- Who are the customers?
- What is important to those customers?
- What is the purpose of the business?
- What is the justification for establishing the business, including the targeted clientele, the location, and the costs?
- Specify the product or service—how is it unique?
- Address contingencies: lawsuits, warranties/lease renewals, economic conditions.

Market Analysis
- Size of the market
- Anticipated market share
- Size of the future market
- Who are your competitors?
- What market share do your competitors have and will you have?
- How are you different from your competitors?
- Are there any barriers to entry (e.g., certificate of need, licenses)?

(Continues)

TABLE 7-9 *Continued*

Capital Requirements
- How much money is needed to start the business and how much to maintain it?
- How will you allocate the money?
- If you need capital, will it be debt or equity? Will you finance it out of your savings or need to borrow money from others?
- If you are seeking investors, what will the investors/creditors get in return?
- Where will you obtain additional capital for expansion or unanticipated events?

Payer Analysis
- Who will pay?
- How much will they pay? What will you charge? What is the going rate of pay?
- Pricing: How will you price the product or service? What is the difference in the price of products or services for a start-up company versus an established company?

Financial Analysis
- Volume projection
- Income statement: projections for 3–5 years
- Balance sheet
- Break-even analysis
- Return on the investment for you and the investors

Sources: Herrick, 2008; Royal College of Nursing, 2007; Schrull, 1997–2006.

TABLE 7-10 Common Mistakes Made by Entrepreneurs

- Undercapitalization
- Not planning appropriately for your income needs
- Expecting the business to grow quickly
- Underestimating how hard you will need to work to succeed
- Organizing and not selling
- Not networking sufficiently
- Not understanding the local market
- Not having an exit strategy
- Not reading the business trends correctly
- Not developing a thorough business plan and marketing plan

Sources: Herrick, 2008; Schrull, 1997–2006.

■ SUMMARY

Developing your own business should be an exciting adventure, where you are the captain of your own ship. Do a self-assessment to determine if you have the personality and skills to be an entrepreneur. Do your homework. Spend time carefully planning your new business. Create an operational (business) plan documenting your planned enterprise and its goals. As part of this plan,

TABLE 7-11 To Do or Not to Do

Do	Don't
Be prepared for a 24/7 venture.	If you have personal problems or little family support, the timing is wrong.
Maintain balance in your life.	If you are not prepared to wear many hats and cannot adapt to many demands, don't do it!
Do as much networking as you possibly can. You must sell yourself as well as your enterprise.	Do not accept more customers than you can handle.
Focus on what is important—establish priorities.	Do not quit your job until you are sure that the new business can sustain you.
Build trust.	Do not misrepresent facts about your product or services to customers.
Challenge your assumptions.	Don't be self-satisfied; always look for ways to make improvements.
Know your limitations.	If you do not have the proper expertise, then don't do it. Establish a business that takes advantage of your knowledge and talents and that you enjoy.
Do your homework. Good preplanning is a "must"! Find something that is unique that your competitors are not providing.	Don't underestimate your competition.
Get a line of credit.	Don't expect an immediate profit.
Hire consultants: a lawyer, an accountant, a business manager, an insurance agent, and any other expert who may be needed.	Don't rely on a partner without a legal agreement, even if you are professional "friends."
Start a business that someone else will be willing to buy. Sell the business when the business is doing well.	Don't sell at the downturn of the business. If the business experiences continuing losses, then cut your losses to a minimum and *get out*. If you can wait it out, sell when there is an upturn in the business or the economy.
Honor your commitments. Keep your promises. Maintain your integrity. Keep your values.	Don't stoop to unscrupulous methods.

Sources: Herrick, 2008; Royal College of Nursing, 2007; Schrull, 1997–2006.

outline the responsibilities of each of the stakeholders and the employees. An organizational chart can illustrate the chain of command.

Chapter 8 addresses marketing as a guide to help you plan your new enterprise. Careful planning will pay dividends in the future:

- Do a feasibility study to assure yourself that this is a venture you really want to undertake.
- Develop business and marketing plans.
- Develop a presentation about your business and marketing plans. Present the plans for the new enterprise to potential supporters (lenders, family and/or investors).

In the future, the growing number of entrepreneurs in nursing will enhance the nursing profession and will be good for the healthcare industry as a whole. Nurses are good ambassadors for physicians, hospitals, home health agencies, and other healthcare institutions. Nurse entrepreneurs are creative thinkers, who are motivated to improve themselves and the nursing profession (Danna, 2006).

■ CASE STUDIES

The Small Business Administration has decided to dedicate both grant and loan funding for nurses to start small businesses within the healthcare arena. Write down two or three business ideas you have and share them with your classmates. Are these ideas unique and feasible?

■ DISCUSSION QUESTIONS

1. Identify advantages and disadvantages to owning your own business.
2. What characteristics do you possess that would pose a challenge to owning your own business?
3. What is the difference between an entrepreneur and an intrapreneur?

■ CLASSROOM EXERCISES

Interview with an Entrepreneur

Interview an entrepreneur of your choice. You may choose a fellow nurse or someone you know who has started a business. Ask the following questions.

1. Why did you start you own business?
2. How long has the business been established?
3. How long was the planning phase?
4. Was a market needs assessment done prior to starting the business?
5. Did you develop a written business plan?
6. Who funded the venture?
7. Did you quit you regular job to establish the business?
8. How did you market yourself?
9. How has the marketing plan evolved?
10. What are the positives about having your own business?
11. What are the negatives about having your own business?
12. How long did it take for the business to become financially viable?
13. Who was the competition?
14. What do you see in the future for the business?
15. What advice would you give to a nurse considering entrepreneurship?

■ REFERENCES

Bergman, P. A. (1998). Invest in yourself: Lessons learned from nurse entrepreneurs. *Nursing Forum, 33*(3), 17–21.

Boling, J. (2009). As a leader in the practice of case management, what new frontiers do you see for case managers? *Case in point: Coordinating care, changing lives, leadership supplement*, pp. 7–9. Retrieved from www.dorlandhealth.com

Danna, D. (2006). Organizational structure and analysis: Entrepreneurship. In L. Roussel, R. C. Swansburg, & R. J. Swansburg (Eds.), *Management and leadership for nurse administrators* (4th ed., p. 143). Sudbury, MA: Jones and Bartlett.

Dayhoff, N. E., & Moore, P. S. (2003). You don't have to leave your hospital system to be an entrepreneur. *Clinical Nurse Specialist, 17*(1), 22–24.

Dayhoff, N. E., & Moore, P. S. (2005). Think like an entrepreneur. *Clinical Nurse Specialist, 19*(2), 65–66.

Elango, B. E., Hunter, G. L., & Winchell, M. (2007). Barriers to nurse entrepreneurship: A study of the process model of entrepreneurship. *Journal of the American Academy of Nurse Practitioners, 19*(4), 198–204.

Finkelman, A. W. (2006). *Leadership and management in nursing*. Upper Saddle River, NJ: Pearson Education.

Harper, S. C. (2003). *The McGraw-Hill guide to starting your own business: A step-by-step blueprint for the first-time entrepreneur* (2nd ed.). New York: McGraw-Hill.

Herrick, C. A. (1990–1995). *Entrepreneurship*. Lectures in a course on consultation [unpublished manuscript]. Mobile, AL: University of South Alabama, College of Nursing.

Herrick, C. A. (2008). Learning modules for a course in Nursing Case Management (NUR 541) [unpublished manuscript]. Greensboro, NC: University of North Carolina at Greensboro School of Nursing.

Mericle, T. (2009). *Can nurses be entrepreneurs?* Retrieved from http://www.jobbankusa.com/CareerArticles/HomeBusiness/ca41204b.html

Mullahy, C. (2004). *The case manager's handbook* (3rd ed.). Sudbury, MA: Jones and Bartlett.

Mullahy, C. (2009). Case management: Entrepreneur to share expertise in Pasadena. Retrieved from http://include.nurse.com/article/20090126/CA02/101260044

Royal College of Nursing. (2007, December). *Nurse entrepreneurs: Turning initiative into independence.* Retrieved from http://www.rcn.org.uk/__data/assets/pdf_file/0018/115632/003215.pdf.

Schrull, J. A. (Fall semesters, 1997–2006). *Entrepreneurship*. Lectures in Case Management (NUR 541). Greensboro, NC: University of North Carolina at Greensboro.

Vollman, K. M. (2004). Nurse entrepreneurship: taking an invention from birth to the market place. *Clinical Nurse Specialist, 18*(2), 68–71.

Webster's new dictionary. (1990). New York: Russell, Geddes and Gossett.

Marketing Your Services as a Case Manager, Consultant, or Entrepreneur

Laura J. Fero
Charlotte A. Herrick

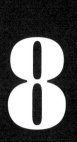

■ OUTLINE

Introduction
Definitions and Concepts: What Is Marketing?
Market Analysis
The Marketing Plan
The Marketing Process
Networking

■ OBJECTIVES

1. Define *marketing*.

2. Describe important marketing-related concepts.

3. Analyze the market for case management services.

4. Discuss the development of a marketing plan.

5. Describe the "four P's" of the marketing plan

6. Compare the marketing process and the nursing process.

7. Discuss the importance of networking.

INTRODUCTION

Marketing is a new subject for many nurses (Finkelman, 2006). Initially, nurse case managers had to market the idea of establishing a case management department to senior hospital administrators (Cohen & Cesta, 2005). Today, most nurses work for institutions that have marketing departments. At the same time, more nurses are establishing their own businesses as case managers, nurse practitioners, consultants, or entrepreneurs; that is, more nurses are going into private practice than previous generations of nurses. Often nurses who work in smaller community agencies, or those who work as managers in these small agencies, are expected to know about marketing concepts and may be expected to conduct marketing activities (Finkler & Kerner, 2000).

But times are changing. As the nursing shortage becomes more acute, nurse recruiters are using marketing strategies to recruit nursing staff (Sullivan & Decker, 2009).

Marketing is a process that drives decisions among competing healthcare organizations as they vie to attract patients or staff. The process includes three elements:

1. A determination of what a target population wants or needs
2. A method(s) for reaching the target population and to deliver what it wants or needs
3. An understanding of the consumers and their needs so as to provide the appropriate services (Finkelman, 2006)

As discussed in Chapter 7, entrepreneurs create an idea, which they then take to the marketplace and sell to consumers (Vollman, 2004). Private practitioners, including consultants and entrepreneurs, need to know how to market themselves and their services as they establish and conduct their own businesses.

This chapter defines the key concepts associated with marketing. Analyzing the market is explored to guide the reader in how to plan a program, develop a product, or provide a healthcare service. The four "Ps" of the marketing process are addressed for planning purposes, and the steps of the marketing process are identified and compared to the nursing process. Finally, the importance of networking is considered as a means to build good relationships with potential consumers and referral sources.

DEFINITIONS AND CONCEPTS: WHAT IS MARKETING?

Table 8-1 summarizes some key definitions related to marketing. In addition, the following concepts are considered important elements in understanding marketing and are discussed further here:

- Exchange theory
- Competition
- Consumer-driven focus
- Segmentation

Exchange Theory and Self-Interest Related to the Marketing Process

Exchange theory—the conceptual framework for marketing—addresses the opportunity between two parties to exchange goods and services at a cost.

TABLE 8-1 Marketing-Related Definitions

Marketing is getting the right message to the right people via the right media, using the right methods.

Marketing is a social and managerial process in which individuals or groups obtain what is wanted by exchanging products and services. The **market** consists of actual or potential buyers of goods, services, and ideas.

Marketing includes advertisements about products and services that are designed to meet people's needs and, therefore, make consumers willing to buy these products or services

Marketing is the exchange of goods and services among individuals and groups.

The **market** is the actual or potential consumer or customer who might need a product or service within a specific geographical area.

Market share is the percentage of the market for a specific product or service that is already captured by another provider.

Sources: Kennedy, 2006; Siegel & Lotenberg, 2007; Sommes & Barnes, cited in Steven, 2006; Woods, 2006.

Each of the parties may have something that will be of benefit to the other party. There is open communication between the two about the delivery of goods and services at a price. Each party negotiates with the other party based on his or her own values and is free to accept or reject the offer. If there is agreement, then each party believes the deal is beneficial to his or her own self-interests. To complete a transaction, the benefit must outweigh the costs to the seller and the buyer or consumer. Under exchange theory, the assumption is made that people will act in their own self-interest (Siegel & Lotenberg, 2007). Consequently, marketing must address the interests of the target population (or audience) and demonstrate how the goods and services will be beneficial and worth the cost.

Competition

U.S. businesses, including those in the healthcare arena, operate in a free enterprise system—that is, in a market economy, where many sellers compete for customers (Austin & Welte, 2008). To sell a product or service, the seller must understand the competition. Frequently, these competitors already have their own niches in the market. They may have more resources, different values, or target a different audience than the seller.

It behooves the entrepreneur to study the competition if he or she wishes to successfully compete in the marketplace. By studying the competition's strategies and population served, the entrepreneur will be able to identify what he or she might be able to offer that is different or unique. Through the research and segmentation phase of the marketing process, the entrepreneur may uncover a group of people who are underserved or a group whose members may be looking for a service that is not currently available in their community. Armed with this information, the entrepreneur might strike gold: A different niche might be found for a new and unique enterprise. Of course, to capitalize on such an opportunity, the entrepreneur must be able to convince the consumer that the benefits of the new product or service are better and more cost-effective than those offered by the competition (Siegel & Lotenberg, 2007).

Consumer-Driven Focus

Marketing is consumer driven. The entrepreneur, consultant, or case manager must understand the potential consumers—that is, their needs, their beliefs and values, and their environment—if he or she hopes to provide a product or service that the consumer will buy. Put simply, the product or service must fulfill a need (Siegel & Lotenberg, 2007). Unlike many consumer products and services, healthcare marketing must also address legislative mandates. The key to success is for the entrepreneur to fully understand the target audience. For example, there is a greater demand in South Florida for a geriatric nurse case manager than there is a demand for a geriatric nurse case manager in a college town, such as Madison, Wisconsin.

The characteristics of the provider may be an important factor when selling oneself to consumers. The characteristics of a provider that are important to consumers are the provider's credentials, including education, certifications, and experience, as well as the location of the business or practice. In a consumer-driven healthcare system, both the characteristics of the provider and the types of services that are offered are frequently determined by the needs and the location of the consumers rather than being dictated by the providers (Hogan & Nickitas, 2009).

Segmentation

Segmentation is a strategy to identify the potential consumer of a product or service. "Segmentation is an automatic sorting of persons into predefined groupings" (Howe, 2005, p. 74). During this process, a segment of the population is defined. The entrepreneur should specialize so that his or her product or service is targeted toward the specific needs of that segment of the population (Siegel & Lotenberg, 2007). In essence, the entrepreneur caters to a narrow group of consumers who have similar characteristics, rather than seeking to sell to the general population (Hiam, 2004). For example, the entrepreneur might specialize his or her consulting service to meet the needs of nonprofit organizations, might target a group of nurse case managers in private practice, or might provide case management services to elderly patients who are chronically ill. The group of potential consumers (i.e., the target population) comprises the group of people who will benefit from the nurse entrepreneur's expertise.

During the segmentation process, increasing smaller portions of the population are examined, until the entrepreneur fully understands the specific characteristics, values, and needs of the targeted segment of the population. The advantage of segmentation is that this strategy allows the entrepreneur to tailor the product or service to a clearly defined population. Constructing a matrix to segment the population will clarify a specific market that is underserved; an underserved population may then be the niche for the new business or practice.

MARKET ANALYSIS

For the would-be entrepreneur, it is essential to analyze the potential enterprise's mission, its values, and the various types of marketing strategies that may be used to "sell" the goods or services. Be clear about the mission and have a vision of the future. Table 8-2 outlines the steps to be taken during the analysis phase of the marketing process.

The more preparation that you do before starting a new enterprise, the greater the chance that you will be successful. The following is a list of other data to analyze:

- Study the specific geographic area.
- Identify the population and the rate of growth.
- Identify the neighborhoods.
- Consider the movement of people in and out of the area.
- Determine the new roads that are in the planning stages that will affect the location of the potential enterprise.

Thoroughly examine all of the documents that may be available in the city or county where you plan to start your new enterprise. The following list of data to be examined will guide you in your analysis of the market in a specific geographical area:

- Census data.
- The county and city data book.

TABLE 8-2 Analyzing the Market

1. **Conduct a situational analysis** of the strengths, weaknesses, opportunities, and threats (SWOT) for the market and the proposed business.

2. **After identifying the targeted population, analyze the potential need for the product or service in the future.** Gather as much data as possible to determine what is happening now regarding a particular service and segment of the population and identify the trends that could affect the potential enterprise in the future.

3. **Identify goals and objectives.** For example, the goal might be to teach health promotion and disease prevention to a group of women ages 30–40 (the target population). A demographic assessment of a specific geographical area might reveal that there is a large population of college-educated women in this age group who are interested in physical fitness.

Source: Schrull, 2006.

- The "Survey of Buying Power" from the *Journal of Sales and Marketing Management*. This instrument reports the median age of the target population and the percentage of people in each age group, the number of households and the average number per unit, the total retail sales and the volume of sales, and the percentage of households with various annual incomes, from less than $20,000 to more than $50,000.
- Records of the chamber of commerce. Use these data to determine the business conditions in general.
- Economic census.
- The demographics of the population whom you plan to serve.
- Data on the competition. How many businesses like the one you are planning to establish already exist in a particular geographical area? What do these businesses offer and where are they located? Can you, as a new entrepreneur, offer something that is unique? (Harper, 2003).

By analyzing the market, you will be in a position to identify the people who will be the consumers of the type of product or services that you wish to offer. Through the process of segmentation, you identify the target population and its characteristics, the geographical areas where they live, and their needs, so that the product or service can specifically meet this population's needs.

Marketing analysis may take a long time, but it is well worth the effort. Its results will guide your path to success. Do your homework so that you are clear about which product or service you plan to provide and to whom. Not only should all of the variables be analyzed, but all assumptions should also be questioned. Identify all of the pitfalls, risks, and potential benefits associated with the proposed business.

Of course, there is no single formula for success. No enterprise can be all things to all people. Concentrate your attention on providing the best goods or services to the people in your target population. Design your product or services to meet specific needs of a particular population. Analyze all of the factors that will influence the target population's ability or desire to buy your product or service (Siegel & Lotenberg, 2007).

THE MARKETING PLAN

The marketing plan is a written description of the enterprise and its plans for the future, whether it is an organization consisting of one provider or many. For example, the organization may comprise a group of nurse consultants made up of experts in several specialties, or it may include a group of case managers from different fields of nursing case management (e.g., a case manager who does life care planning or a case manager who handles worker's compensation claims).

Once the assessment phase—that is, the market analysis—is completed, the next step is planning. Planning targets the potential consumers who were identified by the segmentation process. The analysis of the population provides information about those potential consumers, the competition for the proposed specialty services in this geographical area, and the potential need for this product or service in the future. The marketing strategies should be designed to reach the target population and possibly future groups with similar characteristics.

Necessary Elements of a Marketing Plan

- Identification of the marketing strategy, which is the method to be used to achieve goals and objectives. Strategies may involve use of multimedia technologies as well as personal contacts.
- Establishment of the marketing action plan—a document that describes the actions, responsibilities, accountabilities, and time frames for the marketing efforts.
- Ongoing review, evaluation, feedback, and revision—the control functions of the marketing plan (Schrull, personal communication, class lecture in a course in Nursing Case Management (NUR 541), Greensboro, NC: University of North Carolina at Greensboro, 2006).

Table 8-3 lists the steps to take in developing a marketing plan. Upon completing these steps, evaluate the strategies and the progress made toward achieving the identified goals. Continue to review the plan to evaluate the

TABLE 8-3 Steps in the Marketing Plan

Core Marketing Strategy
This strategy should be the one that will best achieve the goals and objectives and will communicate information to the potential target audience.

Marketing Mix and Budget
1. Determine the "ultimate marketing secret weapon" as a way to explain that your service is unique against the competition. For example, Wal-Mart labels itself as the "low price leader."
2. Answer the consumer's key question: "Why should I choose your business, product, or service versus any other competitive option that is available?" (Kennedy, 2006).
3. Budget for the costs of advertising or other marketing strategies. Radio and television advertisements, pamphlets, brochures, and advertisements in newspapers all cost money. Different media should be examined as potential agents to advertise a product or service. Although presentations are not considered part of media campaigns, there will be a cost if you make national presentations (i.e., transportation, room, and board). Select the most cost-effective method that will reach the most people in the target population, and accept the fact that getting the word out to potential consumers will cost money.

Benchmarks
4. Set benchmarks to measure your progress toward your goals.
5. Identify the strategies that will be most effective to reach the target population in your geographical area.
6. Compare your marketing program and its success with the programs operated by others that may be similar in organization and targeted to similar needs of the population.

---

effectiveness of each of the market strategies. The following strategies should be evaluated as to their effectiveness: media releases; brochures; pamphlets; newsletters; newspaper advertisements; Internet or Web activities; professional endorsements; local, statewide, or national presentations; and personal contacts from networking.

The Four "Ps"

The four P's—product, promotion, price, and place—are the most critical elements covered by the marketing plan (Table 8-4). Nevertheless, they may also be used as a recruiting tool by healthcare institutions to hire new staff, according to Sullivan and Decker (2009).

It is important to identify an effective, eye-catching message during the development of the marketing plan. Brand names evoke images of the product

TABLE 8-4 Product, Promotion, Price, Place: The Four P's of the Marketing Plan

- **Product:** the good or service being developed to meet the consumer's needs. This element includes the quality of the product, special features that make the product or service unique, the brand name, or the reputation of the provider, the product, service, or healthcare institution.
- **Promotion:** the advertising used to promote the use of the product or service. Promotion may occur not only through the media but also via personal contacts through networking; attending local, state, and national meetings; and other public relations strategies, such as use of email or websites. In recruiting nursing staff, both professional meetings and job fairs are good recruiting tools.
- **Price:** the cost of a product or service. In the U.S. healthcare market, the price is dictated by third-party payers and the federal government. If the price is not right, then there is no profit, which poses a problem for the provider. This may explain why so many hospitals are closing their doors. The price related to nursing staff recruitment includes benefits, such as health insurance and retirement benefits and sign-on bonuses.
- **Place:** the location where the products or services will be provided to the consumer and the physical attributes of that location. Place includes the actual physical location, type of location, and wheelchair accessibility to the place where the product is sold or the services are rendered. Transportation and parking are all contributing factors that may either help or hurt a place of business. The type of setting may also contribute to the success of the enterprise—the "warmth" of the waiting room, the friendliness of the staff, and the ease of finding the agency. Easy access to the building is an important factor in recruiting nursing staff and clients. Proximity to a bus stop is another factor that will enhance a place of business.

Sources: Finkelman, 2006; Siegel & Lotenberg, 2007; Sullivan & Decker, 2009; Woods, 2006.

or service. A brand-name identity will boost the image of a product or service and associate it with the provider (Kennedy, 2006).

THE MARKETING PROCESS

The five-step marketing process focuses on identifying the target population's self-interest, so as to "sell" the product or service (Table 8-5). The consumer must believe the product or service is better than anything else that may be available and that it serves the consumer's self-interest—that is, the product or service meets his or her needs.

The marketing process and the nursing process share some similarities, including the fact that both proceed sequentially. Table 8-6 compares the two processes.

TABLE 8-5 The Five Steps in the Marketing Process

The marketing process is a five-step linear process:

1. **Research** (market analysis). Market research is necessary at every stage of the marketing process. Research comprises a systematic process for studying a marketing problem by designing a study, collecting and analyzing data, and using the information from the findings to identify the targeted market. During the evaluation or control phase, the research assesses the outcomes of the marketing efforts.
2. **Segmentation (STP)**. Segmentation targets both the population and the geographical area for marketing purposes. During the planning stage, formative research identifies those segments of the population who could use the product or service and determines the best way to communicate via the media to effectively reach the targeted consumers.
3. **Marketing mix** (MM). The marketing mix includes the identified strategies that are to be used to influence a buyer's decision to use the product or service.
4. **Implementation**. The marketing plan is put into action.
5. **Control** (feedback). Outcomes are assessed, the results are evaluated, and revisions are made to improve the marketing plan.

Sources: Herrick, 2008; Kotler, 2003; Schrull, 2006; Woods, 2006.

NETWORKING

Networking focuses on reciprocal relationships—that is, people meeting people so as to exchange information and support (Sullivan, 2004). It involves contacting others who are potential sources of support and/or future referrals. To build a network of professional and social support, the healthcare professionals should join professional and/or business organizations and perhaps hold an office in the organization. Submitting a manuscript for publication, presenting a paper to a group of colleagues, or conducting a teleconference are ways to extend your professional and business network and enhance your visibility within your profession (Grossman & Valiga, 2009; Kennedy, 2006).

Joining professional organizations, local business organizations, and any other community organizations is a means of making yourself visible to the business and professional community as well as to the general public, which will enable you to market your product or service. When attending meetings, collect names, email addresses, and "snail mail" addresses for future reference. Establish a website, as such a site can provide opportunities for providing customer service, conducting education, and disseminating information about your product or service. Kennedy (2006) recommends using the Internet to advertise your product or service.

When you develop interpersonal relationships locally, statewide, and nationally, you sell yourself, your expertise, and your product or service. The

TABLE 8-6 A Comparison of the Marketing Process and the Nursing Process

Marketing Process	Nursing Process
Perform marketing analysis, research, and segmentation.	Perform assessment.
Determine the marketing mix. Set goals and plan strategies to meet the goals.	Planning and diagnosis: Set goals and identify the nursing interventions. Develop the nursing care plan, multidisciplinary action plan (MAP), or clinical pathway, whichever is currently used in the facility.
Implement the marketing plan.	Implement the nursing care plan.
Control: Get feedback and evaluate the results. Compare the results with the goals and objectives to determine the success of the marketing strategies, or compare the outcomes with agencies that are in the same geographical location and provide services to a comparable population (benchmarking).	Evaluation: Compare the outcomes with the nursing care plan. Determine the patient's progress toward meeting the goals and the identified outcomes. Identify any barriers that might impede the patient's progress.
Redesign the marketing strategies, if necessary, to better meet the goals and objectives and to reach a larger number of people in the target population.	Reevaluate the patient's progress, according to the care plan. Rework the nursing care plan if the outcomes are less than successful and if the patient is not making adequate progress. The new nursing care plan may guide the nurse, other staff, and the patient to achieve expected outcomes.

Source: Herrick, 2008.

people whom you meet may not only be future consumers of your product or service, but may also serve as referral sources.

■ SUMMARY

Marketing takes time and patience, and it can be costly, but is clearly necessary if one wants a successful future as an entrepreneur, consultant, or private practitioner. Analysis of the market is the initial step in developing a marketing plan. Research the potential target population to identify the segment of the population that will be your potential consumers. The new entrepreneur must have a vision for the future and convey that vision to others to sell the product or service. Developing a marketing plan does not preclude also developing a business plan, which should be part of the preparation to launch a new product or service. Market analysis will assist the entrepreneur to pinpoint the niche where the planned service or product is unique. The marketing plan can then help to identify the scope of the practice or service and will guide the development of strategies that will be needed to build the new enterprise. Proper preparation is essential to the future success of a new practice or enterprise.

■ CASE STUDIES

You have decided to start a small business with the mission of caring for elderly clients diagnosed with early-stage Alzheimer's disease. The goal of your program is to keep these individuals as independent as possible, using case managers to assist in the coordination of both their medical and personal needs. The business will target those clients with family members who live out of state and are not present to assist in providing care for their loved ones. Discuss the steps in developing a targeted marketing plan. How would you use this plan to leverage your small business?

■ DISCUSSION QUESTIONS

1. Compare the marketing process with the nursing process.
2. Which step in the marketing process takes the most time and is the most important? Why?
3. How can the four P's of the marketing process guide your marketing plan?
4. Which kinds of networking do you think you might do to market your business?

■ CLASSROOM EXERCISES

Obtain a marketing plan from a local healthcare organization that uses case managers. Review this plan with the other students in your class. Discuss the plan and suggest possible ideas to increase the organization's market share within the community.

■ RECOMMENDED READING

Hastings, G., & Sarenz, M. (2003). The critical contribution of social marketing. *Marketing Theory, 3*(3), 303–322.

Kotler, P., & Armstrong, G. (2004). *Principles of marketing* (10th ed.). Upper Saddle River, NJ: Pearson Education.

Kotler, P., Roberto, E. L., & Lee, N. (2002). *Social marketing: Improving the quality of life* (2nd ed.). Thousand Oaks, CA: Sage.

Roman, K., Maas, J., & Nisenholtz, M. (2003). *How to advertise* (3rd ed.). New York: St. Martin's Press.

Schultz, H. (1997). *Pour your heart into it: How Starbucks built a company one cup at a time*, New York, NY: Hyperion, 1997.

■ RESOURCES/WEBSITES

- www.dankennedy.com
- www.freepublicity.com
- www.instantvoicepromotions.com
- www.theultimatemarketingplan.com
- www.theultimatesalesletter.com

■ GOVERNMENT AGENCIES

- www.commerce.gov
- www.irs.ustreas.gov
- U.S. Small Business Administration: www.sba.gov
- U.S. Small Business Development Centers: www.sba.gov/aboutsba/sbaprograms/sbdc/index.html

■ MAGAZINES/JOURNALS

- *The Entrepreneur:* www.entrepreneur.com
- *Inc.:* www.inc.com
- *Kiplinger:* www.kiplinger.com
- *The American Public Health Association Journal:* www.apha.org/journal
- *Case in Point* (official magazine of the Case Management Society of America): www.dorlandhealth.com

■ REFERENCES

Austin, A., & Welte, V. (Eds.). (2008). The impact of the economy. In *The United States health care system: Combining business, health, and delivery.* Upper Saddle River, NJ: Pearson/Prentice Hall.

Cohen, E. L., & Cesta, T. G. (Eds.) (2005). Internal marketing. In *Nursing case management: From essentials to advanced practice applications* (4th ed., pp. 242–244). St. Louis, MO: Elsevier/Mosby.

Finkelman, A. S. (Eds.). (2006). Organizational structure for effective care delivery. In *Leadership and management in nursing* (pp. 126–156). Upper Saddle River, NJ: Prentice Hall.

Finkler, S. A., & Kerner, C. T. (2000). *Marketing: Financial management for nurse managers and executives*. Philadelphia: W. B. Saunders, pp. 433–458.

Grossman, S. C., & Valiga, T. M. (2009). *The new leadership challenge*. Philadelphia: F. A. Davis.

Harper, S. C. (2003). *The McGraw-Hill guide to starting your own business: A step-by-step blueprint for the first-time entrepreneur* (2nd ed.). New York: McGraw-Hill.

Herrick, C. A. (2008). Learning modules for a course in Nursing Case Management (NUR 541) [unpublished manuscript]. Greensboro, NC: University of North Carolina at Greensboro, School of Nursing.

Hiam, A. (2004). *Marketing for dummies* (2nd ed.). Hoboken. NJ: John Wiley & Sons.

Hogan, M. A., & Nickitas, D. M. (2009). *Nursing leadership and management*. Upper Saddle River, NJ: Pearson/Prentice Hall.

Howe, R. (2005). *The disease manager's handbook*. Sudbury, MA: Jones and Bartlett.

Kennedy, D. S. (2006). *The ultimate marketing plan* (3rd ed.). Avon, MA: Adams Business Publications.

Kotler, P. (2003). *Marketing insights from A to Z*. Hoboken. NJ: John Wiley & Sons.

Schrull, J. (2006). Personal communication, class lecture in a course in Nursing Case Management (NUR 541). Greensboro, NC: University of North Carolina at Greensboro.

Siegel, M., & Lotenberg, L. D. (2007). *Marketing public health*. Sudbury, MA: Jones and Bartlett.

Steven, D. (2006). Strategic planning, goal setting and marketing. In P. S. Yoder-Wise (Ed.), *Leading and managing in nursing* (3rd ed., pp. 125–156). Upper Saddle River, NJ: Pearson/Prentice Hall.

Sullivan, E. J. (2004). *Becoming influential*. Upper Saddle River, NJ: Pearson/ Prentice Hall.

Sullivan, E. J., & Decker, P. J. (Eds.). (2009). Recruiting and selecting staff. In *Effective leadership and management in nursing* (7th ed., p. 203). Upper Saddle River, NJ: Pearson/Prentice Hall.

Vollman, K. M. (2004). Nurse entrepreneurship: Taking an invention from birth to the marketplace. *Clinical Nurse Specialist, 18*(2), 68–71.

Woods, D. (2006). Marketing. In D. L. Huber (Ed.), *Leadership and nursing care management* (3rd ed., pp. 299–311). Philadelphia: Saunders/Elsevier.

Consultation: A Business for Case Managers

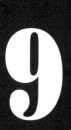

Laura J. Fero
Charlotte A. Herrick

■ OUTLINE

Introduction
Definitions: What Is Consultation?
The Skills and Traits of a Consultant
Reasons That Clients Seek Consultation
The Consultation Process
Types of Consultation
Interventions Suggested by Consultants
Overcoming Resistance
Examining Organizational Dynamics
Choosing a Career as a Consultant

■ OBJECTIVES

1. Define *consultation*.
2. Identify the roles, skills, and personal traits necessary to be a successful consultant.
3. Describe the collaborative process.
4. Discuss the consultation process, including its characteristics and stages.
5. Describe the different types of consultation.
6. Compare internal and external consultation.
7. Describe the interventions prescribed by consultants.
8. Describe the organizational dynamics and the structures of an organization that must be addressed during the consultation process.
9. Discuss the benefits and challenges of being a consultant.
10. Describe the consultee–consultant's collaborative relationship.
11. Identify the formula for effective consultation.

INTRODUCTION

Some nurses, who have become experts in a field of nursing or case management, have founded their own businesses or established their own private practices in consultation. As entrepreneurs, these individuals determine their own destinies. Many nurses use their expertise to consult with other units in their own agencies or they are internal consultants—that is, they are consultants in their own institution. An example is the position of psychiatric liaison nurse, which is a common role for psychiatric nurses in large institutions. Liaisons consult with the nursing staff about coping with difficult or psychiatrically disturbed patients.

Some consultants are external consultants. For example, the nurse who is an expert witness for a lawyer and has established his or her own private practice is an external consultant. If a patient's family files a lawsuit against a healthcare agency, the expert witness—legal nurse consultant—reviews the chart. He or she researches the latest literature and then provides the information to the lawyer representing either the family or the healthcare agency. Later, the expert witness may have to testify in court. According to Milazzo (2008), today legal nurse consultants are in great demand. Types of litigation in which they may play roles include suits related to negligence, malpractice, patient's rights, informed consent, use of restraints, confidentiality, reproductive rights, and timely access to care (Haag & Kalina, 2007). For the lawyer, the legal nurse consultant can bridge the knowledge gap between the law and health care (Milazzo, 1999–2009).

The Association of Perioperative Nurses (AORN, 2009) provides consultation services to healthcare organizations on clinical, practical, and management-related issues. Other external consultants may consult with hospitals to guide nursing administrators through the application process to pursue Magnet status. Some nurse educators consult with schools of nursing that want to apply for the National League of Nursing (NLN) honor, "Excellence in Nursing Education." The NLN has a cadre of nurse educators who review schools of nursing when they apply for NLN accreditation.

Mullahy (2004) described the example of a nurse case manager who is a consultant to a claims department. This individual's knowledge of "clinical needs, medical procedures, and costs can be a significant support toward maintaining cost-effective health care programs" (p. 359). The following is a list of some of the other opportunities for nurse consultants or case management consultants:

- Consultants may work in school nurse and social work programs. For example, consultants may advise public schools to develop case management programs for emotional and behavior disordered children in transition from the juvenile justice system to the public schools.
- Consultants may work in rehabilitation nurse case management. For example, the nurse consultant may act as a liaison between the

inpatient case manager and the worker's compensation case manager, the insurance company and the employer, or the home health case manager or nurse.

- Case managers may develop life care plans in consultation with clients who have experienced a traumatic brain injury, their families, and their attorneys.
- A nurse consultant may provide information to the Public Health Department regarding ethnic disparities. Wisconsin, for example, employs a team of public health nurse consultants who promote the health of Wisconsin's citizens. The Wisconsin Department of Health Services, Division of Public Health (2009) believes that healthy people make healthy communities.

Other examples of external nurse consultants include nurses who are recruited to state agencies—for example, a pediatric nurse consultant provides services to the Michigan Division of Specialized Care for Children (Michigan Civil Service Commission, 2009). Another nurse consultant works for the Pennsylvania Department of Health (2009) in its Diabetic Prevention and Control Program.

Inherent in the role of the nurse case manager is the role of consultant. Nurse case managers rarely provide direct care, but rather consult with the primary care providers, the nursing staff, and other healthcare providers about the care of the patient (Tahan, 2005). They can help the interdisciplinary team adhere to the standards of practice, and can facilitate and coordinate the necessary resources. In addition, they monitor the patient's progress. Nurse case managers consult with the family to understand the family's dynamics and their resources to determine if and how they can take care of the patient when the patient is discharged. They also consult with third-party payers as well as community agencies about potential options that might be applicable for a particular patient's discharge.

DEFINITIONS: WHAT IS CONSULTATION?

Numerous definitions of consultation exist (Table 9-1). However, they all point to a process that occurs within the consultant–consultee relationship, whereby the consultant is the expert who makes recommendations to the consultee, and the consultee seeks the knowledge and advice of the expert.

Several common denominators are apparent among the various definitions, including the fact that consultation is an interactive process. It occurs in stages and has its own characteristics. The consultant must have the expertise to problem solve, to give advice, and to help his or her clients improve their skills

TABLE 9-1 Definitions: Consultation

Cohen (1991, cited in Puetz & Shinn, 1997) defines **consulting** as advising or providing services for others in return for compensation.

Caplan (1970, cited in Herrick, 2008) identifies **consultation** as a process in which the expert is asked to identify ways to handle a problem, involving either the management of clients, the planning of potential interventions, or the implementation of a program.

Curran (2008) defined consultation in terms of the focus of the population on a target population.

- Individual/family example: The consultant assists an obese child and his or her family to plan a healthy diet they may result in weight loss.
- Community example: The consultant works with school nurses to develop a school program focused on good nutrition.
- Population example: The consultant advises health officials and legislators about how to develop a statewide nutrition program to improve the health of the state's population.

Although the target population differs, the goal of the consultation process remains the same: to improve the health of citizens by improving their nutrition.

According to Lange (1987), **consultation** includes common elements such as problem resolution, advice giving, and helping the consultee to improve skills and/ or to make better and more effective plans.

Lippitt and Lippitt (1986) describe **consultation** as a two-way interaction—a process of seeking, giving, and receiving advice. It is a process to assist individuals, groups, or organizations to achieve change.

Loranger (1992, quoted in Caplan, 1970) defines **consultation** as an interaction, whereby the consultant is the expert and the consultee is the person who requests assistance to solve a problem. The consultee usually identifies the problem and initiates the process, while the consultant's goal is to convey information to increase the consultee's skills in managing the problem.

Puetz and Shinn (1997) define **consultation** as a process of providing advice to others. This advice might be in the form of guidance, information, knowledge, or expertise. According to these authors, a consultant can be viewed as a problem identifier and problem solver. The consultant may also discuss a series of options with the consultee that may pave the way for solving the problem.

According to Stichler (2002), the **nurse consultant** is often a recognized leader/ expert who shares knowledge and expertise with clients.

Schien (1997, cited in Herrick, 2008) defines **consultation** as a process involving activities conducted by the consultant to help the client understand the events that have occurred in his or her healthcare environment.

Smith (2008) identifies the **consultant** as a person who assists patients, families, staff, and other healthcare professionals regarding the health care and the available resources to meet their needs.

According to *Webster's Thesaurus* (1991), **"to consult"** is to "confer, discuss, to seek advisement."

TABLE 9-2 Collaborative Relationship Between the Consultant and the Consultee

---

- The relationship is a voluntary relationship between the consultant and client (consultee).
- The consultant attempts to help the client, so as to solve a current or potential problem.
- The relationship is temporary.
- The consultee initiates the relationship.
- The relationship is between peers who are equal.
- The relationship is strictly work related and never personal.
- The relationship may be terminated at any time, upon the recommendation of one of the parties.

Source: Herrick, 2008.

TABLE 9-3 Roles Filled by the Consultant

Leader*
Clinical specialist*
Expert*
Coordinator*
Teacher*
Resource person*
Entrepreneur†
Negotiator†
Independent practitioner†
Salesperson†
Facilitator (conflict resolution)†
Motivator†
Visionary†
Writer†
Group facilitator/leader†
Negotiator†
Researcher‡

---

*Lange, 1987.
†Stichler, 2002.
‡Lange, 1987; Stichler, 2002.

(Lange, 1987). Tables 9-2, 9-3, and 9-4 list the roles of the consultant and the skills and traits that a consultant must have to be effective.

As Table 9-2 indicates, the consultant and consultee work together for a common purpose or mission. They must establish a partnership so that there is both camaraderie and mutual respect.

In addition to the roles shown in Table 9-3, Norwood (1998) has identified other roles of a consultant and divided them into three categories: task, process, and universal. Table 9-4 depicts these three types of consulting roles, characterizing them in terms of the orientation to each role.

TABLE 9-4 Roles of the Consultant and Their Orientation

Task Oriented	Process Oriented	Universal Roles
Fact finder	Joint problem solving	Provider of expertise
Diagnostician	Process counselor	Presenter of information
Problem solver	Change agent	Role model
Educator	Advocate	Leader
Advisor	Motivator	Observer, listener
Coordinator of resources	Support person/confidence builder	Communicator

Source: Norwood, 1998.

THE SKILLS AND TRAITS OF A CONSULTANT

The consultant should enter the collaborative relationship with a clearly defined role to avoid frustration and misunderstandings, role conflict, and failure. The central focus of the consultant–consultee relationship should be the transfer of knowledge and expertise from the consultant to the consultee (Lange, 1987). Table 9-5 lists the consultant's skills that are necessary to be successful, and Table 9-6 outlines the traits that the ideal consultant will have.

It is important that the consultant be certified in a clinical specialty. If the consultant is an expert witness, he or she should be certified both as a legal nurse consultant and in his or her nursing or case management specialty (Milazzo, 1999–2009). The consultant must have a repertoire of skills to carry out a variety of roles, depending on the client's needs, the circumstances, and the desired outcomes.

REASONS THAT CLIENTS SEEK CONSULTATION

People and organizations may request the services of a consultant for many reasons. For example, consultants may be hired to do any of the following tasks:

- Resolve interpersonal conflicts
- Allay feelings of unease or concern that things could be better and to obtain needed objectivity
- Check on how the unit or the organization is doing (i.e., performance appraisal)

TABLE 9-5 Necessary Skills for a Consultant

- Technical skills: The clinical expertise must match the needs of the consultee.
- Interpersonal skill: knowledgeable about the helping process.
- Active listening skills.
- Leadership and management skills: analyzing, planning, organizing, budgeting, controlling.
- Consulting skills: knowledge of the consultation process.
- Integrating skills: knowledgeable about theoretical constructs (e.g., change theory, conflict resolution, leadership theories, communication theories, group dynamics, systems theory, organizational dynamics, theories of motivation). Theoretical constructs are necessary to form a conceptual framework for the consultation process. Each conceptual framework will change with different consultations.
- Clinical expertise.
- Independent learner: self-directed and motivated to succeed.
- Communication skills: speaking, writing, presenting skills.
- Critical-thinking and problem-solving skills.
- Group facilitation skills.
- Negotiation skills.
- Research skills: the ability to gather, analyze, and make judgments about data.

TABLE 9-6 Ideal Personal Traits of a Consultant

- Good listener and communicator.
- Good observer: the ability to observe the obvious and the obscure. The consultant should notice all that is going on in the environment, including the nuances, body language, surroundings (e.g., Is the office neat or messy?), interpersonal relationships among workers, and climate (e.g., Is the administrator/manager a participative and supportive leader or an authoritarian leader? Is the atmosphere positive or negative?).
- Perceptive and sensitive toward others.
- Objective: fair, unbiased, impartial. Listens to all viewpoints. Uses open-ended questions to obtain a full understanding of the problem(s). Is open-minded. Explores all options.
- Flexible: agile, creative; the ability to deal with ambiguity.
- Adaptable: is able to adjust to the unfamiliar.
- Patient: maintains equanimity in the face of conflict, error, or uncertainty.
- Persistent: has endurance, stamina, and tenacity.
- Self-confident: certain of one's skills, knowledge, and abilities.
- Humble: modest.
- Honest and ethical: shows integrity.
- Self-starter: self-directed.
- Trustworthy: maintains confidentiality.

- Facilitate change
- Teach the consultee organizational dynamics and behaviors
- Enhance morale and facilitate cohesion
- Assist with the management of resources
- Improve competency because of a perceived deficit
- Seek information and advice from an expert
- Seek legal counsel and gain information about liability insurance, malpractice and other legal issues
- Save face
- Compete in the marketplace more effectively
- Find constructive ways of disposing of funds by the end of a fiscal year (Lange, 1987; Mullahy, 2004; Norwood, 1998; Puetz & Shinn, 1997)

Frequently, when administrators make a decision that they think will be unpopular or may be met with resistance, they call in a consultant to sell the decision to the stakeholders. Consultants should be aware of and wary of hidden agendas.

THE CONSULTATION PROCESS

Like any process, the consultation process evolves through stages. It comprises an indirect service that is conducted by either an external consultant or an internal consultant. In some ways, the consultation process is similar to the nursing process. The major difference between the consultation process and the nursing process is that the consultant does not implement the plan. Instead, it is up to the primary care provider, the administrator, the program manager, or the nurse to implement the recommendations of the consultant. Of course, the consultee is under no obligation to follow the consultant's recommendations. Table 9-7 addresses the goals of the consultation process.

Stages of the Consultation Process

1. **Gaining Entry**
    - Environmental scanning (learn about the need for consultation)
    - Contracting (identify "mutual wants" and enter a "formal agreement")
    - Gaining physical entry
    - Initiating psychological entry
2. **Problem Identification**
    - Assessment
    - Diagnostic analysis
    - Presentation of findings

TABLE 9-7 Goals of the Consultation Process

- Establish a collaborative relationship
- Assist in problem identification and problem solving
- Facilitate change
- Assist in learning, growth, and development of others by sharing knowledge, providing clinical expertise, and guiding the consultee's learning experiences
- Improve patient care and the delivery of healthcare services

---

3. **Action Planning**
   - Decision making
   - Goals setting
   - Intervention (selection of the proposed options)
   - Developing an action plan
   - Facilitating implementation
4. **Evaluation**
   - Formative-evaluation: occurs midway through the process to determine the process's adherence to the timeline, barriers have been encountered, identification of new problems, the potential need to alter the plan resistance to change, ability to meet needs and issues, and so on
   - Process evaluation: an ongoing evaluation at periodic times during the consultation process
   - Summative evaluation: evaluates the final outcomes or the end product
5. **Disengagement**
   - Determining readiness to disengage
   - Maintaining change
   - Managing the psychodynamics of disengagement
   - Presenting the final report
   - Achieving closure (Lippitt & Lippitt, 1978, 1986; Norwood, 1998)

Although the consultation and nursing processes are similar, each stage is labeled differently. Table 9-8 compares the two processes.

TYPES OF CONSULTATION

Four types of consultation are distinguished, each of which depends on the focus of the consultation process.

Client-Centered Consultation

The focus of the consultation process is on the client or family and planning for their care. The consultant is an expert or specialist in managing health care or mental healthcare problems.

TABLE 9-8 A Comparison of the Consultation Process and the Nursing Process

Consultation Process	Nursing Process
Entry	Assessment
Data analysis and problem identification	Diagnosis
Action planning	Planning
Monitoring	Implementation
Evaluation	Evaluation
Report writing and disengagement	Documentation and termination (due to transfer or discharge)

Consultee-Centered Consultation

The focus is on the consultee and his or her problem, due to the consultee's lack of knowledge, skill, or confidence. The consultant provides guidance to improve knowledge and skills, serving as an educator, trainer, and expert.

Program-Centered Consultation

The focus is on the system or organization and the delivery of services. The consultant gathers and analyzes data and assesses the readiness for change, prior to recommending solutions. The consultant makes recommendations for the implementation of specific strategies for program change(s). In this role, the consultant acts as a change agent.

Administration-Centered Consultation

The focus in this type of consultation is on problem relationships within the organization, particularly among managers/administrators and staff, and/or on problems of programming. The consultee may lack skills in leadership, communication, or the ability to build a cohesive work team. The consultant assists the administrator with leadership skills, helping the consultee to establish a vision and convey it to his or her work group. The consultant also encourages the administrator to examine the allocation and budgeting of resources (both human and material resources) to benefit the program. In this role, the consultant acts as the expert (Caplan, 1970; Caplan & Caplan, 1993; Loranger, 1992; Odom, 1994, cited in Herrick, 2008). As mentioned earlier in this chapter, consultants may be involved in either external consultation or internal consultation. External consultants come from outside of the organization. Internal consultants come from

TABLE 9-9 Advantages and Disadvantages Associated with External and Internal Consultants

Advantages

External Consultation	Internal Consultation
• Can be more objective.	• Is familiar with the organization and its structure and climate.
• Makes suggestions for a new approach and provides a new perspective. • Rapport must be established so that trust can develop.	• Knows the norms, values, and culture. Is aware of points of tension and conflict. • Trust is already established.
• Regarded as the expert → more power.	• May not be regarded as the "expert" → less power. May be perceived as part of the problem rather than the solution.

Disadvantages

External Consultation	Internal Consultation
• Doesn't know the culture. • May not fully understand the problem(s). May not fully understand the needs and the concerns of the agency personnel.	• May have additional duties without adequate compensation.
• May not understand the organizational dynamics including the interpersonal conflicts.	• May have role conflicts.
• Is costly.	• Is cost-effective.
• May be inaccessible for follow-up.	• May be biased (not immune to organizational influences). May have a preconceived opinion, although the consultant is available for follow-up.

within the organization, but usually from a different unit. The skills needed by both types of consultants are the same, but the advantages and disadvantages of these types of consultation services differ (Table 9-9).

INTERVENTIONS SUGGESTED BY CONSULTANTS

Numerous interventions may be in the toolbox of many consultants. Table 9-10 lists some of the most common options.

TABLE 9-10 Interventions Performed by Consultants

- **Receiving:** The consultant establishes rapport and gathers data.
- **Informing:** The consultant educates the consultee(s) as the expert.
- **Energizing:** The consultant handles the resistance to change while motivating the consultee to embrace change.
- **Facilitating:** The consultant provides a smooth pathway for transitions by clarifying issues, providing information about the consequences of change, examining options, and identifying strategies to achieve goals.
- **Reflecting:** The consultant evaluates the outcomes.

Specific characteristics or labels associated with the consultant's focus for these interventions may be found in the literature. According to Blake and Mouton (1989), these labels characterize the activities of the consultant.

Acceptant Consultation

In acceptant consultation, the consultant provides clients with a sense of personal security so that when working with the consultant, the consultee feels free to express thoughts without fear of adverse judgments or rejections. He or she promotes catharsis. The consultant is an advocate, supporting the client in making his or her own decisions. He or she is an active listener, helping the client to clarify the situation. The consultant uses a nondirective style.

Catalytic Consultation

In catalytic consultation, the consultant assists clients in collecting data and information to reinterpret their perceptions as to how things are. Giving specific suggestions is avoided. The consultant increases the rate at which a process of change is occurring, while setting specific goals to assist those within the status quo to do what they are already doing, albeit better. He or she acts as a facilitator and resource person, helping the consultee to redefine the problem. The consultant is a motivator and leader, conveying a vision of the future. However, the client or consultee chooses his or her own path.

Confrontational Consultation

A confrontational consultation challenges clients to examine how the current foundations of thinking may be distorting their perceptions. The consultant assists the client to explore the consequences of value-related behaviors as a first step toward implementing change. The consultant creates awareness of a discrepancy between generally accepted values and self-defeating assumptions. He or she challenges the client's thinking and provides counter-arguments. In this way, the consultant acts as a change agent.

Prescriptive Consultation

In a prescriptive consultation, the consultant analyzes the situation and tells the client what to do to rectify the situation. The client relies on the expert skills of the consultant to identify a problem, diagnose it, and recommend a solution (medical model). The consultant uses an authoritative and directive style. The consultant is the expert.

OVERCOMING RESISTANCE

Resistance is a common response to change (Sullivan & Decker, 2009). Such behavior represents an attempt to cope with change or to avoid change. Resistance may be difficult for the consultant to deal with, yet should be an expected event. Table 9-11 lists some interventions that the consultant may use to deal with the expected reactions to change.

EXAMINING ORGANIZATIONAL DYNAMICS

Frames of Reference

During the initial assessment, multiple frames of reference may be used to examine the factors that make up an organization and its personnel. Understanding the organizational structure and dynamics is essential to identify the problem areas that may need to be addressed. The following outline can serve as a guide for the consultant (Norwood, 2008):

TABLE 9-11 Ways to Overcome Resistance

- Treat the persons involved with respect as individuals.
- Involve those affected by the change in the planning process.
- Provide accurate and complete information.
- Give time for people to air objections.
- Always take group habits and norms into account.
- Make only essential changes. Be open to potential revisions.
- Learn to use problem-solving techniques effectively.
- Gain support of top officials and the important stakeholders before initiating the change.
- Make provisions for feedback.
- Provide emotional support.

1. Structural Frame

    a. Roots, rules, policies

    b. The managerial hierarchy and the division of labor

    c. The structure, environment, and technology (Is the structure "in sync" with its internal and external environments?)

    d. The organizational chart

2. Human Resources Frame

    a. Relationships (interdependence)

    b. Cohesion and sense of belonging

    c. Human resources and social psychology

    d. Interpersonal communication channels (What are they, and how open or closed are the channels?)

    e. The degree of autonomy experienced by the staff

    f. Decision making (Who makes the decisions, and who monitors and supervises how the decisions are carried out?)

    g. The goodness of fit between the needs of the organization and the needs of its personnel (How could organizational processes or structure be changed to better meet the needs of the members of the organization?)

3. Political Frame

    a. Political relationships; power, conflict, concentration of power (where it resides, and with whom)

    b. Delegated power; coalitions; resources

    c. Handling of problems related to scarce resources (Conflict, compromise, negotiation?)

4. Symbolic Frame

    a. The culture, organizational rituals, and behaviors of management and staff; relationships among personnel.

    b. The spiritual and expressive side of the organization (Do the personnel identify with the organization?)

    c. Values reflected in the organization's identity?

Description and Assessment

1. *Organization*: name, type, primary purpose, services or products; organizational structure (organizational chart).
2. *Clients*: characteristics.
3. *Environment:* the environmental forces influencing the organization and the nature of the impact (federal laws, funding sources and contingencies, political events and their influence on the organization).

4. *Location:* characteristics of the immediate neighborhood and its influence on the organization. What is the access to resources?
5. *Physical plant:* The salient characteristics and their impact on productivity and morale.
   - *Services technology:* the major features of the service delivery processes.
   - *Administrative structure:* leadership styles, communication patterns, decision making; leader–follower relationships (the power structure).
   - *(CAO):* Background—professional training and experience; dominant values and concerns; support networks; leadership skills and styles; the leader's vision; the leader's ability to communicate with staff.
   - *Staff:* Background: professional training and experience; dominant values and norms. Who belongs to which subgroups and support groups? What are the rewards and incentives for "good" work? How cohesive are the interpersonal relationships among the staff and with administrators? How well do people work together? Which communication skills are evident in the organization and within the workgroups or teams? What is the work ethic?
   - *Growth opportunities:* What are the opportunities for growth and change for both the organization and personnel? What are the strengths, weaknesses, opportunities, or threats (SWOT)? How can the agency or organization best use a consultant?

Source: Gallessich, 1982.

Process Observations

Table 9-12 summarizes the facets of the organization and its processes that may be observed by the consultant. Once rapport has been established, the consultant should use a more directive style of leadership, asking direct questions to discern relevant information from the client (Table 9-13). This next stage of the consultation process is known as the problem identification and data analysis phase.

CHOOSING A CAREER AS A CONSULTANT

Many nurse case managers see consultation as an opportunity to influence the delivery of health care and to determine when and how work will be accomplished to meet the needs of a target population, a healthcare program, or an

TABLE 9-12 Process Observations

- Interpersonal relationships
- Administrative procedures
- The structure and organizations of the agency, the responsibilities of the employees, the authority, the planning procedures
- Communication patterns
- Methods for decision making, including those who are involved and those who must implement the decisions
- The administrator's leadership style
- The organizational values and norms
- The rewards and incentives to perform well and produce a quality product
- Openness and flexibility of administrators and staff versus resistance to change
- The organizational climate (the degree of cooperation versus conflict)
- The life cycle of the organization (i.e., the stage of growth and development)
- The responses to crises
- The use of resources
- Methods for conflict management

TABLE 9-13 Probing Interview Questions to Ask Clients

- What is the major problem that this organization faces?

- Which problems do you face that are shared by the rest of the healthcare agencies or professionals in similar organizations or professions?

- Which problems confront these organizations that are unique to this geographical area?

- In what ways has inadequate planning affected the success of this organization?

- Has this organization been hurt or made less profitable by government laws or regulations?

- How does this organization rank in terms of sales, quality of care, or whatever the focus is for this agency? Identify benchmarks and compare the organization to its peers on that basis.

- What has been the rate of staff turnover? Is the trend up or down? If turnover is a problem, which strategies have been implemented to solve this problem?

- What did your assessments of employee satisfaction and productivity suggest for future personnel policies?

- What do you see as the organization's strengths? What do you see as its weaknesses?

Table 9-14 The Benefits of Choosing Consulting as a Career Path

- The opportunity to work with a variety of clients in different healthcare settings
- The opportunity to be independent and set one's own priorities and work schedule
- The opportunity to work on proactive projects rather than reactive problem solving
- The ability to work creatively without the constraints of institutional politics
- The opportunity to influence the directions and convey a vision for a program, another professional, or a healthcare organization
- The diversity of multiple clients in different settings
- The opportunity to travel and meet leaders of healthcare organizations.
- The chance to make real and tangible differences in healthcare delivery
- The opportunities to observe, address, and learn from a wide range of challenging situations
- A sense of accomplishment when the client actually implements the recommendations and is successful in accomplishing its goals

Source: Stichler, 2002.

organization. Like any role in nursing or nursing case management, there are both benefits and challenges in the consultant role. Table 9-14 identifies the benefits that the consultant may experience.

Some of the challenges or risks involved in establishing a consultation practice derive from the fact that there is no support system for independent consultants. Consequently, consultants must establish their own network of supportive relationships, but ultimately they are on their own. There is no steady paycheck with this type of practice—and the consultant must pay the office personnel and bill collectors first. It may take a significant amount of time to reach the break-even point when establishing a consulting business (or any independent practice, for that matter). Initially, another source of income other than a paycheck is necessary to stay afloat until the break-even point is reached.

Consultants who have their own practices will usually work longer and harder than they did while working for an institution—but it is satisfying to be your own boss. All too often, however, there is a tendency to focus on the business or enterprise to the exclusion of all other interests. The consultant must remember to keep a balance between the consulting practice and other interests, most importantly paying attention to his or her family, who serve as the consultant's main support system.

■ SUMMARY

Case managers are consultants to patients and their families, as well as to other professionals on the interdisciplinary team, and to program developers. They

TABLE 9-15 Effective Consultation: A Formula

The effective consultant is:
Oriented toward personal and professional growth
+
Knowledgeable about the consultation process
+
Has excellent human relations skills (especially listening and communication skills)
+
Has clinical or administrative expertise
=
Effective consulting skills

Source: Herrick, Jenkins, & Odom, 1995.

may also consult with other healthcare teams, schools of nursing, departments other than their assigned department in an acute care setting, staff from other agencies, and even insurance companies.

Case managers serve as a resource for information such as healthcare benefits, the location of available resources, the usual course of an illness, the best way to develop a care map or pathway, or any other healthcare issues that may be of concern to patients, their families, or other professionals. Because consultants frequently work in a variety of settings with diverse groups across the healthcare continuum, they must have a broad base of nursing knowledge, and they need access to available resources and information about community resources that may be useful to both the consultant and the consultee. Table 9-15 summarizes the consultation process in an easy-to-remember formula.

Frequently nurse case managers act as internal consultants. The internal case manager can be a rich source of information for patients and staff. According to Tahan (2005), the nurse case manager as an internal consultant in an inpatient setting should be well versed in institutional policies and procedures, operations, and systems and the most recent standards of care, so that the nurse case manager can provide the interdisciplinary team with the most up-to-date information (Tahan, 2005). As a consultant to the healthcare team, the case manager can identify those practices that best support efficient, cost-effective, high-quality care. The external consultant can do the same, but may offer a somewhat fresher perspective and perhaps greater objectivity.

More and more case managers are setting up their own practices to serve the healthcare community. For example, many legal nurse consultants provide consultation services to law firms, insurance companies, healthcare facilities, government agencies, and private corporations. If a nurse case manager has the entrepreneurial spirit, there are numerous opportunities in the healthcare community to establish a consulting practice (Milazzo, 2008).

■ CASE STUDIES

Because of your clinical expertise, you have been asked to consider a consulting job to assist healthcare organizations in achieving Magnet status. Answer the questions in the following self-assessment tool to assist you in making your decision.

1. Do I enjoy working in situations where I need to use my persuasive and influencing skills without vested authority?
2. Am I comfortable interacting with chief executives, boards of directors, legislators, community leaders, and others in powerful roles?
3. Do I have good writing and presenting skills? Do I like putting papers and presentations together?
4. Am I comfortable with conflict negotiation situations, including dealing with people who are emotional, posturing, or protecting their staff?
5. Do I like the challenge of thinking critically, strategically, and analytically?
6. Do I enjoy working with different types of people in different situations?
7. Am I a self-directed, self-managed, self-confident, risk-taker?
8. Do I have a body of knowledge, a set of skills, a vision and the ability to convey that vision, and the ability to market and sell myself?
9. Am I comfortable with ambiguity, uncertainty, and not being in control of situations?

Based on your results, would you undertake this new career opportunity? Why or why not?

■ DISCUSSION QUESTIONS

1. What is the current local market for the kind of consultant I would like to be? Who are my competitors?
2. Why is it important for a consultant to understand group and organizational dynamics?

■ CLASSROOM EXERCISES

Select a local restaurant in which to enact this observational experience. Plan to participate in this exercise with another person. After placing your order, unobtrusively observe the events that unfold among employees and customers, including interactions, conversations, organizational climate, efficiency in serving the public, productivity, and anything else that may seem pertinent. Describe your observations as clearly as possible so that your description would help a second party picture the workings of the system. Jot down your findings on a piece of paper and review them at a later date. To check for the influence of subjectivity, after you have made notes, share your findings with your peer and compare your observations. What were the similarities and differences?

1. Describe the organization.
2. Describe the clientele.
3. Describe the salient features of the restaurant's working, including how they affected the employees and customers.
4. Describe the type of food served, efficiency of the service, and quality of the food.
5. Describe the relationship between the employees and management and the employees and the customers.
6. Describe the employee motivation level, rapport with customers, and communications skills.

After the observational experience, briefly answer the following questions.

1. Compare the two observations between you and your peer, identifying similarities, differences, and anything you missed (and why you might have missed this observation).
2. Describe which skills you would need to enhance to become an effective consultant.
3. If you were actually a consultant, describe how you would plan to consult with the manager and staff at this restaurant. What would be your initial focus?
4. List the recommendations to improve the facility that you might give to the manager and staff.

▪ RECOMMENDED READING

Blake, R., & Mouton, J. S. (1989). *Consultation* (2nd ed.). Menlo Park, CA: Addison-Wesley.

Caplan, G. (1970). *The theory and practice of mental health consultation*. New York: Basic Books.

Caplan, G., & Caplan, R. (1993). *Mental health consultation and collaboration*. San Francisco: Jossey-Bass.

Gallessich, J. (1982). *The profession/practice of consultation*. San Francisco: Jossey-Bass.

Lange, F. C. (1987). *The nurse as an individual, group or community consultant*. Norwalk, CT: Appleton Century Crofts.

Lippitt, G., & Lippitt, R. (1978). *The consulting process in action*. San Diego, CA: University Associates.

Lippitt, G., & Lippitt, R. (1986). *The consulting process in action* (2nd ed.). San Diego, CA: University Associates.

Loranger, N. (1992). The clinical nurse specialist as a consultant for play on the pediatric bone marrow transplant unit. *Clinical Nurse Specialist, 6*(4), 176–178.

Norwood, S. (1998). *Nurses as consultants: Essential concepts and processes.* Menlo Park, CA: Addison-Wesley.

Puetz, B. E., & Shinn, L. J. (1997). *The nurse consultant's handbook.* New York: Springer.

■ REFERENCES

Association of Perioperative Nurses (AORN). (2009). *Perioperative nursing consultation: A member benefit.* Retrieved from http://www.aorn. org?PracticeResources/NurseConsultation

Blake, R., & Mouton, J. S. (1989). *Consultation* (2nd ed.). Menlo Park, CA: Addison-Wesley.

Caplan, G. (1970). *The theory and practice of mental health consultation.* New York: Basic Books.

Caplan, G., & Caplan, R. (1993). *Mental health consultation and collaboration.* San Francisco: Jossey-Bass.

Curran, C. (2008). Theoretical foundations for community health. In M. J. Clarke (Ed.), *Community health nursing: Advocacy for population health* (5th ed., pp. 61–81). Upper Saddle River, NJ: Pearson/Prentice Hall.

Gallessich, J. (1982). *The profession/practice of consultation.* San Francisco: Jossey-Bass.

Haag, A. B., & Kalina, C. (2007, March). Professional practice: What role does the case manager play in a litigated case? *AAOHN Journal, 55*(3), 93–95.

Herrick, C. A. (2008). *Nurse case managers in private practice* [unpublished learning module for students taking a Case Management course]. Greensboro, NC: University of North Carolina at Greensboro.

Herrick, C. A., Jenkins, T., & Odom, S. E. (1995). *Consultation in nursing practice* [unpublished manuscript]. Mobile, AL: University of South Alabama.

Lange, F. C. (1987). *The nurse as an individual, group or community consultant.* Norwalk, CT: Appleton Century Crofts.

Lippitt, G., & Lippitt, R. (1978). *The consulting process in action.* San Diego, CA: University Associates.

Lippitt, G., & Lippitt, R. (1986). *The consulting process in action* (2nd ed.). San Diego, CA: University Associates.

Loranger, N. (1992). The clinical nurse specialist as a consultant for play on the pediatric bone marrow transplant unit. *Clinical Nurse Specialist, 6*(4), 176–178.

Michigan Civil Service Commission. (2009). *Job specifications: Nurse consultant.* Retrieved from www.michigan.gov/documents/NurseConsultant_12960_7.pdf

Milazzo, V. (1999–2009). *The Vickie Millazzo Institute, a division of Medical–Legal Institute Inc.* Retrieved from http://www.legaln nurse.com

Milazzo, V. (2008, July 20). *Demand for legal nurse consultants is at an all time high.* Retrieved from http://www.americanchronicle.com/articles/view/11688

Mullahy, C. M. (2004). *The case manager's handbook* (3rd ed.). Sudbury, MA: Jones and Bartlett, pp. 259–373.

Norwood, S. (1998). *Nurses as consultants: Essential concepts and processes.* Menlo Park, CA: Addison-Wesley.

Odom, S. E. (1994). *Consultation* [notes from a lecture and paper submitted for partial fulfillment of a doctorate in nursing science]. Birmingham, AL: University of Alabama at Birmingham.

Pennsylvania Department of Health, Diabetes Nurse Consultants. (2009). *Diabetes prevention and control program.* Retrieved from http://www.portal.state.pa.us/portal/server.pt/community/diabetes/14160

Puetz, B. E., & Shinn, L. J. (1997). *The nurse consultant's handbook.* New York: Springer.

Smith, D. L. (2008). Advocacy in action: Case management. In M. J. Clark (Ed.), *Community health nursing* (5th ed., pp. 276–295). Upper Saddle River, NJ: Pearson/Prentice Hall.

Stichler, J. F. (2002). The nurse as consultant. *Nursing Administration Quarterly, 26*(2), 52–68.

Sullivan, E. J., & Decker, P. J. (Eds.). (2009). Initiating and implementing change. In *Effective leadership and management in nursing* (7th ed., pp. 66–77). Upper Saddle River, NJ: Pearson/Prentice Hall.

Tahan, H. (2005). The role of the nurse case manager. In E. L. Cohen & T. G. Cesta (Eds.), *Nursing case management: From essentials to advanced practice applications* (4th ed., pp. 288–289). St. Louis, MO: Elsevier/Mosby.

Telephone-Triage Consulting, Inc. (2009). *Consultation.* Retrieved from http://www.telephone-triage.com/index.php?option=com_content&task=view&id=26

The new Webster's thesaurus: The vest pocket edition. (1991). Hartford, CT: Lewtan Line, p. 29.

Wisconsin Department of Health Services, Division of Public Health. (2009, January). *Public health nurse consultant.* Retrieved from http://dhs.wisconsin.gov/phnc

New Trends in the Evolution of Case Management: Faith Community Nursing

Jacqueline DeBrew
Leila Moore
Sandra Blaha
Charlotte A. Herrick

10

■ OUTLINE

■ OBJECTIVES

1. Describe the vision of Granger Westberg, which contributed to the development of faith community nursing (parish nursing), and the history of nurses functioning in churches.

2. Discuss the philosophy of faith community nursing.

3. Address the importance of caring and reflective practice as conceptual frameworks to guide faith community nurses when working with church congregations.

4. Identify the members of the faith community nurse's team who are important to the nurse's "collaborative practice."

5. Define the roles, functions, and skills of the faith community nurse.

6. Compare the roles, functions, and skills of the faith community nurse with the community nurse case manager.

7. Address the importance of standards of practice.

8. Define quality and its relationship to the effectiveness of faith community nursing programs.

9. Discuss why this model of case management is spreading across churches and communities.

INTRODUCTION: HISTORICAL PERSPECTIVES

A Pastor's Vision of Providing Holistic Care to Hospital Patients

In the 20th century, Granger Westberg envisioned a collaborative partnership between the hospitalized patient, the chaplain, the physician, and the nurse to provide holistic care. In 1944, he became one of the first hospital chaplains in the United States. Westberg also developed a course for nurses at Augustana College in Illinois called Religion and Health; teaching that course led him to write his first book, *The Nurse, Pastor and Patient*, which was published in 1955. Decades later, he published *A Personal Historical Perspective of Whole Person Health and the Congregation*, originally written in 1990 and rewritten in 1999 (Solari-Twadell & McDermott, 2006).

In 1955, Westberg developed Clinical Pastoral Education (CPE), which focused on disease prevention and the whole person's health. The CPE program was developed to educate ministers and priests to become hospital chaplains, with the ultimate goal being for ministers and priests to provide pastoral care to hospital patients and to integrate health care into their church ministries. During a CPE course, pastors are taught counseling skills and learn about health-related topics. They examine ethical issues and explore philosophical and theological questions.

As part of the CPE movement, a health cabinet was formed within a congregation in Lombard, Illinois, in 1979 to explore the development of health ministries and to determine the structure of a health ministry within a congregation (Patterson, 2003). In 1985, Lutheran General Hospital created the Parish Nurse Resource Center, later to become the International Parish Nurse Resource Center, under the direction of Ann Solari-Twadell. This center originated in Park Ridge, Illinois, but was transferred to the Deaconess Parish Nurse Ministries in St. Louis, Missouri, in 2002. "This center provides support and education for parish nurses in America and around the world" (Leila Moore, Personal communication, May 28, 2007; Patterson, 2003).

Westberg firmly believed that people need "wellness care," which focuses on prevention, rather than strictly "illness care," which is historically what the healthcare system has provided. In the early 1980s, Westberg recognized that managed care would have a significant impact on the U.S. healthcare system. He believed that the country would not have enough healthcare dollars to support the model of acute, episodic care in the 21st century with the aging of the baby boomers. Instead, Westberg felt, congregations could provide an optimal environment to promote wholeness. To this end, he established health centers in churches, staffing the centers with doctors and nurses. Unfortunately, the costs of funding these clinics proved prohibitively expensive for churches.

During this time, Westberg found that the nurses were instrumental in caring for and teaching congregations about healthy lifestyles and noted that they had a unique ability to interpret the meaning of medical jargon for pastors and parishioners. Their community health background provided a framework for working with other agencies in the community so they could become brokers or referral agents. From there, the idea of working with church congregations grew to its current case management model. Westberg developed the idea of parish nursing, later renamed congregational nursing and now called faith community nursing (FCN). In addition, he championed the idea of whole-person wellness.

A Pilot Project: Faith Community Nursing

In the 1980s, Westberg approached the administrators of Lutheran General Hospital (LGH) in Park Ridge, Illinois, about developing a pilot study that would place nurses on the staff of congregations. By 1985, six churches were participating in the original pilot project. Each church helped to pay for a part-time nurse. During the first year, the church paid 25% of the nurse's salary and LGH paid 75%. In the second year, the church increased its contribution to 50% of the nurse's salary, with this share increasing again to 75% in the third year. In the fourth year, each church was responsible for paying the entire salary for the parish nurse. Although there were no formal educational courses or workshops for nurses at that time (there are continuing education opportunities now), the nurses from the six churches in the pilot project met for 3 hours each week to share their experiences.

Westberg believed that churches are the one organization in the United States that is best suited to becoming the leader in preventive medicine. The history of parish nursing is closely tied to an understanding that churches are dedicated to keeping people healthy in mind, body, and spirit (Solari-Twadell & McDermott, 2006). "FCNs now serve in hundreds of churches across the country and in many foreign countries" (Leila Moore, Personal communication, May 28, 2007). Their focus is on wellness, health promotion, disease prevention, and referrals for early intervention. Salvation is defined as being whole in mind, body, and spirit (Brown & Magilvy, 2001; Solari-Twadell & McDermott, 2006). The underlying assumption is that a faulty belief system affects the body's functioning and well-being, and that people must integrate the domains of the body, mind, and spirit to achieve whole health.

Catholic Churches: A Historical Perspective

The ministry of FCN has its roots in the Roman Catholic traditions of the past, whereby religious communities of women served the poor. These women provided nursing care and spiritual consolation. This historical precedent of home care established by churches to provide nursing care to the poor guides FCN programs today.

The Daughters of Charity of St. Vincent de Paul was established in the 1600s in France. This society of wealthy women was sponsored by the Roman Catholic Church, and its members visited the sick in their homes and provided nursing care and spiritual comfort. To assist in establishing similar charities in Paris, St. Vincent de Paul recruited country girls with good reputations to work with the sick out of Parisian churches (Solari-Twadell & Egenes, 2006). Thus the Daughters of Charity was developed, and served as the forerunner of FCN. In 1642, the first four Daughters of Charity took their vows to devote their lives to provide nursing care to the sick poor.

Rationale for Placing Nurses in Churches

Proponents of FCN cite several reasons for placing nurses in churches:

- Churches are found everywhere where people live; as a consequence, churches are an accessible healthcare resource.
- Churches have a long history of serving communities through social and educational programs.
- Churches symbolize the need to take seriously the problems of the human spirit that can cause an illness.
- Churches can provide a reservoir of people who are willing to volunteer their services.
- Churches have members who have a growing appreciation for the opportunity to model the need for cooperation between scientific medicine and religion.

More and more of today's nurses have the desire to integrate human caring with medical care—that is, to combine "high touch" with "high tech." FCN is a form of case management, in that many of the roles, functions, and necessary skills are similar between FCN and nursing case management (NCM). These commonalities include prevention and health education, teaching self-care, coordination of healthcare delivery systems and access to care via the broker role, counseling, providing emotional and social support, advocacy, and collaborative practice with other professional disciplines. The focus of both FCN and NCM is broader than the individual client: It includes the family and the community as well. FCN saves healthcare dollars by identifying health problems early and assisting patients to access the right resources at the right time. NCM is also concerned with keeping costs down as much as possible, while ensuring that patients receive quality health care. FCN serves a special population—namely, members of a congregation belonging to a church denomination. Thus nurses working under the aegis of FCN programs have the opportunity to integrate the humanities and the sciences to improve the quality of these parishioners' lives.

THE PHILOSOPHY OF FAITH COMMUNITY NURSING

FCN is an emerging area of specialized nursing practice, which is continually evolving (as noted by the frequent name changes). Its key characteristics are summarized in Table 10-1.

TABLE 10-1 The Characteristics of Faith Community Nursing

- The inclusion of the spiritual dimension is central to FCN practice; FCN encompasses the physical, psychological, social, and spiritual domains. The American Nurses Association (ANA) recognizes FCN as a specialty practice of nursing based on the role expectation of the intentional care of the spirit, while providing nursing care.
- FCN balances knowledge of nursing science with knowledge of theology and the humanities. It balances service with worship. Nursing care functions are balanced with providing pastoral care.
- The historical roots of FCN lie in the traditions of monks, nuns, traditional healers, and the nursing profession, particularly community health nursing (e.g., the Henry Street Settlement in New York City, Hull House in Chicago, and the New York Visiting Nurse Association).
- The target population consists of the parishioners in a faith community. The nurse works in collaboration with the pastoral care staff and the members of the congregation. FCN transforms the faith community into a healthy community through partnerships with other community health professionals, using various healthcare resources. The nurse ministers to the congregation regarding their healthcare concerns.
- FCN services are designed to build on and strengthen the capacities of individuals, families, and congregations to understand and care for one another in the light of their relationship to God, and to encourage them to care for themselves and the broader society. FCN respects people's beliefs and treats each individual with dignity. It educates the congregation about healthcare issues, which empowers them to become active partners in the management of their personal health care.
- FCN acknowledges that health is a dynamic process that embodies the spiritual, psychological, physical, and social dimensions of an individual. Spiritual health is central to an individual's well-being and influences a person's quality of life. A sense of well-being and illness can occur simultaneously. However, healing may exist in the absence of a cure.

Source: Solari-Twadell & McDermott, 1999.

CONCEPTUAL FRAMEWORKS FOR FAITH COMMUNITY NURSING

The Concept of Caring

Caring is the foundation of both general nursing practice and FCN practice. In both types of practice, a circle of care is developed that centers on the nurse respecting the patient's religious beliefs and practices, listening to the patient, and providing emotional support. During the initial phase of the nursing process, spiritual needs are assessed, by picking up on religious cues (e.g., references to "the man upstairs") and emotional cues (Why me?). An assessment tool to identify the patient's spiritual needs has been developed and is available from the Health Ministries of the Lutheran Church of the Missouri Synod (Schnoor, 1999).

In FCN, the nurse holds the spiritual dimension as central to nursing care. He or she balances theology with the science of nursing. The target population is a religious congregation and its ministry. FCN's services are strength based, empowering individuals for self-care. The nurse partners with individuals, families, other healthcare professionals, and ministers to provide a healing environment for church members. He or she understands that health is a dynamic process that embodies all of the personal domains of mind, body, and spirit. In addition, the nurse invites volunteers from the congregation to minister to others in the congregation. He or she trains the volunteers and coordinates their activities. The nurse facilitates support groups and counsels individuals to meet their healthcare needs (Solari-Twadell & McDermott, 2006). The emphasis is on holistic health.

Reflective Practice

A key focus for the faith community nurse is reflective practice (Table 10-2). Table 10-3 outlines some of the activities that may be used to promote the introspection needed to ensure truly reflective practice. Other spiritual self-care practices might include rest, exercise, yoga, tai chi, or any activity that nourishes the mind, body, and spirit. Nurses in FCN programs must be aware that self-care must come first, so that they can effectively nurture members of their congregations.

COLLABORATIVE PRACTICE: BUILDING PARTNERSHIPS

Partnerships Between Faith Community Nurses and Pastors, Physicians, Other Nurses, and Congregations

Collaborative practice is an integral function of FCN, so much so that it is written into the standards of practice (discussed later in this chapter).

TABLE 10-2 Reflective Practice: Strategies for the Faith Community Nurse

Self-Care: FCN Nurturing the Self

- *Self-reflection through the arts:* Painting, music, and dance are all avenues to express oneself so as to nurture the soul and to experience self-awareness.
- *Self-reflection through theology:* Spirituality requires deep introspection. Solitude, prayer, and meditation are strategies that the faith community nurse may use to experience introspection.
- *The waterwheel model of spiritual leadership for parish nurses:* This model is a comprehensive framework for the practice of the faith community nurse. The nurse must have the capacity to be self-aware. Self-awareness encourages the faith community nurse as a spiritual leader to be open to new ideas, which may alter his or her core beliefs and values. Spiritual leaders should be reflective learners, continuously seeking new perspectives. Lifelong learning challenges the nurse to continue to learn new ideas and new ways of thinking. The faith community nurse values integrity, openness, wholeness, trust, honesty, hope, and prayer, to name a few of the values mentioned by Solari-Twadell and McDermott (2006).

TABLE 10-3 Activities for Reflection

- **Small Groups:** sharing ideas and beliefs. Small groups provide intellectual stimulation to expand one's knowledge and a milieu in which to offer mutual encouragement and support. Feedback from group members is a way of staying centered, becoming more self-aware. The group facilitator may be the faith community nurse or someone else who is selected by the group. The main function of the faith community nurse is to establish support groups.
- **Journal Writing, Speaking, or Writing about a Personal Experience:** examining a distressing event, a memory, a conversation, or a life event, through journal writing. Writing about daily events fosters self-awareness. The journal may include daily events or an outstanding event, as well as the writer's responses. Thoughts and feelings should be freely expressed. Quotes, dreams, readings, interpersonal relationships, idea maps, meaningful clippings, and pictures may be included.
- **Reading:** Something inspirational may provide insight and enhance understanding, such as reading a Bible passage, a theological text, or a story about a devout person.
- **Imaging While Meditating and Reflecting on an Experience:** Questions that introspection may answer include "What does the image indicate?", "What is the meaning of the experience?", and "What can be learned from it?"
- **Prayer:** to replenish the faith community nurse's energy and guide his or her activities. Taking time to reflect on the activities of the day, the needs of the congregation, and the nurse's own needs through prayer may help the FCN to understand the past and the present and to anticipate and plan for the future.
- **Exploring the Matter:** comparing the experience alongside the wisdom of others, including ethicists, philosophers, religious leaders, and religious authors.
- **Identifying the Themes:** comparing the themes with religious thought.

Collaborative practice means working together and, according to Blanchfield and McLaughlin (2006), encompasses three essential elements:

- *Communication.* Communication may take the form of meetings, phoning, worshiping, emailing, attending retreats, letter writing, and attending congregational and community gatherings.
- *Connections.* Faith community nurses need to be actively involved in developing and maintaining connections across the community over time. Connections require networking skills.
- *Cooperative Goal Setting.* Collaborative team members should share their thoughts and talents to work toward common goals. When connecting with organizations outside of the faith community, the missions of those organizations must be respected. There should be ongoing relationships between the faith community nurse and healthcare providers in healthcare and community organizations and with nurses in other churches, mosques, or synagogues. When planning collaborative interventions, common goals must be developed conjointly. (See Chapter 6 on building collaborative relationships with patients.)

Networking

Faith community nurses must reach out to other organizations to provide a comprehensive healthcare ministry. In doing so, they network with others to make available health initiatives that foster preventive care, self-care, and wellness. These nurses must build a network of support connecting three institutional cultures—the nursing profession, the faith community, and the healthcare community. When acting as a networker, the faith community nurse builds bridges to foster understanding and to develop resources that are needed to create a "whole-person" FCN program.

Networking with federal state and local programs is also necessary. For example, the National Institutes of Health, Centers for Disease Control and Prevention, Health Resources and Services Administration, Substance Abuse and Mental Health Services Administration, Children's Defense Fund, and Administration on Aging are all institutions that can provide resources for FCN programs. The local health department, the department of social services, and other local organizations such as the Women, Infants and Children (WIC), as well as universities and schools of nursing, may also be valuable resources for programming.

Collegial Partnerships

The faith community nurse can maintain positive working relationships with his or her peers by attending meetings, working with members of the health

TABLE 10-4 The Qualities That Pastors Expect of a Faith Community Nurse

The FCN is:
- A self-starter
- A communicator who is able to network among different church groups as well as meetings of other organizations outside of the church
- Able to attend church functions and services
- Available as needed
- A good listener
- A leader and program organizer

and nursing cabinets, actively participating with sponsoring agencies, and participating in the local faith community network and other healthcare networks. In addition, he or she should develop collegial partnerships with the parishioners and members of a family and community.

Collaborating with the Pastor

The pastor should be a primary consideration on the faith community nurse's agenda. Each partner must respect the competence of the other. The pastor must articulate the role of the faith community nurse to the congregation, and both the pastor and the nurse must support each other and plan programs together. Along the way, they should provide ongoing feedback to each other. Pastors typically hope that the faith community nurse will exhibit the qualities listed in Table 10-4.

Collaborating with God

Caring for the spiritual needs of members of the church is a challenge. Faith community nurses can minister to the spiritual needs of individuals through prayer as well as being able to offer whole-person nursing and health care.

Collaborating with the Congregation

The faith community nurse should invite parishioners who have specific skills and competencies to serve in the whole-health nursing ministry as volunteers. The nurse can empower people to be alert and respond to the needs of the sick, aged, or infirm, and can coordinate and guide their activities in ministering to those individuals.

Collaborating with Physicians

Physicians may support the faith community nurse by participating on the health cabinet, as either members of the church or consultants. In addition, a doctor (MD or DO) may consult with the faith community nurse about chronic disease management, disease prevention, ethical issues having to do with end-of-life care, suicide prevention, substance abuse, care of the frail elderly, well-child health, and safety. The physician can provide the faith community nurse with information about available resources to meet the mental health and general healthcare needs of the congregation. In addition, the doctor may formally partner with the nurse to provide whole-person health care.

Collaborating with Other Ministries, Faith Community Nurses, and Directors of Nurse Ministries

Working together with other churches will help the parties involved avoid duplicating programs. If one church provides a food program, participation by other churches will make the program stronger so that it may serve the needs of the entire community, while another church may offer a program of supportive volunteers for new immigrant families. When churches band together, costs are contained and efforts are not duplicated.

Nurses who work with faith communities from different congregations should also work together to make their resources available to as many people as possible, deciding on a common goal and then working toward that goal. To date, collaboration among faith community nurses has resulted in some of the initiatives listed in Table 10-5.

Collaborating with Individuals and Families

The faith community nurse does not provide direct nursing care for an individual patient, but rather cares for the congregation as a whole in terms of their health and wellness. If the nurse counsels individuals, maintaining confidentiality is essential.

The questions listed in Table 10-6 should be addressed when establishing a one-on-one counseling relationship. Laying these questions on the table, so to speak, will assist the faith community nurse and the individual parishioner to establish a collaborative counseling relationship, so that a partnership can be formed and trust established.

Collaborating with Schools of Nursing

Schools of nursing and FCN ministries both have a great deal to gain by working collaboratively. The FCN program can provide students with learning opportunities in community health nursing with a focus on fostering health, wellness, and primary prevention. Schools of nursing, in turn, can provide

TABLE 10-5 Faith Community Nursing Initiatives

- Developed shared retreats and prayer services
- Mentored new faith community nurses
- Created interdenominational walking programs
- Participated in research to study and document the outcomes of FCN programs
- Cosponsored programs on topics such as ethics, cardiovascular health, and end-of-life issues.
- Developed continuing education programs for faith community nurses
- Advocated for accessible and affordable health care
- Written grants for congregational health initiatives
- Collaborated with faculty in schools of nursing, in program development, and in authoring books and articles on FCN
- Developed programs for the underserved in the community (e.g., the homeless, immigrants, the working poor, others who have no health insurance)
- Established health fairs to deliver screenings to identify pending illnesses, such as high blood pressure, depression, and other health or mental health problems, so as to accomplish early interventions
- Provided flu shots and immunizations for the prevention of communicable diseases

Source: Blanchfield & McLaughlin, 2006.

TABLE 10-6 Counseling Parishioners: Guided Questions

- Who else, including family members, does the individual want involved?
- Does the parishioner know that the faith community nurse documents their meetings?
- How are these documents kept secure?
- Why is documentation necessary?
- What is confidentiality?
- Does the faith community nurse have permission from the parishioner to collaborate with his or her healthcare provider?

opportunities for the nurse who works exclusively in a church to obtain grant writing and research skills. Collaboration between nursing schools and FCN programs can enrich both the school and the FCN program. This collaborative relationship can be a "win-win" for nursing faculty and for faith community nurses.

Collaborating with Community Agencies

Besides providing healthcare resources, community health organizations can help the faith community nurse to better understand the community's needs and its resources. Ongoing communication, connecting, and networking all take time and effort, but are well worth it. For example, collaborative efforts have led to outcomes such as mass immunizations to prevent the spread of infectious diseases, well-children physical examinations, and screenings for depression, osteoporosis, diabetes, vision, and hearing, to name a few of the programs conducted by faith community nurses. The collaborative relationships between community agencies and churches provide ample opportunities for both in terms of reaching more people for health promotion and early case finding, breaking down barriers that might limit citizen participation, reducing the duplication of efforts, and expanding the missions of both the community's endeavors and the church's ministry to provide holistic healthcare services to the greater community and its citizens (Blanchfield & McLaughlin, 2006; Loyd & Ludwig-Beymer, 1999).

The Nursing Cabinet

Nurses from other organizations often collaborate with the faith community nurse in bringing health information to educate parishioners, and by contributing ideas to bring prevention programs to the community (such as flu shots for older citizens). The efforts of the members of the nursing cabinet may also help the faith community nurse provide better access to healthcare resources, thereby assisting in early case finding and subsequent intervention. The nursing cabinet provides an opportunity for brainstorming and creative thinking, so that new initiatives can be developed to improve the overall health care delivered to the community and to provide needed resources to members of local churches.

The healthcare cabinet includes a variety of professionals with an interest in health care, including physicians, nutritionists, counselors, elected officials, paramedics, and congregational leaders. It provides the faith community nurse with valuable community resources. Table 10-7 lists some of the outcomes that may be achieved through the efforts of the healthcare cabinet.

FAITH COMMUNITY NURSING: ROLES, FUNCTIONS, AND SKILLS

The faith community nurse integrates faith and health into nursing practice. He or she provides spiritual care, while teaching holistic health strategies. The first parish nurses identified five roles for this position; more roles have been developed over the course of time (Brown & Magilvy, 2001). Table 10-8 compares the roles of the faith community nurse and the nurse case manager. As shown in the table, many of their roles are similar but are performed in different settings, focused on different populations. For example, the nurse case manager may work in a hospital, clinic, or community setting, whereas the faith community nurse functions in a parish setting (see Chapter 4).

TABLE 10-7 Outcomes of the Collaborative Efforts of the Healthcare Cabinet

- Develops brochures, articles, and speaking opportunities
- Provides formal introductions, so as to facilitate collaboration with healthcare agencies, community agencies, and local businesses
- Establishes advocacy training programs
- Provides information about the various healthcare services in the community that each member represents, which enhances the collaborative relationships among the members of the healthcare cabinet, making for a stronger support system for the FCN program

Table 10-9 summarizes the skills needed by both faith community nurses and nurse case managers. All of the skills are the same for both types of professionals, with the exception of grant writing skills—not all nurse case managers write grants. Funding for an NCM program generally comes from managed care companies or insurance companies, which usually do not require grant writing skills. Funding for FCN programs comes from grants, church funds, and donations; thus it is often necessary for the faith community nurse to write grants to ensure the ongoing viability of this program.

The faith community nurse must understand organizational dynamics from a systems perspective so that he or she can understand the interface between the church and the community. The nurse must be cognizant of current medical and healthcare systems in the community where the church resides. He or she must have a complete picture of how the church (or churches) and community healthcare services can collaborate to provide holistic care across the healthcare continuum to those most in need of medical and nursing care. Understanding the case management process can prepare the faith community nurse to enact the roles that are comparable to the roles filled by the nurse case manager— namely, assessing a population, brokering and facilitating access to healthcare resources, and monitoring and evaluating the quality and cost-effectiveness of care.

STANDARDS OF PRACTICE

Standards were developed to identify the scope of practice for what were originally called parish nurses, now known as faith community nurses. The development of the standards and the definition of the scope of nursing practice reflect the commitment of the Health Ministries Association to work with the American Nurses Association (ANA) to promote an understanding of the role of the faith community nurse in the community and addressing the fact that the faith community nurse's role is a specialized area of nursing practice.

TABLE 10-8 A Comparison of the Roles and Functions of the Faith Community
Nurse and the Nurse Case Manager

Faith Community Nurse	Nurse Case Manager
Health educator: Teaches patients and families self-help skills and provides information about the parishioner's illness. The faith community nurse develops educational programs and special courses, provides articles for the church bulletins and newsletters, maintains a health ministry bulletin board and a literature rack for parishioners' information and education, and arranges for church facilities to provide space to conduct educational activities. Prevention is the goal.	**Health educator:** Teaches patients and families self-help skills and empowers the patient to obtain the highest level of wellness. The focus of education is usually on an individual or family, rather than on a group. The health educator may provide the patient and family with literature to help them better understand the illness and the healthcare system. Monitoring the patient's progress is a vital role for the nurse case manager. The goal is to maintain the highest level of wellness possible (Tahan, 2005). Both the faith community nurse and the nurse case manager participate in workshops or courses in nursing practice, health promotion, and current healthcare issues for continuing education. Both also attend educational programs that are required by the sponsoring agency.
Health counselor: Advises parishioners and families about self-care, and listens to their concerns about their health. The faith community nurse, as a health consultant, conducts home assessments at the request of parishioners, provides for health screenings, and assists with visitation and follow-up in homes, hospitals, and long-term care facilities when parishioners become ill. As a coach, the faith community nurse may select a parishioner to closely monitor the person's progress as he or she moves forward toward health. The nurse conducts home assessments and visits the patient when he or she is in the hospital, a long-term care facility, or a nursing home.	**Health counselor:** The nurse case manager advises patients and families about self-care and listens to their concerns about their health. He or she is a health consultant/coach. The nurse case manager conducts home or agency assessments prior to a patient's transfer and accepts appropriate referrals for follow-up care in the patient's new setting— either the home, nursing home, or long-term care facility. He or she monitors the patient's progress (Tahan, 2005).

TABLE 10-8 *Continued*

Faith Community Nurse	Nurse Case Manager
Referral agent (broker): Provides information about community healthcare resources and refers parishioners to healthcare providers across the healthcare continuum, according to their needs. The nurse may refer parishioners to pastors, physicians, or healthcare agencies, such as a public health clinic. The faith community nurse serves as the liaison between the congregation and the community. He or she maintains information about community resources as needed to make appropriate referrals. The broker ensures that the patient and family receive the right care from the right healthcare professional at the right time.	**Referral agent (broker):** Provides information about community healthcare resources and refers patients to the appropriate healthcare professionals, according to their needs. Because of his or her continuing use of community resources, the nurse case manager maintains collegial relationships with many of the healthcare providers in various community agencies. He or she ensures that the patient and family receive the right care from the right healthcare professional at the right time (Cohen & Cesta, 2005; Tahan, 2005).
Coordinator: Of volunteers and other resources to serve the healthcare needs of church members. The faith community nurse coordinates the volunteers' activities after recruiting them to participate in the FCN ministry. The faith community nurse provides orientation and education for the volunteers and supervises their activities. He or she provides feedback about the volunteers' performance.	**Coordinator:** Of healthcare resources. The nurse case manager ensures that the healthcare professionals are able to provide cost-effective, high-quality health care. He or she facilitates access to the appropriate resources needed across the healthcare continuum to avoid fragmentation of services (Tahan, 2005).
Support group leader and developer: Assesses the need for support groups, facilitates their development, and arranges for the appropriate leadership. The faith community nurse evaluates the effectiveness of the support group in meeting the healthcare needs of the participants.	**Support group leader and developer:** May or may not enact this role. If the nurse case manager does develop a support group and provide its leadership, the group members usually all have the same illness, such as breast cancer, rather than belonging to a religious denomination. The nurse case manager evaluates the effectiveness of the support group in meeting the healthcare needs of the participants.
Mentor: Mentors the church's staff and the congregation.	**Mentor:** Mentors other healthcare providers, the patient, and family (Tahan, 2005).

(Continues)

TABLE 10-8 *Continued*

Faith Community Nurse	Nurse Case Manager
Team member: Other team members include the church staff, the congregation, and other healthcare professionals, who are frequently also members of the congregation.	**Team member:** Other team members are healthcare providers, including physicians, social workers, and physical therapists, among others. The patient's family is also considered part of the team. Together they collaborate, using each person's unique knowledge and skills to provide comprehensive health care (Koenig, 2005).
Advocate: Acts as the spokesperson about health issues on behalf of the congregation. The faith community nurse assists people to understand and effectively use healthcare and social services systems. He or she is a resource person for church committees and community organizations, and makes the churches—both the staff and the congregation—aware of social and legislative issues affecting health care (e.g., the recent and continuing debate over healthcare reform).	**Advocate:** Acts as the spokesperson for patients and their families. The nurse case manager advocates for the overall health of the community, as well as for his or her assigned patients. Nurse case managers are advocates for their patients, as well as stewards of healthcare resources, assisting patients and families to navigate the complex, confusing, and fragmented healthcare delivery system that is in place today. The nurse case manager may also address healthcare issues publicly; for example, he or she may contact a legislator regarding healthcare reform (Carter, 2009; Tahan, 2005).
Administrator/leader/manager: Is in charge of assigning the volunteers to serve the needs of the parishioners. Even if the faith community nurse is not in charge of evaluations, he or she is still responsible for organizing and directing the healthcare programs conducted at the church. The faith community nurse organizes and administers these healthcare programs.	**Administrator/leader/manager:** Is frequently in charge of coordinating services provided by other healthcare professionals, but has no direct responsibilities for assigning them to a particular patient. The nurse case manager monitors the patient's progress and does evaluate the effectiveness of other providers' work. He or she is not directly in charge of other members of the team, but is responsible for organizing and directing the patient's health care. The nurse case manager is the coordinator and facilitator of the healthcare team. He or she is a leader rather than a manager (Powell & Carr, 2009; Tahan, 2005).

(Continues)

TABLE 10-8 *Continued*

Faith Community Nurse	Nurse Case Manager
Researcher: Demand for outcomes studies is tied to fiscal concerns. Both the nurse case manager and the faith community nurse must document their outcomes so that their work will continue to be funded. Funds for FCN programs often come from several sources, including grants, donations, and churches.	**Researcher:** Outcome data are necessary to prove the viability of a NCM program. Funding for nurse case manager's work comes from hospitals, nursing homes, home health agencies, and government programs, such as the Children's Health Insurance Program, Medicare, and Medicaid (Powell & Carr, 2009). Research is important in planning patient care based on the best evidence that is available (Tahan, 2005).
Evaluator—quality assurance: Participates in evaluations of the quality and effectiveness of the FCN program and documents the outcomes. Brown & Magilvy (2001) believed that more evaluation of FCN on the health of the congregation and the community is needed.	Evaluator—quality assurance: Participates in evaluations of the quality and effectiveness of the NCM program and documents the outcomes (Patterson, 2003; Tahan, 2005). Anecdotal evidence is not enough to adequately provide evidence of quality and effectiveness (Carter, 2009).

The nurse is a member of a multidisciplinary team who functions in an arena of different faith communities (e.g., Catholic, Protestant, Moslem, and Jewish communities). The 15 standards that guide nursing practice include standards that refer to the nursing process. Many of the standards are similar to standards for nursing practice in other fields of nursing (Bickford, Humes, & Carson, 2005). The scope and standards for faith community nurses state that these nurses will collaborate with parishioners, various healthcare delivery systems, church leaders, and healthcare providers in various community agencies to promote clients' health (Health Ministry Association/ANA Scope and Standards of Parish Nursing Practice, cited in Blanchfield & McLaughlin, 2006). Currently, the standards of practice are being revised to be inclusive of the current activities of faith community nurses' practice (Leila Moore, Personal communication, May 28, 2007). Every faith community nurse should be familiar with the scope and standards of practice for faith community nurses.

TABLE 10-9 Skills Needed by Faith Community Nurses and Nurse Case Managers

---

- Communication & interpersonal skills
- Clinical skills
- Teaching skills
- Counseling skills
- Coaching skills
- Critical-thinking and problem-solving skills, along with the knowledge of community resources
- Group process skills*
- Mentoring skills
- Collaborative and networking skills
- Leadership skills
- Organizational skills
- Research skills†

---

*Although the nurse case manager may not facilitate a support group, both the faith community nurse and the nurse case manager need group process skills to build collaborative teams.
†Outcomes studies are important to future funding, no matter where the funds come from—a grant, a church, a hospital, or an insurance company. Today, more nurses from all areas of nursing practice are developing research skills so that they can answer clinical questions and provide nursing interventions that are evidence based.
Source: Tahan, 2005.

QUALITY OF CARE

Concepts concerning quality have gained widespread acceptance within Christian churches. The benefits of addressing quality in FCN programs include empowering congregations for healthy living and whole-person care, evaluating processes, documenting excellence in FCN ministry, emphasizing God's mission, providing a vision for the congregation, keeping the focus of care on the parishioners, preventing health problems, and creating an atmosphere conducive to both spiritual health and physical health. To ensure that these goals are achieved, quality data are collected to make good decisions and to evaluate the faith community nurse's delivery of quality health care (Loyd & Ludwig-Beymer, 1999; Tahan, 2005).

■ SUMMARY

Faith community nursing is a relatively new and a growing model of case management that is unique to nursing practice. Like the nurse case manager, the faith community nurse facilitates the patient's ability to access healthcare resources and coordinates those healthcare resources to meet the individual's or family's needs. Nurse case managers view themselves as advocates for the patient and family—and so do faith community nurses. The focus of the faith community nurse is on health education and illness prevention, which is similar to the focus of many community-based nurse case managers. What is unique about the faith community nurse is that this professional combines the functions of nursing care and the functions of pastoral care, integrating spiritual care with all of the other aspects of health care to provide holistic nursing care (Westberg, 2006).

■ CASE STUDIES

In the area in which you live, an increasing number of people are being diagnosed with type 2 diabetes. The community is heavily engaged with the local church. Describe the steps you would take to approach the church about the implementation of an FCN program with the goal of diabetic education and management.

■ DISCUSSION QUESTIONS

1. What is the philosophy behind faith community nursing?
2. Which members of the faith community are necessary participants for working successfully with church congregations in FCN programs?
3. Compare the role of a faith community nurse with that of a traditional case manager.

■ CLASSROOM EXERCISES

Read an article on faith-based nursing and then, with your classmates, discuss your thoughts on program implementation, collaboration necessary for success, and outcomes measured. Discuss the barriers to implementation and ideas on program integration in the community.

■ RECOMMENDED READINGS

Loyd, R., & Ludwig-Beymer, P. (1999). Listening to faith communities: Collaborations with those served. In P. A. Solari-Twadell & M. A. McDermott (Eds.), *Parish nursing*, (pp. 107–122). Thousand Oaks, CA: Sage.

Solari-Twadell, P. A., & Egenes, K. (2006). A historical perspective of parish nursing: Rules for the sisters of the parishes. In P. A. Solari-Twadell & M. A. McDermott (Eds.), *Parish nursing: Development, education and administration* (pp. 9–16). St. Louis, MO: Elsevier/Mosby.

▪ REFERENCES

Bickford, C., Humes, Y., & Carson, W. (2005). *Scope and standards of nursing informatics practice.* Silver Spring, MD: American Nurses Association.

Blanchfield, K. C., & McLaughlin, E. (2006). Parish nursing: A collaborative ministry. In P. A. Solari-Twadell & M. A. McDermott (Eds.), *Parish nursing: Development, education and administration* (pp. 65–82). St. Louis, MO: Elsevier/Mosby.

Brown, N. J., & Magilvy, J. K. (2001). Parish nursing as community focused case management. In E. L. Cohen, & T. G. Cesta (Eds.), *Nursing case management* (3rd ed., pp. 155–163).

Carter, J. (2009). CCMC news and views: Finding a place at the discussion table: Case management and health care reform. *Professional Case Management, 14*(4), 165–166.

Cohen, E., & Cesta, T. G. (2005). *Nursing case management: From essentials to advanced practice applications* (4th ed.). St. Louis, MO: Elsevier/Mosby.

Koenig, E. (2005). Collaborative models of case management. In E. L. Cohen & T. G. Cesta (Eds.), *Nursing case management: From essentials to advanced practice applications* (4th ed., pp 79–86). St. Louis, MO: Elsevier/Mosby.

Loyd, R., & Ludwig-Beymer, P. (1999). Listening to faith communities: Collaborations with those served. In P. A. Solari-Twadell & M. A. McDermott (Eds.), *Parish nursing* (pp. 107–122). Thousand Oaks, CA: Sage.

Patterson, D. L. (2003). *The essential parish nurse: ABCs of congregational health ministry.* Cleveland, OH: Pilgrim Press.

Powell, S. K., & Carr, D. D. (2009). Editorial: Case managers as leaders. *Professional Case Management, 14*(4), 163–164.

Schnoor, M. (1999). Spiritual care giving: A key component of parish nursing. In P. A. Solari-Twadell & M. A. McDermott (Eds.), *Parish nursing: Development, education and administration* (pp. 43–44). St. Louis, MO: Elsevier/Mosby.

Solari-Twadell, P. A., & Egenes, K. (2006). A historical perspective of parish nursing: Rules for the sisters of the parishes. In P. A. Solari-Twadell & M. A. McDermott (Eds.), *Parish nursing: Development, education and administration* (pp. 9–16). St. Louis, MO: Elsevier/Mosby.

Solari-Twadell, P. A., & McDermott, M. A. (2006). *Parish nursing: Development, education and administration.* St. Louis, MO: Elsevier/Mosby.

Tahan, H. A. (2005). The role of the nurse case manager. In E. L. Cohen & T. G. Cesta (Eds.), *Nursing case management: From essentials to advanced practice applications* (4th ed., pp. 277–295). St. Louis, MO: Elsevier/Mosby.

Westberg, G. (2006). A personal perspective of whole person health and the congregation. In P. A. Solari-Twadell & M. A. McDermott (Eds.), *Parish nursing: Development, education and administration* (pp. 3–10). St. Louis, MO: Elsevier/Mosby.

Disease Management

Jacqueline DeBrew
Charlotte A. Herrick

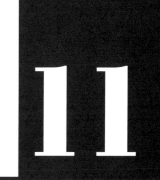

■ OBJECTIVES

1. Define terms associated with disease management.

2. Discuss the evolution of disease management (DM) from a historical perspective, as an outcome of case management (CM), and in terms of managed care and the increasing numbers of people who require long-term services.

3. Compare DM with CM models with newer models, such as telehealth, used in a managed care environments.

4. Identify the roles and the necessary skills of the disease manager, as well as the functions, settings, and populations served by DM.

5. Describe the various components of DM.

6. Discuss the strategies used frequently by disease managers.

INTRODUCTION

Case management continues to evolve. The next two chapters examine the more recent trends in the evolution of various case management models of healthcare delivery, including disease management, telephonic disease management, and telehealth. These more recent models will continue to grow as the U.S. population ages, more people develop chronic health conditions, and costs continue to skyrocket, necessitating an emphasis on cost containment. As the U.S. budget deficits expand, the ability of the federal government to fund Medicare, Medicaid, and the Children's Health Insurance Program will be further threatened. Today, the big question is healthcare reform—specifically, how to fund health care for all American citizens. It will be necessary for economists, healthcare providers, legislators, and policymakers to continually examine the delivery of health care so as to provide the best quality for the least amount of money.

INTRODUCTION TO DISEASE MANAGEMENT

Disease management (DM) evolved during the 1990s as a means to deal with the rising costs of caring for people with chronic diseases and to improve the quality of care. DM has grown rapidly over the last few years. By 2010, it is expected that there will be 10,000 disease managers in the United States, including nurses, social workers, pharmacists, dieticians, health educators, and counselors (Howe, 2005). DM concentrates on people with chronic conditions, who require long-term care and close monitoring to prevent complications or acute exacerbations of a chronic disease (Huber, 2005). It was developed to coordinate services, lower costs, and improve outcomes for these populations (Huber, 2006). DM programs came into existence at the request of health insurance companies and large self-insured employers that sought to deal with the spiraling costs of health care (Howe, 2005). Huber (2005) has stated that the rapid growth of DM is the result of a "perfect storm"—that is, the coming together of a number of forces that have combined to make sweeping changes in the delivery of health care. Table 11-1 identifies the forces that have been instrumental in developing the disease management model.

Like case management (CM), this emerging healthcare delivery model evolved to contain costs by helping people to take better care of themselves, thereby preventing complications from a chronic disease. Thus DM programs seek to avoid emergency room visits and repeated hospitalizations for partici-

TABLE 11-1 Forces Influencing the Development of Disease Management

- The aging of the U.S. population
- The maturing of the baby-boom generation
- High medical and pharmaceutical costs
- Advancing medical technology
- Dramatic increases in the number of chronic health conditions
- U.S. government budget deficits

pants. Proactive outreach and patient education, as well as healthcare advising and counseling, are major strategies, among others that will be addressed in this chapter. DM strategies aim to improve the quality of care and, therefore, the quality of life for patients with chronic conditions. Empowerment strategies for self-care are the center of the disease manager's interventions. Healthy living and lifestyle changes are taught. Emphasis is on the coordination of preventive care. DM strategies are coordinated across the healthcare continuum and are continued during the remainder of the patient's life. A DM program offers coordination, consistency, and customization of care for people at risk of a relapse due to noncompliance with their medical regimens (Huber, 2006).

The Disease Management Association of America (DMAA) was founded in 1999 as a professional organization for disease managers in the United States. It represents the members of all DM disciplines. As part of its mission, it has standardized definitions, program components, and outcomes measures and offers support services and educational materials. DMAA offers healthcare providers and patients the following services:

- Supports the healthcare provider/patient relationship.
- Emphasizes prevention of complications, using evidence-based practice guidelines (EBP).
- Continually examines clinical and economic outcomes with the goal of improving the overall health of the nation (DMAA, 2004, cited in Huber, 2005).

Currently there is no disease management certification. Many disease managers take the Case Management exam given by the Commission for Case Management Certification (CCMC).

Table 11-2 defines the most important terms used in DM.

HISTORICAL PERSPECTIVES: DISEASE MANAGEMENT'S EVOLUTION AND FUTURE

Disease Management in the 1980s and 1990s

Disease management emerged from case management, utilization management, and managed care. Its purpose is to control costs and coordinate the healthcare delivery system for people with chronic illnesses, who were often costly members of managed care organizations. Pharmaceutical companies established DM programs to support patients' compliance with their medication regimens.

By 1996, several DM companies offered services generally focused on three medical conditions: diabetes, asthma, and heart failure. The patients with these

TABLE 11-2 Disease Management: Definition of Terms

Clinical information system (CIS): a software program that disease managers use to track and record their work.

Continuum of care: a linkage of health services across the healthcare delivery system, including health promotion, disease prevention programs, outpatient clinics, public health, primary care, diagnostic centers, pharmaceutical companies, ambulatory care clinics, acute inpatient settings, rehabilitation/chronic long-term care institutions, home health services, and palliative care, such as hospices (Huber, 2005). The disease manager coordinates care for the patient with a chronic disease across the continuum of care.

Economic modeling: a process by which the disease manager determines if a program is cost-effective. Cost–benefit ratios are determined to examine the economics and viability of a program and its value to patient care and to society.

Health promotion: the science and art of helping people change their lifestyle to move toward a state of optimal health. Health promotion is a DM strategy to help the patient achieve maximum health and wellness, within the confines of his or her chronic condition.
Optimal health: the balance of physical, emotional, social, spiritual, and intellectual health domains.
   Physical: Fitness, nutrition, medical self-care, control of substance abuse.
   Emotional: Care for an emotional crisis, stress management.
   Social/intellectual: Educational, achievement, career development.
   Spiritual: Love, hope, charity (*American Journal of Health Promotion*, 1989, cited in Huber, 2005, 2006).

Population: a selected group of people, based on a specific disease; may also be referred to as the *target population.*

Target population: a group of people who share a specific characteristic, either environmental or personal (Howe, 2005; Huber, 2006).

Predictive modeling (PM): a narrowly segmented population or group of people who are at risk for complications due to their chronic illness, and who most likely will incur high medical costs (Meek & Citrin, 2005).

Behavior change: the goal and primary outcome of DM. Change is not limited to the patient, but also includes the healthcare team, facilities, risky organizational practices, and government agencies.

Evidence-based medicine (EBM): the framework for DM interventions. EBM may also be referred to as *evidence-based practice* (*EBP*). EBM is the application of research findings to practice—the "conscientious, explicit and judicious use of current best evidence in making decisions about the care of individual patients" (Sacketts & Associates, cited in Howe, 2005, p. 60). EBM is not a rigid set of guidelines but rather combines clinical expertise with research evidence to make the best decisions. Prior to applying the research findings to practice, the disease manager must first formulate a question that considers the patient, the interventions, the alternatives, and the results from available research (Terra, 2007).

Population health approach: an approach that aims to improve the health of the entire population and to reduce health inequities (disparities) among population groups. It has a broad perspective, examining a range of factors that affect a population's health (Huber, 2005).

TABLE 11-3 Disease Management Target Populations: People with Chronic Diseases

---

- Congestive heart failure
- Diabetes mellitus
- Asthma
- Special populations: the frail elderly and children with special healthcare needs
- Substance abuse
- Depression and other chronic mental health conditions, such as post-traumatic stress disorders (PTSD) and schizophrenia.
- The medically indigent
- High-risk pregnancies
- Occupational health/worker's compensation recipients
- AIDS
- COPD
- Hypertension (high blood pressure)
- Catastrophic injuries, requiring long-term rehabilitation as a result of a complications, leading to a chronic disability
- Traumatic brain injury (TBI)

---

conditions, who were at the highest risk of generating costs for the payers, were the target population. What has finally evolved is a healthcare model that focuses on maintaining people's health through wellness and prevention programs (Huber, 2005).

The chronic conditions addressed by DM are those that are characterized by high rates of prevalence, high costs, and a significant role for the patient as a result of his or her lifestyle. Behaviors play an important role regarding the patient's health and his or her ability to manage the disease (self-care). The focus of DM, according to Howe (2005) and Huber (2005), is on the people who have one or more of the chronic diseases listed in Table 11-3.

Several trends have led to DM:

- People are living longer with chronic diseases
- Increasing healthcare costs, which demand efforts aimed at cost containment
- The growth of managed care companies as the main sources of healthcare delivery
- A greater demand by the public for improved safety and access to quality care (Huber, 2006)

Table 11-4 lists some of the specific features that characterize DM. Some are similar to the features found in nursing case management (NCM); others are unique to DM.

TABLE 11-4 Features That Characterize Disease Management

- Population management
- Care coordination*
- Consistency of care for "at-risk" populations
- Encouragement and counseling to achieve patients' compliance*
- Proactive interventions, outreach, and early case finding*
- A focus on prevention and early interventions
- Patient education: empowerment strategies for self-care *
- Improved access to care*
- Providing continuity of care over the length of the life of the patient
- Establishing a data management system for patient identification and management

*Features also found in nursing case management.

Disease Management in the 2000s and Beyond

In the United States, there has been an explosion of DM programs over the last 5 to 10 years. DM has made a concerted effort to prove its worth and has collected enough data to prove that DM, when delivered to a specific population of people with a chronic disease, can have positive effects on both clinical and financial outcomes (Howe, 2005). DM can be found across a variety of settings and many chronic conditions. Advanced technology and data handling have improved the ability to provide DM to many people across geographical areas. The success of DM as a commercial enterprise has far exceeded the expectations of healthcare providers, policymakers, and economic analysts (Howe, 2005).

Technology has proved to be invaluable to the continuing development and the increasing use of DM (Eisenberg, 2009; Randall, 2009). DM uses remote home monitoring systems, telephonic and home visitation services, email communication, Web interfaces, telemonitoring, and telephonic communication to keep in touch with patients. For example, the Orlando Visiting Nurse telemanagement program monitors 300 patients' vital signs using technological devices installed in their homes and counsels the patients daily by phone (Randall, 2009).

The future of DM will depend on four factors:

- Continuing advances in technology and the ability to identify and stratify high-risk populations
- The professionalism of the disease manager through the development of educational programs in colleges and universities
- The ability to document models that provide savings in terms of healthcare costs
- The development of new strategies that will translate into cost savings in the future

Continuing research that links specific interventions with improved outcomes and cost savings is key to determining the future of DM (Howe, 2005). Predictions are that DM will continue to grow as the population of people who experience a chronic illness proliferates (Huber, 2005). The future challenge will be to move current practices to newer paradigms that will further improve the quality of health care, enhance the quality of patients' lives, and improve financial outcomes (Howe, 2005).

Disease Management and Nursing Case Management: Similarities and Differences

Case management (CM), nursing case management (NCM), and DM are complementary strategies. Each is unique, though all share certain common areas of practice. The case manager provides access to the right healthcare resources in a timely and cost-effective manner, while the disease manager works with a specific population to improve patient self-care and to provide education to maximize the efficacy of treatment (Owen, 2004). The disease manager addresses specific clinical conditions. The nurse case manager facilitates access to treatment for both acutely and chronically ill patients. Both the nurse case manager and the disease manager coordinate comprehensive care. According to Owen (2004), when the CM model is combined with the DM approach, the result can be better, more responsive, and more cost-effective care. The case manager is focused on the more acutely ill patient, whereas the disease manager's focus is on the chronically ill patient. The goals are the same, however: better outcomes at lower costs. The disease manager's expertise is specific to a disease or a group of diseases, while the nurse case manager's expertise is broader than on a specific disease. Table 11-5 lists the similarities and differences between the two models.

CHARACTERISTICS OF A DISEASE MANAGER

The roles and skills of a disease manager require knowledge of the nursing process. He or she must be an expert about a limited number of diseases, must be knowledgeable about the latest research evidence, and must be skilled in various nursing interventions. Technological skills are required as well.

Today, many Americans are living longer with chronic and complex problems, suffering from more than one medical condition, as well as social and/or psychological problems. Disease managers work closely with physicians to keep these patients as healthy as is possible. They have frequent patient contacts by phone, email, or monitoring devices, thereby ensuring that disease

TABLE 11-5 Similarities and Differences Between Disease Management and Nursing Case Management

Similarities
- Goals are similar: cost-effective, quality care.
- Both use strategies that involve health promotion, illness care, care coordination, resource management, case finding, and patient education. Both work with an interdisciplinary team.
- The case manager and the disease manager view their relationships with the patient and family as a partnership, and both view themselves as advocates.
- The case manager and the disease manager are both outcomes oriented, rather than process oriented.
- Both DM and CM use strategies and interventions based on EBM.

Differences
- The case manager and the disease manager serve different populations. The nurse case manager coordinates care for one patient or group within a specific setting, such as the hospitalized patient. The relationship of the NCM to the patient is usually time limited or episodic. The disease manager studies a population, while serving each patient individually or a group of patients with the same illness—for example, an underserved population of poor children suffering from obesity with diabetes. The disease manager–patient relationship frequently takes place over time.
- The case manager is viewed as a generalist, while the disease manager may be considered a disease specialist.
- The intensity of the interpersonal relationship may be greater for the disease manager than for the nurse case manager because of the length of time over which the disease manager serves the patient.
- Although clinical pathways (CPs) are still used in some NCM settings, CPs are not used in DM because CPs are viewed as too restrictive, are considered too time limited, and do not take into consideration comorbidities or individual patient responses (Howe, 2005).

Summary
The population focus of each model is different and some of the strategies differ, although many of the strategies used by the disease manager and the nurse case manager are similar (e.g., coordinating healthcare resources, facilitating the healthcare team, documenting outcomes, and teaching self-care.)

managers can better meet the challenges of these complex patients, while the patients remain in their own homes.

Table 11-6 lists the various roles of the disease manager and defines the necessary skills that are required to enact the role. Table 11-7 addresses the functions, interventions, and settings that are characteristic of the disease manager.

Some of the strategies differ between DM and NCM, while many of them are similar. The focus of the disease manager is on aggregates or a target population; the setting of the DM program is usually the community. Contact with

TABLE 11-6 Roles and Skills of a Disease Manager

Roles of the Disease Manager
- Advocate*
- Broker* (matches resources to identified patient needs)
- Care planner, facilitator, and coordinator*
- Clinician* (The disease manager is an "expert" in specific diseases. Although the nurse case manager must also be a clinician, his or her expertise focuses on healthcare resources for patients who suffer from a variety of different diseases.)
- Source for clinical assessments*
- Observer and healthcare monitor* (face-to-face or using technology at a distance)
- Communicator* (Both the nurse case manager and the disease manager communicate face to face. The disease manager also communicates with patients by phone.)
- Educator*
- Counselor/health coach*
- Motivator*
- Change agent*
- Cognitive/behavior or behavioral therapist (conducted more by the disease manager)
- Supervisor*
- Resource/utilization manager*
- Documenter*
- Data collector and analyst*
- Evaluator*
- Researcher*

Skills of the Disease Manager

- **Clinical skills***

The disease manager must have extensive knowledge of the disease process and treatments, the expected outcomes, and the self-care skills that the patient and family will need to be taught. The disease manager is expected to be the "expert" of the diseases to which the disease manager has been assigned. The nurse case manager's skills are those that are necessary to care for a broader group of people who have a variety of diseases. He or she must have knowledge of the treatments, the expected outcomes, and the necessary self-care skills for people with a variety of diseases.

- **Communication skills***

The disease manager must perfect his or her telephone communication skills to include the ability to (1) effectively make "cold calls"; (2) conduct telephone assessments and interventions; (3) identify at-risk patients (early case finding); and (4) be skilled at coaching and counseling (Howe, 2005). Both the disease manager and the nurse case manager must also have good communication skills to interact with families and to build an interdisciplinary, collaborative team with all of the involved stakeholders. (See Chapter 6 on collaboration.)

(Continues)

TABLE 11-6 *Continued*

- **Knowledge and skills to guide decision making***

Disease managers participate in decision making regarding interventions based on (1) clinical expertise, (2) patient values, and (3) the best evidence. Both disease managers and nurse case managers are expected to translate complex medical knowledge into meaningful information for patients and families via verbal instructions, educational materials, and (sometimes) videotapes. The best way to determine if the patient or family understands the message is to request a restatement of the message.

- **Skills to facilitate DM structures**

Once the population is identified, the disease manager puts in place the following structures, which are designed to ensure best practices across populations:

  - *Inputs* (Clinical assessment, utilization data, laboratory values, and so on
  - *Throughputs* (Rules are the criteria to develop and implement the care plan, according to established protocols and EBM)
  - *Outputs* (Outcomes include the patient's progress, the quality of the program, and system outcomes, such as continuity of care).

- **Knowledge of skills related to behavior modification**

Behavior modification is an important DM strategy for changing behaviors to a healthier lifestyle.

- **Outcomes management skills***

Identifying and documenting outcomes in DM is as important as it is in CM. (See Chapter 13 on outcomes management.)

- **Interpersonal skills***

These skills are necessary to work with the other disciplines on an interdisciplinary team. It is important to include physicians and other healthcare providers, the patient and family, the chaplain, the regulatory agencies, and third-party payers in the DM program. Networking with all of the stakeholders requires these skills. The disease manager, like the case manager, must coordinate the necessary resources and facilitate acquisition of needed healthcare resources.

- **Technological skills**

Disease managers will increasingly rely on technology. New monitoring devices are introduced daily. The disease manager will be required to handle technological data, and to be able to apply those data to patient care. Technological devices are common tools in today's DM programs, and there will be more to come. Examples include implanted cardiac defibrillators, information from EKG monitors that are sent to a phone, tiny blood samples that can detect a potential cardiac event, and monitors that measure a patient's vital signs (respirations, pulse, and temperature), daily weights, and oxygen saturation levels and send these data to a central monitoring station. Technology will provide the tools to allow patients to do more for themselves in their own homes, in consultation with the disease manager and physician. Smart technology is an integral part of DM now and will remain so in the future (Eisenberg, 2009; Randall, 2009).

*Also required for the nurse case manager.

TABLE 11-7 Functions, Interventions, and Settings for Disease Managers

---

Functions and Interventions of a Disease Manager
- Use EBM guidelines.*
- Identify the population with a disease and coordinate those persons' care.
- Stratify the population by the degree of risk. Develop a plan of care, according to acuity levels.
- Match the interventions with the patient's and family's needs.*
- Develop a plan to meet the patient's needs.*
- Interventions: Educate, advise, coach, counsel, and support the patient and family in self-care activities. Apply counseling and nursing strategies.*
- Evaluate the patient's progress and examine the outcomes.*

Settings for Disease Management
- Acute care disease management/hospital-based*
- Primary care clinics*
- Pharmaceutical companies
- Insurance companies*
- Call centers for telephonic disease management
- Hospital-outpatient continuum-of-care programs that are focused on a special population, such as The Heart Center" at High Point Regional Hospital, High Point, North Carolina; the COPD Rehabilitation Program at Forsyth Hospital, Winston Salem, North Carolina; and the Cancer Center at Wesley-Long Hospital, Greensboro, North Carolina

---

*Also required for the nurse case manager.

the patient can occur in the home, by telephone, by email, or by a monitoring device that sends the information to the disease manager's office. The disease manager follows a group of patients over each patient's lifetime In contrast, the nurse case manager serves many different patients, who suffer from a variety of illnesses, in different settings across the continuum of care and across institutional boundaries. Contact is usually on a person-to-person basis for a limited period of time. The DM may be considered the specialist and the NCM the generalist.

THE VALUE OF HEALTHCARE DELIVERY BY A DISEASE MANAGER

DM has demonstrated its value. The disease manager prevents exacerbations and subsequent hospitalizations for patients with chronic and complex diseases by improving patients' abilities to care for themselves. By carefully monitoring the patient, the disease manager can identify early signs of a relapse, thereby preventing emergency room visits and hospital readmissions; consequently, healthcare dollars are saved. Table 11-8 lists the value dimensions that are the result of a DM program, including the cost–benefit ratio. Although most

TABLE 11-8 The Value Dimensions of Disease Management

- Clinical Value: Examples of clinical value include improved laboratory values, reduction in pain scores, and improved ability for self-care. The ability of the disease manager to assess, plan, and move the patient to more positive outcomes is of clinical value.
- Financial Value: Lower costs in general include lower medication costs, fewer procedures, reduced clinical visits, reduced emergency room visits, and fewer hospital days.
- Educational Value: The value of education is that it may lead to better clinical, financial, and satisfaction outcomes. Education empowers patients for self-care.
- Satisfaction Value: The advocacy role for the disease manager leads to satisfaction among all stakeholders, including the patient and family (Howe, 2005).
- Cost–Benefit Ratios: The benefit of the program, divided by the cost, which indicates the return on the investment. For every dollar that is invested, the typical DM program's income is $1.76 (i.e., the return on the investment). According to Howe (2005, p. 34), most DM programs have a 2:1 return on investment.

disease managers don't worry about cost–benefit ratios as much as they worry about their patients' progress, Howe (2005) believed that disease managers could enhance their effectiveness by understanding cost–benefit ratios that determine the financial outcomes, thereby demonstrating the value of DM both to patients and to the larger society.

THE COMPONENTS OF DISEASE MANAGEMENT

Six components of a DM program are listed below, which have been identified by the DMAA. Some of these components will be explored in this chapter, some are self-explanatory, and others been defined elsewhere in this textbook:

1. Population identification
2. Evidence-based medicine
3. Collaborative practice, including physicians and other healthcare team members (see Chapter 6 on collaboration).
4. Patient self-management education (primary prevention, behavior modification, and other counseling strategies and close monitoring for compliance).
5. Process and outcomes measurement and outcomes management (see Chapter 13 on outcomes management).
6. Providing feedback and reporting to the patient, family physician, and other provider (Huber, 2006)

Predictive Modeling

Predictive modeling (PM) is a statistical process that looks into the future and quantifies the likelihood of high healthcare costs for one person in comparison to others. It is a computerized method of identifying those people who would benefit the most from DM. This set of tools is used to stratify a population according to its risk for poor outcomes and provides opportunities for an early intervention, based on statistical data (Meek & Citrin, 2005; Calhoun, Admire, & Casey, 2005). Disease managers use a trigger list, developed from PM, to identify potential patients who would benefit from DM. PM is a statistically valid tool that improves providers' ability to identify and treat high-risk, high-cost patients earlier and more effectively (Calhoun et al., 2005). It allows DM organizations to focus on specific populations of patients and, therefore, to use their resources wisely.

Segmentation and Stratification

Segmentation is another way to identify a population—in this case, by categorizing people into predefined groups based on cost parameters or clinical patterns. This technique is used in conjunction with PM. The sorting takes place after the initial identification but before the first contact with a disease manager. Segmentation uses percentiles. For example, 10,000 diabetics might be identified based on the scores developed by the PM tool. The top 5% might then be targeted for DM.

Next, people are stratified from the segmentation so that care plans can be identified for them. **Stratification** relies on assessments, laboratory values, documentation of specific events regarding a health crisis, and a collection of other data. People are divided into levels of care that require different levels of interventions (Howe, 2005). Stratification serves several purposes: (1) developing a clinical picture, (2) assigning the degree of the frequency and intensity of the treatments, and (3) matching a patient to the appropriate disease manager and his or her expertise (Howe, 2005). Patients are divided into levels; for example, there might be three levels in a diabetes program. Stratifying patients assists the DM program to determine acuity levels and the costs of care.

DISEASE MANAGEMENT STRATEGIES

Caregiving in DM is comprehensive and spans boundaries across the patient's lifetime. It includes planning, life care planning, implementing interventions, coordinating resources, monitoring and evaluating the quality and costs of care, and counseling and educating patients about healthy lifestyles.

Patient Education

Patient education is central to DM, to enable patients to develop the skills for self-management. Education promotes compliance. Part of DM education involves instituting a system of reminders for patients to manage their self-care activities. The health educator's goal is to motivate patients to be active participants in their own care.

Motivational Interviewing

Disease managers encourage people to do the right thing for the sake of their health. Robert J. Botelho has developed a Web-based program to help disease managers hone their skills in motivational interviewing (www.motivate healthyhabits.com). Ideally, disease managers will use change-related language with their patients as part of this process. The steps in motivational interviewing are as follows:

1. Listening
2. Recognizing and affirming that the person has real issues and barriers to changing behaviors
3. Pointing out the patient's current desires to change behaviors to meet healthy goals
4. Instilling hope by conveying a positive outlook
5. Goal setting

Goal Setting

Goal setting challenges the patient to succeed and keeps the individual on task. It identifies activities that a patient must do to meet the identified goal(s). Table 11-9 addresses considerations to guide the disease manager when negotiating patient goals.

The patient and family are more likely to work toward goals that are set through a shared decision-making process. Table 11-10 lists some motivational strategies that can be useful to the disease manager in moving the patient and family toward these ends.

Patient and Family Counseling

Advising, coaching, and counseling require attention to helping the patient to understand both the disease and his or her skills and resources to cope with that disease. After the initial assessment, the disease manager provides advice, guidance, and emotional support. He or she shares information about the

TABLE 11-9 Guidelines to Establish Goals with a Patient

- Invite the patient's active participation.
- Goals should have a timeline.
- Goals should be easily identified as either met or unmet.
- The language needs to be clear, concise, and well written.
- Goals should be realistic and achievable.
- A patient should not have too many goals at one time.
- Goals should be SMART:
  Specific
  Measurable
  Attainable
  Realistic
  Tangible with a target date

Source: Howe, 2005, p. 97.

TABLE 11-10 Motivational Strategies

- Problem solve with the patient and family, rather than "telling" or instructing them about what to do.
- Discuss the reasons for making a change and the possible strategies to effect a change.
- Be positive, and provide encouragement and compassionate support as the patient strives to make changes.
- Listen more and talk less.
- Be concise, be clear, and convey an understanding of the patient's thoughts and feelings. Convey empathy.
- Provide positive feedback as the patient strives to make lifestyle changes.
- Be available as an expert. Create an aura of "expert advice, on demand." Be flexible. Change strategies as needed.

Source: Howe, 2005.

potential tasks to cope with the lifestyle changes. The disease manager must take care to apply "the right approach to the right situation, at the right time" (Howe, 2005, p. 93).

Counseling Strategies

Declarative (telling style) approach. Once trust has been established, the declarative approach can be used with simple bold statements, such as, "You need to exercise more and lose weight."

Information sharing (selling style) approach. Delay providing information or education, until the patient is ready to hear the information. The clue as to when the patient is ready is when he or she starts asking questions. The patient must be motivated to learn.

Patient/disease manager discussion (persuasive approach). A discussion format should be used when educating the patient about new information. It should be focused and concise, and stated in simple language. The disease manager should ease the patient into examining new ideas. Discussion provides an opportunity for persuasion.

Shared decision making (participative style approach). Informed and shared decision making is a process for the patient to gather relevant health information from his or her clinician, the disease manager, and other clinical and nonclinical sources, and to assess that information in conjunction with the patient's values and beliefs. Together the patient and the disease manager make decisions in planning interventions.

Counseling Process

The counseling process involves the following steps:

1. The patient understands the risk or seriousness of the disease or the condition to be prevented.
2. The patient understands preventive services, including the risks, benefits, alternatives, and uncertainties.
3. The patient has weighed his or her values regarding the potential benefits and harms associated with each type of intervention.
4. The patient has engaged in the shared decision-making process so that he or she feels comfortable with the decisions.

Benefits of Counseling

- Improved understanding
- Is effective when there are difficult choices to make
- Involves a partnership rather than a patriarchal relationship that is authoritarian (the traditional parent–child or the expert doctor–patient relationship)
- Enhances compliance because of the patient's "buy-in" to healthcare decisions (empowerment)

Negatives of Counseling

- It is time-consuming. Telling is less time-consuming than counseling.
- Some patients want a "quick fix" or to be told what to do.
- Informed and shared decision making requires that the patient has a certain amount of knowledge about medical treatments and alternatives, and must be able to understand the language of medicine.

Health Advocacy

The disease manager, as an advocate, focuses on individuals who either have a chronic illness or are at risk for developing one or at risk for having an exacerbation of a disease (e.g., a smoker is at risk for chronic obstructive pulmonary disease [COPD] or a smoker who already has asthma and continues to smoke and, therefore, is at high risk for COPD). The disease manager–patient relationship is a partnership, in which the disease manager enacts the roles of an educator and change agent.

The health advocate uses the following four strategies:

1. Patients are coached about how to deal with stress.
2. Patients are taught about their medical condition(s) so that they understand their treatment plans.
3. Psycho-education and behavior change techniques are used to help patients who currently engage in high-risk behaviors adopt healthier lifestyles to better manage their condition(s).
4. Individuals with chronic conditions are assisted to effectively use the healthcare system and are taught how to access the appropriate level of care (Huber, 2005).

The Health Belief Model

The disease manager, as an advocate, is a spokesperson for the patient if he or she is unable to speak for him or herself. The advocate uses the **Health Belief Model** as a framework to guide DM interventions. The disease manager considers the patient's view of his or her chronic condition. The Health Belief Model can be divided into five constructs:

1. Perceived susceptibility: the person's opinion of the chances of getting a certain condition.
2. Perceived severity: the person's opinion of how serious this condition is or will be.
3. Perceived benefits: the person's opinion of the effectiveness of some actions, upon the advice of the health advocate, to reduce the risk(s) regarding the seriousness of the current or possible future condition(s).
4. Perceived barriers: a person's opinion of the concrete and psychological costs of the advised action to deter a possible negative health consequence.
5. Self-efficacy: the confidence the person has that, upon accomplishing a specific health goal(s), improved health will be the outcome (Howe, 2005).

Behavior Modification

A key role for the disease manager is to motivate patients to change poor habits and life styles to benefit their health. Disease managers need to understand the "stages of change"—including the fact that behavioral changes occur gradually and over time. Relapses are inevitable and are part of the process of working toward lifelong changes.

Individual behavioral change is a process that occurs in six stages:

1. *Pre-contemplation.* The person is aware that there is a problem, but has not seriously thought of making a change. The disease manager provides information in terms of written educational materials to inform the patient of the possibilities for change and the potential consequences of continuing on "as is."
2. *Contemplation.* The person is seriously thinking about making a change. Ambivalence is central to this phase. Giving up an enjoyed behavior causes a sense of loss, despite a perceived gain. The disease manager and the patient together examine the benefits and the barriers and then weigh the costs versus the benefits.
3. *Preparation.* The person plans to take action. He or she makes some lifestyle adjustments prior to making an overall change. The patient is ambivalent, but prepares to make specific lifestyle changes. Patients may experiment with small changes. Making a small change may signal that a decision has been made to make a major change.
4. *Action.* The person implements an action plan to modify his or her behavior. During this phase, the person needs a great deal of positive feedback and emotional support. He or she has demonstrated that a lifestyle change is desirable.
5. *Maintenance and relapse.* The person continues the new behaviors but may struggle with lapses or relapses.
6. *Termination.* There is zero temptation and the person has the ability to resist the temptation to relapse. The "habit" or "addiction" or the previous lifestyle is no longer a part of the person's identity (Herrick, Herrick, & Mitchell, 2010; Howe, 2005; Huber, 2005).

Several behavior modification models are available that can guide the disease manager when undertaking this type of counseling. Cognitive-behavioral therapy is described here briefly. If the reader is interested, further reading is suggested.

Cognitive-Behavioral Therapy

This cognitive-behavioral model focuses on the patient's thoughts and behaviors. Negative thoughts are reframed to attain a more positive outlook. The patient disputes the distortions that are barriers to changing behaviors. For example, in a smoking cessation program, triggers that stimulate the desire to smoke are identified and potential rationalizations to continue smoking are disputed. Healthier coping behaviors are identified and planned for the next time there is the temptation to smoke. When patients feel better as a result of the changes they have made in their thinking and behaviors, the positive results reinforce the changes and healthy behaviors are repeated. The disease manager provides the patients with positive feedback (reinforcement) to maintain the changes.

■ SUMMARY

Disease managers integrate healthcare services into a system of care, coordinating resources and advocating for people with chronic conditions to ensure that their care is appropriate and timely. Identifying populations in need of DM services requires risk identification, using information technologies and computerized data, including predictive modeling, stratification, and segmentation. To be effective, the disease manager needs access to clinical, administrative, and financial information, as well as access to logistical and epidemiological data. DM strategies involve telemanagement, educational counseling, behavior therapies, and motivational interviewing. Evidence-based medicine and the nursing process represent the framework for decision making in a DM program. Interventions include comprehensive health and mental health care. The goals are to prevent exacerbations of a chronic illness among high-risk populations by encouraging healthy lifestyles, thereby the quality of life for patients with chronic diseases while containing costs.

■ CASE STUDIES

You are a case manager in a clinic that specializes in the treatment of patients with congestive heart failure. You have been following Mr. Brown for nearly 6 months, without much success. He has been readmitted to the hospital twice in the past 45 days for fluid overload. You have tried to engage him to empower him to manage his disease process. Unfortunately, Mr. Brown continues to reject a change in his diet. Discuss which techniques you could use to engage Mr. Brown in his own care and begin to understand the rationale for the prescribed diet restrictions.

■ DISCUSSION QUESTIONS

1. Discuss the historical evolution of disease management and how it is being utilized in the current healthcare system in the United States.
2. Which types of populations can benefit from disease management programs, and why?
3. Which reportable outcomes are necessary to ensure the effectiveness of disease management programs?

■ CLASSROOM EXERCISES

Identify a high-risk population in your community. Discuss the process for identification, implementation, evaluation, and engagement of the local hospital in supporting such an endeavor. Identify who would make the decision on the implementation of a disease management program and strategies to maintain the program.

■ RECOMMENDED READINGS

Eisenberg, S. S. (2009). What does the future holds for disease management? *Managed Care, 18*(2), 26–31.

Owen, M. (2004). Disease management: Breaking down the silos to improve chronic care. *Case Manager, 15*(3), 45–47.

Terra, S. M. (2007). An evidence-based approach to case management model selection for an acute care facility. Is there really a preferred model? *Professional Case Management, 12*(3), 147–157.

■ REFERENCES

Calhoun, J., Admire, K., & Casey, P. (2005). Implementing a predictive modeling program, Part I. *Lippincott's Case Management, 10*(4), 185–189.

Eisenberg, S. S. (2009). What does the future holds for disease management? *Managed Care, 18*(2), 26–31.

Herrick, C., Herrick, C., & Mitchell, M. (2010). *100 questions and answers about how to quit smoking.* Sudbury, MA: Jones and Bartlett.

Howe, R. (2005). *The disease manager's handbook.* Sudbury, MA: Jones and Bartlett.

Huber, D. L. (2005). *Disease management: A guide for case managers.* St. Louis, MO: Elsevier/Saunders.

Huber, D. L. (Ed.). (2006). Disease management. In *Leadership and nursing care management* (3rd ed., pp. 361–382). Philadelphia: Saunders Elsevier.

Meek, J., & Citrin, R. S. (2005). Predictive modeling and its application to disease and case management. In D. L. Huber (Ed.), *Disease management: A guide for case managers* (pp. 21–31). St. Louis, MO: Elsevier/Saunders.

Owen, M. (2004). Disease management: Breaking down the silos to improve chronic care. *Case Manager, 15*(3), 45–47.

Randall, B. (2009, August/September). New dimensions in disease management: Best practices in telemanagement. *Case in Point*, pp. 30–31. Retrieved from http://www.dorlandhealth.com/Best-Practice/new-dimensions-in-disease-management.html

Terra, S. M. (2007). An evidence-based approach to case management model selection for an acute care facility. Is there really a preferred model? *Professional Case Management, 12*(3), 147–157.

Telehealth

Jacqueline DeBrew
Charlotte A. Herrick

■ OBJECTIVES

1. Define the terms found in the e-health literature.

2. Describe the evolution of e-health and various technological strategies in disease management (DM) during the last 20 years.

3. Identify the various chronic conditions and populations of patients who may benefit from medical care and DM that includes high-tech strategies.

4. Discuss how technology can enhance the quality of care and the quality of DM, based on the research that addresses evidence-based medicine.

5. Identify the issues and challenges that DM faces in using technology.

6. Discuss "on-demand" telephonic disease management.

7. Describe the skills and steps in the DM process, using telephonic DM as a way of delivering DM services.

8. Describe the use of remote patient monitoring technology for home care, including its challenges, the obstacles, and the reimbursement issues.

9. Identify the goals, benefits, and limitations of a well-designed disease management/case management information system.

INTRODUCTION

Increasingly, technology is being used in a number of ways to enhance the abilities of case managers, nurse case managers, and disease managers to provide services to patients. E-case management, telehealth, telephonic case management (CM)/disease management (DM), remote patient monitoring, and case management information systems that comprise computerized data analysis systems are all addressed in this chapter. Both the benefits and the challenges of these technologies are described, and the way in which each of the technological strategies is used in CM/DM is identified. Technology is proving to be valuable in numerous aspects of CM, including "beyond-the-walls" case management, nursing case management (NCM), and DM. Although technology was briefly described in Chapter 11 in relation to DM, technology will be explored in more depth at this time.

According to Marineau (2007), telehealth can be a tremendous resource to meet the healthcare needs of our society. Technological advances have been developed so that monitoring devices can be installed in the homes of sick people who otherwise would have needed to be hospitalized (i.e., without technology), thereby reducing healthcare costs. A number of factors are contributing to the technology-driven changes in healthcare delivery, including wider adoption of DM/CM, the growing number of baby boomers who are reaching retirement age and have chronic diseases, society's greater comfort with technology, the desire for home care instead of hospital care, the need to curb healthcare costs, and the fact that technology can be quicker and more accurate than human monitoring in some cases (Eisenberg, 2009; Marineau, 2007).

Table 12-1 defines the various terms found in the literature about technology-driven DM.

HISTORICAL PERSPECTIVES

In 1879, during a measles epidemic, subscribers belonging to a telephone service were assigned telephone numbers to access information about their child's illness so that they could better care for the child at home. Also, during the 1870s, a telephone exchange was set up among 10 physicians and a local drug store for prescription assistance.

In another early example of telemedicine, as cited by Skiba et al. (2005), a closed-circuit TV system was used to educate psychiatric healthcare professionals working in a state psychiatric hospital in a remote area of Nebraska and to allow for consultation with the staff about patient care issues; these services were provided by the Nebraska Psychiatric Institute.

TABLE 12-1 Medical Technology: Definition of Terms

e-Health: the use of electronic technologies and telecommunications in the practice of providing clinical care, patient education, and professional health education. Another definition for *e-health* is the application of Web-based technologies to organize disease management (Skiba, Sorensen, McCarthy, & Brownrigg, 2005; Cohen & Cesta, 2005). The purpose of using technology is to facilitate the patient's ability for self-care and to improve the support offered to patients by their healthcare providers.

Telehealth: the delivery of healthcare services when barriers exist because of time and distance. These technologies may include telephones, computers, and interactive video transmissions and monitoring devices. *Telehealth* is a term that encompasses many technologies, including telemedicine, telenursing, disease management (DM), telepsychiatry, video conferencing, and more. *Telehealth* is the use of technology, including computers, to exchange information and to provide services to clients in DM programs (Park, 2006) *Telehealth* includes the fields of telemedicine, medication information systems, electronic patient records, disease monitoring, supply chain management, and biotechnologies (Mullahy, 2004).

Telephonic Case Management/Disease Management: providing CM/DM services over the phone. Telephone work is necessary to keep open lines of communication without driving up costs. This approach is effective in implementing strategies for prevention, screenings, case findings, and monitoring of patients who are in recovery and progressing well, and who do not need intensive CM services. It is especially effective in the delivery of health care to remote areas with limited healthcare facilities. Case managers and disease managers can oversee large caseloads in geographically distant areas (Mullahy, 2004). However, many DM programs use the telephone exclusively for disease management, monitoring each patient's progress and evaluating the outcomes of the patient education about self-care. Mullahy (2004) has questioned the quality of care when the phone is used exclusively.

Remote Patient Monitoring (RPM): application of technological devices to patient care so as to determine a patient's progress by collecting and analyzing reliable and valid clinical data from a distant site. RPM-collected information has proved to be more factual then self-recorded data. Today, devices are available that can monitor a patient's weight, blood pressure, pulse, and heart rate in the patient's home (Howe, 2005).

Case Management Information System (CMIS): a central storage space in which to save patient data. Services providers can use a CMIS to build more complete and accurate records, including the patient's history, that can be easily retrieved and shared with other providers. Critical data such as medication allergies and previous life-threatening conditions can be filed in a manner that calls attention to them. These data can be used to support the decision-making process, remind patients of self-care interventions, and flag important information for providers (McGonigle & Mastrian, 2007).

Massachusetts General Hospital also used television cameras and monitors for patient care during the 1950s and 1960s. Some years later, Willemain and Mark coined the term "telemedicine" to describe this sort of technologically driven practice (Skiba et al., 2005). During the 1980s, triage nurses based in hospitals used the telephone for assessments to determine priorities for seeing a patient either in the physician's office, in the outpatient clinic, or in the emergency room.

STRATEGIES FOR APPLYING TECHNOLOGY TO CASE MANAGEMENT

E-Case Management/Telehealth

Applications

Currently, technology is becoming pervasive in the healthcare arena, owing to the ongoing development of health information networks and infrastructures. It is predicted that medical technology will continue to proliferate in the years to come. A national information network will link nursing information systems, so that nurse case managers and disease managers can have ready access to the latest evidence-based medicine and nursing. The driving forces that have influenced the use of telehealth technology are similar to the driving forces that were influential in the development of CM/DM. Specifically, these changes in the delivery of health care stem from the following factors:

- The movement from provider-centered care to patient-centered care
- The movement from hospital-based care to community-based care with the point of service in the patient's home
- The movement from an authoritarian provider–patient relationship to a partnership between the patient and the healthcare provider
- The movement from health care managed by the healthcare providers to self-care managed by an empowered patient and family, supported by CM/DM (Park, 2006)

With the use of technology, nurse case managers and disease managers can monitor patients in their homes, conduct ongoing assessments, teach patients self-care strategies, and oversee the outcomes of patients' self-care activities. Voice or sound computer-generated reminders or alarm systems can remind patients to take their medications, change their dressings, and make follow-up appointments with the physician or nurse practitioner. Although technology can never replace the personal relationship between a case/disease manager and the patient, it can decrease the number of interpersonal contacts, which saves time and money. Technology can also provide more accurate data than self-reports. Thus technology can be a means of monitoring patients' progress more closely, thereby improving outcomes by both identifying potential problems early and improving the quality of health care.

Insurance companies and other third-party payers are developing healthcare information networks to collect data related to patient care, perform variance analyses, and identify benchmarks for outcomes. The goal is to determine the best quality of care, while at the same time containing costs (Simpson, 2005). Simpson (2005) predicted that it might be 10 years or more before a pervasive network of informational systems will have the ability to communicate with all patients.

Information technologies are a critical part of DM, including gathering patient data, integrating and analyzing the information, and then disseminating the results (Huber, 2005). Databases that include clinical, financial, and administrative information can be analyzed to determine current trends and identify how they are affecting DM interventions. Claims information provides data for using predictive modeling, which can be used to determine costs based on the analysis of demographics, diagnoses, medication/pharmaceutical claims, and survey data (Huber, 2005). Predictive modeling identifies patients in need of DM services and the probable costs of providing care to each of those patients.

Technological support is available to healthcare providers as well as to their patients. Table 12-2 lists some of the health-related conditions that are frequently addressed by DM programs, as identified in the literature on technology.

Applications of technology as part of case management of other conditions will continue to occur. The variety of diseases and conditions subjected to the technology will also grow across the healthcare continuum as telehealth tech-

TABLE 12-2 Conditions and Special Populations That May Benefit from Telehealth

Chronic Conditions	
Congestive heart failure (CHF)	Diabetes
Hypertension	Asthma
Morbid obesity	Cancer
Catastrophic injuries and conditions	Chronic obstructive pulmonary disease
Substance abuse and other mental health	(COPD)
problems, such as post-traumatic stress	High-risk pregnancies and other
disorder	women's health issues
Special Populations	
"At risk" children	The frail elderly

nology is perfected and research studies demonstrate its cost-effectiveness (Huber, 2005; Mullahy, 2004). Marineau (2007), for example, found that patients hospitalized with an acute infection were successful in transitioning to home care supervised by a nurse practitioner with the aid of telehealth, including devices that could monitor their vital signs, oxygen saturation, daily weights, and blood sugars.

Evidence-Based Telehealth Practice

Skiba et al. (2005) reviewed several studies that examined telehealth interventions, including their efficacy, safety, and the quality of outcomes, along with costs. They concluded that a growing body of evidence supports the use of telehealth programs, although more evidence is needed to quantify this value.

Issues and Challenges

- *Privacy and Confidentiality.* The Health Information Portability and Accountability Act (HIPAA) is national legislation that was passed to improve the efficiency and effectiveness of information systems in the healthcare arena and to establish standards and requirements for exchanging electronic information, taking confidentiality about sharing healthcare information into consideration. The Privacy Rule of the legislation defines how patient information can be disclosed; the Security Rule sets baseline standards for ensuring the confidentiality, availability, and integrity of patients' healthcare information (Skiba et al., 2005).
- *Standards of Practice.* In 1998, the American Nurses Association published "Core Principles on Tele-health"; in 1999, it published "Developing Tele-health Protocols: A Blueprint for Success." Both of these documents outline standards of practice in relation to telehealth. The American Telehealth Association (ATA) has also produced guidelines for healthcare professionals and patients using e-health care (http://www.ihealthcoalition.org/ethics/ehealthcode0524.html). All of these publications are aimed at clearly identifying and defining standards of practice for all healthcare providers who use telehealth strategies— case managers, nurse case managers, disease managers, physicians, nurses, social workers, and more (Skiba et al., 2005).
- *Licensure and Legal Jurisdiction.* The current licensing system for healthcare professionals in the United States is very complex. Essentially, each state licenses its own nurses and other healthcare providers. This system is not only complex but can be confusing when

it comes to NCM/DM programs, which may cross state boundaries using telehealth strategies. The nurse case manager and the disease manager must abide by the laws and licensing requirements of the state in which the patient resides, as well as his or her own state.

The National Council of State Boards of Nursing has proposed an interstate licensing model, known as the "Interstate Nurse Licensure Compact," to ensure that the quality of all nurse providers in telehealth meets national and state standards (Skiba et al., 2005) (http://www.ncsbn.org). More than 15 states have passed legislation that would allow them to become part of the Compact agreement, but many more states still need to pass this legislation for the welfare of telehealth care providers and for patients in need of DM services (Skiba et al., 2005).

Although more outcomes studies need to be conducted, sufficient evidence exists to prove that the use of technology in medical and nursing care, as well as in CM/DM, saves lives and dollars and improves the quality of home health care for patients and their families.

TELEPHONIC CASE/DISEASE MANAGEMENT: AN OVERVIEW OF THE "ON-DEMAND" MODEL

Telephonic CM/DM has continued to grow, with call centers being established across the United States, serving people in both urban and rural areas. The costs of telephonic CM/DM are relatively inexpensive, and the adoption of such programs has had a positive impact on outcomes. Mullahy (2004) reviewed an "on-demand" CM service that used the phone exclusively. In this service, patients were triaged according to their immediate needs. For example, after assessing the patient's needs on the phone, the nurse determined whether the patient should go to the doctor's office tomorrow morning or whether the patient should make an immediate emergency room visit tonight. The purpose of an "on-demand program" is to give the patients enough knowledge to identify potential problems and to understand and seek out the most appropriate level of treatment. "On-demand" coverage for chronic diseases can be a 24-hour-per-day proposition. As part of such a service, the disease manager integrates strategies of patient education, advising and counseling, and empowering patients and families to make their own decisions regarding their health and their medical treatment (Mullahy, 2004).

Mullahy (2004) expressed doubts about how effective the quality of the care is if all communication among the patient, the family, and the physician occurs strictly over the phone, especially in a scenario involving a noncompliant or poorly educated patient. Park (2006) believed that there are too many opportunities for miscommunication over the phone.

THE TELEPHONIC CASE/DISEASE MANAGEMENT PROCESS

Howe (2005) described the telephonic DM process, including the interpersonal interactions between the disease manager and the patient, and the assessment and intervention techniques and strategies used that have proved to be successful in achieving positive outcomes. Before describing the process, however, Howe identified a series of challenges with this approach. The biggest challenge for the disease manager is to use only one sense—hearing—to provide patient care; this restriction can be very frustrating for the disease manager, who traditionally uses all five senses in doing assessments.

Engagement: The First Call

Many authors recommend that an introductory letter be sent to the patient prior to the initial telephone contact. Engagement is the focus of the first call, which is probably the most challenging call that the disease manager makes. The patient may be hesitant to talk on the phone to a stranger about personal health issues. The necessary skills that were identified by Howe (2005) were those of a salesperson. As shown in Table 12-3, he suggested use of a variety of techniques borrowed from specialists in selling.

Gathering Clinical Information to Develop a Clinical Picture: The Second Call

The second call requires "reselling, reconfirmation, and reminding" (Howe, 2005, p. 42). This call will focus on developing a clinical picture of the member/patient. The disease manager should first find out the patient's perceptions of his or her condition. The disease manager will seek information about the patient's current health status and any medications taken (both prescription and over-the-counter drugs, and any alternative therapies that he or she may be using; if the patient has a list of his/her medications the DM should acquire a copy). If necessary, the disease manager can have the patient read medication labels over the phone to clarify which agents are being used. The disease manager needs to ascertain key information about the medications, as suggested in Table 12-4.

Developing the Problem/Asset List

The purposes of the problem list are fourfold:

- To develop a snapshot of the person's medical status
- To identify the strengths and resources available to the patient for self-care

TABLE 12-3 Guidelines for the First Call in a Disease Management Program

---

The disease manager needs:
1. To have a thick skin in response to resistance—lack of trust is common.
2. To be confident. Convey confidence to the patient.
3. To tailor his or her voice to gender (men react to a warm compassionate voice differently than do women).
4. To sound casual. Do not read the introduction from a script.
5. To identify himself or herself clearly and slowly as a registered nurse and state the name of the disease management company.
6. To say nothing more until you get a response from the patient, using silence.
7. To introduce the purpose of the call—for example, "the purpose of my call is to let you know about a *free service* that is designed to provide health support to the members of United Health Care" (Howe, 2005). Because most disease management programs are sponsored by parent organizations, they are free. The person you are calling needs to know this immediately.
8. To listen. Allow the member (patient) to engage you in a conversation. Be an active listener.

The DM should:
1. Encourage the person to reveal medical information.
2. Assume that finally the patient will cooperate.
3. Ask open-ended questions.
4. Keep the nature of the DM program general. Cover broad topics, such as education and support services, help the patient think about health-related activities, and support the physician's treatments with helpful clarifications.
5. Not talk a lot on the first call. Let the patient know that you assume that he or she will be an active participant. Be brief.
6. Introduce the idea of the second call and schedule a date and time for that call. Remind the person to put the date and time on his or her calendar.
7. Document information about the member that you learned during the telephone communication, including personal information, such as the name of the dog that you heard barking in the background, demographic information, and any health-related issues that may have been discussed.

Source: Howe, 2005.

- To assess the patient's understanding of his or her medical condition
- To determine the patient's relationships with medical care providers

Utilization Review

Most disease managers have access to utilization data that the DM company provides. Review with the patient the utilization data for emergency room visits, hospitalizations, and other medical office visits. This discussion provides the disease manager with an opportunity to teach what is the appropriate use of each level of medical care.

TABLE 12-4 Gathering Information About Medications as Part of a Disease
            Management Program

• The prescription, including its name and the dose
• The availability (Is it currently present in the house?)
• Adherence to a medication regimen
• The patient/member's knowledge about his or her medications, their purpose,
  special instructions, and his or her understanding about how the medications
  work in the body
• Medication reactions, effects, and side effects
• Nonprescription medications: drug–drug interactions
• Poly-pharmacy evaluation
• Medication abuse
• Alternative therapies: vitamins, chiropractor, massage therapists, and so on

Assessment

Most programs require the disease manager to fill out an assessment form. The
disease manager should introduce the assessment as a way of getting to know
more about the person. For example, he or she might say, "I have a 12-question
assessment that will be helpful to both of us and for me to get to know you
better and how I can be of help to you" (Howe, 2005, p. 48). According to Howe,
keeping the patient on track may prove to be difficult during the assessment.
Do not take any longer than 15 minutes to complete this tool, or the patient
will lose interest. Offer words of encouragement during the assessment. Often
the assessment provides an opportunity for a teachable moment; even so, the
disease manager should refrain from teaching at this point and leave it for
another call. Opportunities will occur later. Teaching in the middle of the
assessment may prevent the disease manager from finishing the assessment.

Care Planning

Many DM programs have preset care plans based on disease-specific protocols
and evidence-based practice. When developing the care plan with the patient/
member, it must make sense to the person. The format used to do so should
include demographic data, a prioritized list of issues, goal setting, a list of
recommended interventions, note taking, and any reference materials for use
by the patient and/or the disease manager. The following example shows one
recommended format for care planning:

▪ Name:
▪ Status: active
▪ Demographic data

- Problem/asset list
- Medication list
- Goals: list the met or unmet goals
- Planned interventions and the patient's progress
- Note: educational materials sent to the patient on (date); follow-up call (date)

Caregiving

The care plan may include patient education, telephone interactions, advising, counseling, coaching, supportive interventions, educational materials sent to the patient, classes and/or support groups suggested by the disease manager for the patient to attend, home visits, and clinic or doctor visits (Howe, 2005).

Telephonic disease management is a process that can be extremely challenging. The communication and listening techniques that are essential to using the phone effectively as a DM strategy are not easy to master. The goals for a telephone DM program are the same as in other CM, NCM, and DM programs, however:

- To improve the health status of the patient/member
- To prevent exacerbations of disease processes
- To ensure that the patient is receiving quality care
- To reduce costs by decreasing the number of unnecessary office or emergency room visits or repeated hospitalizations (Howe, 2005)

REMOTE PATIENT MONITORING: TECHNOLOGY IN HOME CARE

Overview

Remote patient monitoring (RPM) has been used for more than 20 years, yet it is supposedly "just here" (Howe, 2005, p. 109). In 1986, the Glucometer was introduced to monitor patients' blood glucose levels; this device contained a memory chip to record data. A year later, Bayer released a personal computer software application that, through a cable that connected the meter to a computer, could capture the meter's data and view it in several ways. The introduction of this software represented a revolutionary event in managing a chronic disease.

Today, a wide array of technological strategies exist to monitor a patient's weight, blood pressure, peak blood flow readings, pulse, oximetry, blood glucose meters, apnea (breathing), and lab data including cholesterol, HIV, and urine albumin levels. These data are stored in clinical information systems and used by the disease manager to decide upon timely interventions. Other home care devices subject to remote monitoring include ventilators and nebulizers, wheelchairs, and infusion pumps. Park (2006) has suggested that home surveillance tools, such as video cameras or sensors, might eventually be used to track the patient's movements in the home.

The U.S. Food and Drug Administration (FDA) ultimately decides whether these remote monitoring devices and devices warrant the agency's approval when used in the home. As such, the FDA undertakes to evaluate different designs and regulates medical devices to provide reasonable assurance of their safety and effectiveness. According to Eisenberg (2009), these kinds of information and communication technologies and monitoring devices will revolutionize health care in the future, decreasing the costs and increasing our ability to improve health care. The DM call center will be the hub where information from such devices is collected, collated, analyzed, stored, and eventually routed to the appropriate healthcare provider.

Definitions

- A **medical device** is any product or equipment used to diagnose a disease or other conditions, or to cure, to treat, or to prevent disease.
- A **home healthcare medical device** is any product or equipment used in the home by persons who are ill or have disabilities. Both providers and users may need education, training, or other health care-related services to use and maintain the devices safely and effectively in the home or in other places, such as work, school, and church. (Howe, 2005).

The Process: Patient Identification

- High-risk patients: RPM devices are primarily intended for use by the highest-risk patients, because close monitoring will help to determine when to intervene as the patient decompensates.
- Frequent flyers: The repeated use of the emergency room, or frequent hospitalizations in the past year, qualifies a patient for the use of a RPM device.

The Purpose

- The disease manager can objectively track the patient's health status and use the data to guide planning and interventions in a timely way.
- The patient can monitor himself or herself for self-care and can get immediate feedback about the progress he or she is making toward identified goal(s).

HOME CARE AND TECHNOLOGICAL DEVICES

The transition from a primary focus on hospital care to greater use of home care has largely been made possible by advances in technology. Dialysis, intravenous therapies, blood transfusions, chemotherapies, HIV-related services, continuous positive airway pressure (CPAP) devices, ventilators, and other RPM devices have all made home care safe for severely compromised patients. Even with the use of technology, however, the patient's condition must be relatively stable to warrant being cared for at home. In addition, the family must have the necessary skills be able to care for the patient and manage the technological devices. Patients recover faster in the home setting and maintain a higher level of functioning at home; consequently, home care is generally preferable to hospital care.

In recent decades, home health care has evolved into a billion-dollar industry. The case/disease manager is the pivotal link between the physicians, the patient and family, at-home services providers, and the payer. Issues around each of these entities must be addressed and the efforts of each entity coordinated. The use of technology makes this kind of seamless operation possible, albeit not without some challenges in using technology effectively (Table 12-5).

TABLE 12-5 Challenges Related to Home Care

- Identifying the appropriate criteria for patient selection.
- Separating the high-risk patients from other patient populations.
- Connecting to existing clinical information systems.
- Establishing policies and procedures that are necessary for the disease manager to mentally process and integrate information from the streams of data so as to react appropriately, according to the outcome data and in a timely manner.
- Monitoring and reading the data and reacting to an alarm. The presence of an alert in the monitoring software should be clearly identified, so that the disease manager who is monitoring the software can respond immediately and appropriately to data that are "abnormal."
- A lack of technological savvy among disease managers. It is vitally important that the disease manager has a clear understanding about how the device works and how the information is to be used. Some operational problems may arise because of human errors, committed by either the patient, the family, or the disease manager. The disease manager should assess the patient's and the family's knowledge and understanding of the use of the device and its management, and then provide an educational session and document it. A list has been developed for users about the do's and don'ts of using a RPM device. The FDA has highlighted important information for patients, using a remote device. Instructions come with each device and should be read carefully.

The Demand for Research Data Regarding RPM Devices

■ Determine the best design for each device to ensure the best effectiveness and accuracy.
■ In terms of measurements, the data should have appropriate validity and reliability, and be accurate; the transmission of data must be timely; and the data should be of high quality and durability.
■ Although research studies have demonstrated the cost-effectiveness of home care using RPM, more research is necessary to convince payers to reimburse the costs of using RPM devices, which will result in further cost savings.

Reimbursement Issues

Payment for these RPM devices is still to be determined. Questions that remain to be answered include who should order these devices, for whom and for how long, and who should pay (i.e., the patient, the hospital, the third-party payer such as Medicare and Medicaid or other insurance payers). Until reimbursement issues are settled, the technological aspects of DM may stagnate at its current levels for the time being.

CASE MANAGEMENT INFORMATION SYSTEMS

An automated case management information system (CMIS) has the following goals:

■ To improve the collaborative relationship between case/disease managers and patients and their families
■ To provide a central storage space for patient-centered data
■ To assist service providers to build a more complete and accurate database of information about the patient
■ To identify critical information such as medication allergies
■ To improve the decision-making process
■ To facilitate communication among providers
■ To determine population trends by tracking aggregate data for benchmarking, conducting research, and demonstrating the effectiveness of the interventions for an aggregate population

The Benefits

■ A CMIS may be able to improve the case/disease manager's workflow, improve patient care, and improve patient outcomes.

- The patient's progress can be tracked along the healthcare continuum.
- Interventions can be linked to specific outcomes to determine best practices.
- Noncompliant patients can be quickly identified, which may reduce future complications and hospital readmissions for those individuals.
- Patient outcomes can be improved.
- Quality of care can be improved.
- Cost containment becomes possible.

Limitations

- No system can replace the intuitive clinical judgments of the healthcare provider.
- Interpersonal relationships can never be replaced in terms of the integrity and the effectiveness of healthcare delivery. The patient–provider relationship is of utmost importance
- The lack of standardized terminology continues to impede the development of information systems for health care.

Important Considerations

- Determining the performance, reliability, security, stability, availability, backup and recovery, maintainability and usability of a CMIS
- System flexibility that allows the CMIS to be customized to the organization's needs
- Scalability that allows for a seamless system to meet organizational needs for continuing changes
- Portability that allows for data sharing with another authorized user in a different organization (McGonigle & Mastrian, 2007, pp. 239–240)

THE BENEFITS OF TELEHEALTH FROM THE PATIENTS' PERSPECTIVE

Marineau (2007) conducted a qualitative study in patients' homes, except for one patient who was interviewed in the hospital during chemotherapy treatments. The interview questions were open ended. Ten themes emerged from the interviews. Notably, the patients expressed confidence in their primary physician's recommendations for telehealth and the relief they felt when they found that they could remain at home and still be connected with a healthcare provider. They felt cared for by the healthcare team after experiencing daily telehealth visits. They thought that telehealth care was quality care and believed that it was provided in a timely manner. They enjoyed not having to attend the clinic, as many had difficulties with both mobility and transportation. A couple of patients said they thought that they were sent home too early and at the time felt too sick to go home. Overall, however, the impressions of the majority of patients regarding their telehealth experiences were positive.

■ SUMMARY

The explosion of technological advancements has led to rapid changes in the delivery of health care. More outcomes studies regarding telehealth are needed to support the use of technological devices in managing patient care, although the initial data are positive. One thing is certain: Practitioners in all fields of nursing must develop technological skills and understand information systems so that they can be a part of the ongoing advances in medical/nursing technology.

Technology has affected the healthcare delivery system in myriad ways, and may be both a blessing and a curse for the nurse case manager or disease manager. The blessings include improved access to care for many more patients, especially those living in remote geographical areas; shorter lengths of hospital stays because of the ability to monitor patients at home; and the potential to improve the quality of care with careful monitoring, which can also save expensive healthcare dollars. Today, there is better access to medical information for patients, families, and healthcare providers, including DMs.

The down side is that technological advances have actually increased some costs rather than containing them; for example, the use of surgical robots has required major investments. The advances in technology will require nurses, nurse case managers, and disease managers to learn new skills so that they can use the information to best advantage and manage the devices appropriately. Also, patients and families may find RPM devices difficult to manage. Ready access to health information is beneficial to nurse case managers and disease managers, which in turn benefits their patients. Unfortunately, some patients may misinterpret information found on the Internet, which means that nurse case managers and disease managers must perfect their teaching skills to clarify the misinformation.

Cox (2006) believed that developing expertise in new technologies will enable nurses to become indispensable to the healthcare team. Tomorrow's nurses must be skilled in the use of computers, understand computerized information systems, and be open to acquiring new technological skills to be used across state boundaries. Thurkettle (2003) advised nurse case managers to stay up to date about technological advancements. Technology will provide the means by which home health care will be delivered to more patients, which will not only help improve the quality of patients' lives but also serve the best interests of patients and families, communities and society, by delivering cost-effective, quality care.

■ CASE STUDIES

Many telephonic programs have evolved that employ nurses who work from their homes. Discuss some of the benefits and barriers to such programs. Would you have the self-discipline to be highly productive in managing your caseload? If not, why not? Do you believe that telephone-based case management strategies are as effective as face-to-face interaction?

■ DISCUSSION QUESTIONS

1. Discuss both the pros and the cons of using technology in managing patients with chronic conditions.
2. Which reimbursement issues do companies providing telephonic patient support face?
3. Describe the skills necessary to be an effective home-based case manager.

■ CLASSROOM EXERCISES

Read an article on the effectiveness of telephonic case management. Discuss the population, program details, implementation strategies, and outcomes of the program profiled in the article. What are the benefits and the barriers to this program? Which specific skills are necessary for a case manager to be highly productive in a virtual environment?

■ RECOMMENDED READINGS

Eisenberg, S. S. (2009). What does the future hold for disease management? *Managed Care, 18*(2), 26–31.

Marineau, M. (2007). Special populations: Telehealth advance practice nursing: The lived experiences of individuals with acute infections transitioning to the home. *Nursing Forum, 42*(4), 196–208.

Thurkettle, M. A. (2003). Information management as a process and product of case management. *Lippincott's Case Management, 8*(3), 117–121.

■ REFERENCES

Cohen, E. L., & Cesta, T. G. (2005). *Nursing case management: From essentials to advanced practice application* (4th ed.). St. Louis, MO: Elsevier/Mosby.

Cox, K. B. (2006). Power and conflict. In D. L. Huber (Ed.), *Leadership and nursing care management* (3rd ed., pp. 501–542). Philadelphia: Saunders/Elsevier.

Eisenberg, S. S. (2009). What does the future hold for disease management? *Managed Care, 18*(2), 26–31.

Howe, R. (2005). *The disease manager's handbook.* Sudbury, MA: Jones and Bartlett.

Huber, D. L. (Ed.). (2005). Overview of disease management and case management. In *Disease management: A guide for case managers* (pp. 1–13). St. Louis, MO: Elsevier/Saunders.

Marineau, M. (2007). Special populations: Telehealth advance practice nursing: The lived experiences of individuals with acute infections transitioning to the home. *Nursing Forum, 42*(4), 196–208.

McGonigle, D., & Mastrian, K. (2007). Tips, tools & techniques: Information systems and case management practice: Part II. *Professional Case Management, 12*(4), 239–240.

Mullahy, C. M. (Ed.). (2004). The case management work format and process: Telephonic case management; industry directions. Demand management: A self-care management model: 24 hour coverage. In *The case manager's handbook* (3rd ed., pp. 13–14; 193–245; 569–576; 583–584). Sudbury, MA: Jones and Bartlett.

Park, E.-J. (2006). Telehealth technology in case/disease management. *Lippincott's Case Management, 11*(3), 175–182.

Simpson, R. L. (2005). Case management and information technology. In E. L. Cohen & T. G. Cesta (Eds.), *Nursing case management: From essentials to advanced practice application* (4th ed., pp. 380–384). St. Louis, MO: Elsevier/Mosby.

Skiba, D. J., Sorensen, L., McCarthy, M. B., & Brownrigg, V. J. (2005). Telehealth applications for case management. In E. L. Cohen & T. G. Cesta (Eds.), *Nursing case management: From essentials to advanced practice applications* (4th ed., pp. 384–397). St. Louis, MO: Elsevier/Mosby.

Thurkettle, M. A. (2003). Information management as a process and product of case management. *Lippincott's Case Management, 8*(3), 117–121.

Outcomes Management

Laura J. Fero
Charlotte A. Herrick

13

■ OUTLINE

■ OBJECTIVES

1. Discuss the roles and functions of the nurse case manager regarding outcomes.

2. Define concepts related to outcomes management.

3. Define concepts related to outcomes measurement.

4. Discuss outcomes management and its purposes.

5. Identify outcomes measures and indicators.

6. Discuss the historical perspectives of outcomes measurement that influenced the change from a process orientation to an outcomes orientation.

7. Discuss outcomes measurement and management.

8. Describe the cultural and environmental influences on quality outcomes.

9. Identify the most frequently used tools, instruments, and indicators to evaluate effectiveness.

10. Describe program evaluation.

INTRODUCTION

The era of managed care, with its mandate to provide cost-effective yet quality care, has changed the perspective of healthcare providers from a process orientation to an outcomes orientation. It is essential for healthcare disciplines and systems to evaluate their performance so as to provide the public with documented evidence of their ability to deliver high-quality, cost-effective care.

Outcomes measurement is the process of determining the indicators that are valid and reliable measures of outcomes, gathering the data, analyzing the data and interpreting the results, making changes in nursing care, and evaluating effectiveness (Huber, 2006). It has also been defined as the assignment of numbers to determine the different outcomes among various subjects (Duffy & Korniewicz, 2002).

The driving force for the measurement of outcomes has been the necessity to have a financially solvent healthcare system, which relies on documenting the costs of care. The current managed care environment is making the documentation of outcomes critical. Driving forces for outcomes measurement include the need for quality improvement, financial incentives, capitation, and competition among healthcare organizations, the demand for information by employers and consumers, and the demand for documentation by accrediting agencies. Case management in today's healthcare environment is outcomes and goal driven.

Outcomes management is a multidisciplinary endeavor that is designed to improve quality of health care, decrease fragmentation, enhance the results of medical and nursing interventions, and contain costs (Foster, 2003; Huber, 2006).

Outcomes research is conducted in clinical settings to improve patient care by combining outcomes measurement and management with research so as to link quality to patient care (Wright, 2006). Ongoing systematic studies are reviewed and applied to clinical settings to improve patient care (Hogan & Nickitas, 2009).

Effective case management moves the patient through the care delivery process toward goals and outcomes, which must be clearly defined and measurable (Rossi, 2003). Rossi purported that when it comes to outcomes, the cost constraints that affect decisions made by the government, administrators of managed care organizations, businesses, and others will continue to tighten. As outcomes data become more readily available and reliable, these data will be used increasingly in making decisions to improve the quality of care.

Three types of outcomes measures are distinguished. First are *diagnostic-specific* measures—for example, critical pathways and care maps. The second type of outcomes measures is *system-specific* outcomes, which include adverse factors such as medication errors, infection rates, and patient falls. Other measures of organizational effectiveness are costs and productivity. Measures found in total quality management are system measures. Systemwide outcomes must be multidisciplinary. Other system indicators measure the hospital care environment based on staffing ratios, educational levels of the staff, and staff retention and turnover rates. The third type of outcomes measures is *discipline-specific* outcomes, which include performance, practice processes, and quality of practice. With these measures, for example, rates of burnout and job dissatisfaction are measured for each discipline.

Kleinpell (2007) developed some specific outcomes measures to help promote evidence-based care by advanced practice nurses (APNs). The following list identifies five nursing outcomes for the APN:

- Nursing knowledge
- Patient and family education
- Nurse satisfaction
- Hand hygiene compliance
- Rates of adherence to best practice

Kleinpell also listed other outcomes, such as length of stay, resources used, and patient satisfaction. She pointed out that many outcomes measures are possible, but that no one set of indicators is inclusive for all APNs' practice. Instead, measurement of outcomes depends on the specific setting and on the target population; that is, the APN will measure outcomes that reflect the setting and the population being served.

Nursing outcomes have been identified by the American Nurses Association (ANA) in several publications, and are also addressed in new reimbursement initiatives proposed by the Center for Medicare and Medicaid Services (CMS). Under this proposal, for example, hospitals, nursing homes, and home health-care agencies will no longer be paid for preventable complications (Rosenthal, 2007).

The nurse case manager, along with the nursing manager of an acute care unit, must be proactive in understanding patient care expenses and the costs of each of the services that are provided. They must collaborate to identify patient care problems and the necessary resources to ensure that patients get what they need at the time when they need the resources. Measuring outcomes can assist both the case manager and the nurse manager to evaluate issues related to patient care, such as staffing, cost management of products and services, and the coordination of care, as well as encouraging them to ensure that preventive measures are in place and operational.

TABLE 13-1 Nursing Outcomes

- Improved quality of care
- Decreased length of stay (LOS)
- Improvement of the patient's health status
- Decreased costs
- Improved adherence to the plan of care
- Better coordination of care
- Improved patient involvement in his or her care
- Patient and family empowerment

Source: Aliotta, 2006.

THE ROLES AND FUNCTIONS OF THE CASE MANAGER

The Role of the Nurse Case Manager

Key functions of the case manager include assessor, planner, facilitator, coordinator, educator, and advocate. Table 13-1 lists the outcomes that are a result of the work of the nurse case manager.

A study recently published in the *Journal of the American Medical Association* found that coordination and close collaboration between the primary care physician and a nurse reduced Medicare costs for chronically ill patients. The findings in this study supported the supposition that coordination among professionals reduces the cost of care ("Field Trends," 2009, p. 16).

CONCEPTS RELATED TO OUTCOMES MANAGEMENT AND MEASUREMENT

Quality Indicators

Quality is the striving for excellence (Pelletier & Albright, 2006).

Quality health care is the degree to which health services and performance of healthcare professionals result in an increased likelihood of positive outcomes and are consistent with current standards of care (Pelletier & Albright, 2006).

Quality assurance (QA) includes activities that are designed to monitor, prevent, and correct quality deficiencies. The QA system identifies opportunities to improve care, based on collecting information related to errors that have met a predetermined set of criteria. Specific factors contributing to incidents, the systems that influence errors, and a specific process to improve quality are not identified (Cohen & Cesta, 2005).

TABLE 13-2 The Purposes of Quality and Outcomes Management

- Determine the effectiveness of care so as to improve the quality of care
- Identify better educational interventions so as to teach patients and families self-care
- Determine the most productive interventions so as to improve the patient's health status
- Determine the costs of sources needed for care to assess costs and make decisions
- Improve access to care
- Determine institutional outcomes and the delivery of care

A **continuous quality improvement program (CQI)** involves an analysis that studies potential strategies for improving the delivery of quality health care. This process includes examining the hospital system, personnel, the management of clinical services, and the financial structure. It is an ongoing multidisciplinary process of measurement and evaluation, along with proposing potential changes (Pelletier & Albright, 2006).

A **quality improvement program** is an umbrella program that extends into many areas for the purpose of accountability. Such a program represents an ongoing measurement and evaluation process that includes structure, process, and outcomes. Values and standards are used to evaluate care with the purpose of improving it (Pelletier & Albright, 2006).

Total quality management (TQM) involves the evaluation of all systems so as to improve the quality of goods or services by reducing costs and ensuring customer satisfaction. Such a process involves all of the staff in the improvement of quality. The goal of TQM is to ensure that the organization has a culture of care, committed to patient satisfaction, including the encouragement of innovation and a commitment by all of the staff (Hogan & Nickitas, 2009). CQI falls under the realm of TQM, which was originally developed many years ago by W. Edwards Deming (Cohen & Cesta, 2005; Pelletier & Albright, 2006; Sullivan & Decker, 2009).

Table 13-2 identifies reasons to embark on a quality management program.

OUTCOMES MEASURES AND INDICATORS

Outcomes are the result(s) that are obtained from the interventions that are accomplished toward patient care goals (Huber, 2006). They may be measured at reference points along the measurement process, during the patient's recovery (Whitehill, 2005). **Effectiveness** can be defined as the degree to which the positive outcomes are achieved (Goode, 2005).

Case management outcomes are those indicators that reflect the quality of care that are measured in terms of met or unmet goals and the outcomes that result from the patient care plan and the healthcare team's interventions (Daniels & Ramey, 2005). The indicators must be valid and measure accurately the indicators that are supposed to be measured.

Outcomes data provide the information necessary to plan for the future, so as to provide better health care for the public at lower costs. Outcomes are the documented end results of goals attainment (Huber, 2006).

Outcomes monitoring is the continuing review of data related to the patient's progress, the allocation of resources, and the application of the best interventions so as to achieve optimal patient outcomes as a result of quality care.

Outcomes measures (indicators) are indicators of effectiveness of the healthcare providers; examples include improved health status, improved quality of life, and meeting client preferences. Nursing outcomes should continuously be evaluated, so that modifications can be made to the care plan (Austin & Wetle, 2008). Quality of health care is measurable, and nurses and nurse case managers in all settings are increasingly being expected to actively participate in identifying and measuring patient outcomes. Outcomes measures are the quantifiable indicators that are assessed to ensure that health care is provided safely, in a timely manner, and by competent and compassionate healthcare providers, using the best available evidence (White, 2004).

Outcomes indicators are valid and reliable measures related to the results of nursing and medical interventions (Huber, 2006). Mateo, Matzke, and Newton (2002) listed six steps for identifying relevant measures (indicators), as shown in Table 13-3.

Many of the proposed outcomes indicators have been categorized into the following types of measurements:

- Staff satisfaction
- Patient satisfaction

TABLE 13-3 Steps to Identify Relevant Outcomes Measures

1. Conduct a literature review.
2. Compare the data with those for other organizations (*benchmarking*).
3. Determine which outcomes to measure.
4. Use gap analysis (identifying a gap between current and ideal systems for the purposes of managing data).
5. Develop new data sources.
6. Establish a system for data collection, measurement, and management.

Source: Mateo, Matzke, & Newton, 2002.

- Improved quality of care
- Better communication and collaboration
- A decrease in costs or cost containment

Staff satisfaction measures rates of nurses', nursing assistants', and physicians' job satisfaction, as well as their rates of burnout. Also under the heading of staff satisfaction are indicators such as rates of absenteeism and turnover as well as the ability to recruit qualified personnel. Staff satisfaction ratings may be obtained by survey, at the time of the yearly evaluation, or during exit interviews.

Patient satisfaction is usually measured after discharge. It includes patient satisfaction, family satisfaction, and the number of registered complaints.

Improved quality of care is documented through ongoing quality measurements. These measurements focus on the following issues:

- Data documenting quality
- Readmission rates (one day, one week, or one month)
- Consistency of therapeutic interventions from case to case
- The quality of patient education
- Improved patient outcomes
- Variance analysis (which ideally will demonstrate fewer variances)
- Continuity of care, such that there are smooth transitions from one level of care to another

Improved communication and collaboration among disciplines translates into improved teamwork through better lines of communication and the development of collaborative practice among team members. The interdisciplinary team develops the case management plans or multidisciplinary action plans (MAPs), along the way sharing documentation of the patient's progress (Cohen & Cesta, 2005).

Improved financial outcomes measures result in several types of cost containment:

- Reduced length of stay (LOS)
- Fewer third-party payer denials
- Reduction in the preoperative and postoperative LOS
- Improved use of resources (both products and personnel)
- Reduced costs of care
- Decreased delays in waiting for tests and procedures
- Reduced wait times in the emergency room and transfers to a hospital bed
- An adequate ratio of nurses and ancillary staff per patient so that there are fewer errors that cost more

Goal-driven outcomes are those outcomes that are favorable for both the patient and the organization, such as improved quality of care, decreased LOS, better resource utilization, and improved continuity of care (Cohen & Cesta, 2005).

HISTORICAL PERSPECTIVES ON OUTCOMES MANAGEMENT

Prior to the 1960s

The process of outcomes management has evolved over time. Initially, medical outcomes were collected, such as morbidity and mortality rates, rates of procedures and surgeries, and LOS in the hospital. Outcomes management then moved to structural outcomes such as the number of hospital beds, technologies available, and the number of providers.

The 1960s

During the early 1960s, clinical endpoints were collected, such as functional status, well-being, and patient satisfaction. During this period, measurements included the number of hospital days (LOS), type and doses of medication, functional status related to health and the time that the patient spent in certain activities, morbidity rates, disabilities, discomfort, and dissatisfaction (Huber, 2006).

The 1970s

In the 1970s, nursing audits were developed and definitions of the quality of nursing care shifted to focus on the client's knowledge of his or her illness and treatments, medications, the client's adaptive behaviors and self-care skills, and the client's improved health status. A classification system was developed by the Visiting Nurses Association (VNA), called "The Omaha System," which collected data on three types of outcomes: knowledge, behavior, and health status (signs and symptoms).

The 1980s

In the 1980s, the development of Medicare and Medicaid changed the focus of health care from process to outcomes. This decade saw a number of new developments, including the establishment of new agencies that developed criteria to measure cost-effective, quality care. Table 13-4 identifies the developments that occurred during the 1980s, which established criteria to measure the quality of care.

TABLE 13-4 Developments Related to Outcomes Management in the 1980s

---

- **Medicare** and **Medicaid** developed a database to review outcomes.

- The **Agency of Health Care Policy and Research** (AHCPR) was established in 1989. It developed a system to review the effectiveness of various treatments.

- The **Joint Commission** (formerly the Joint Commission on Accreditation of Healthcare Organizations; JCAHO) developed outcome indicators to evaluate the quality of care (the Indicator Measurement System), which later became Oryx. Participating hospitals, when seeking accreditation, had to choose an outcomes measurement and submit the data quarterly to The Joint Commission.

- The **Minimum Data Set** (MDS) was developed for long-term care, which includes a resident's physical and cognitive functioning, medical, emotional, and social status.

Source: Huber, 2006.

The 1990s

The quality of home healthcare services came under intense review during the 1990s. Consequently, a number of programs were developed, including the **Outcomes and Assessment Information Set (OASIS)**. Medicare demanded that home health agencies collect outcomes data.

The 2000s

The Magnet Recognition Program

The Magnet model seeks to identify those hospitals that are recognized as having excellent nursing staff, who provide quality nursing care. These hospitals have been designated by the American Nurses Credentialing Center as outstanding based on "empirical outcomes." The recognition program, called Magnet status, traditionally has used the following criteria to determine the nursing staff's excellence:

- The nursing leadership is transformational.
- The organizational structures empower staff to actively participate in decisions to improve patient care.
- The nursing staff exhibit exemplary practice related to their roles with patient, families, communities, and the interdisciplinary team.
- The hospitals have developed innovative strategies to improve patient care.
- They have made visible contributions to the science of nursing.

A later model for Magnet status added another criterion, which has to do with outcomes. Prior to the introduction of the new criterion, the Magnet model focused primarily on structure and process rather than outcomes. Today, however, hospitals seeking Magnet recognition must use quality data to measure outcomes, including benchmarking. They must also be able to demonstrate that they have found solutions to the problems identified during data analysis (American Nurses Credentialing Center [ANCC], 2008)

Pay for Performance

Pay for performance (P4P) was originally conceived as a means to provide incentives for people and corporations to perform at their best, so as to attain excellent results (Roussel & Swansburg, 2006). Examples of strategies that have been used include merit pay, bonuses, and stock ownership plans. In contrast, the CMS has taken a more negative approach by *not* paying for poor performance (Rosenthal, 2007).

Since 2000, the CMS has been conducting demonstration projects across the United States with both public and private healthcare agencies, in collaboration with healthcare providers and other stakeholders, to find out if financial incentives can improve the quality of health care and reduce unnecessary healthcare costs due to preventable complications that increase the costs of hospital care. The preventable complications from patient hospitalizations include nosocomial infections, pressure ulcers, patient falls, urinary tract infections associated with catheters, and pneumonias acquired during the use of ventilators (CMS, 2005/2007).

As of October 1, 2008, hospitals were no longer eligible for compensation by Medicare for preventable complications during a patient's hospitalization (Rosenthal, 2007). Many of these complications are directly related to poor-quality care. The National Quality Forum (a nonprofit agency that measures quality in various disciplines) has identified a series of specific nursing-related outcomes that healthcare organizations can use as guidelines for improving care. The incentives for hospitals to comply with standards of practice are guided by best practices and are focused on prevention. By eliminating reimbursements for complications due to poor performance, it is thought, the quality of care will improve and costs will be reduced (Kirchheimer, 2008).

Kirchheimer (2008) believes that focusing on the link between quality outcomes and nursing care will provide an opportunity to highlight nurses' contributions to quality patient care. Apparently, data collection for nursing outcomes has not been a priority for many hospitals, largely data collection is time consuming and expensive. However, P4P will emphasize the nurse's role in preventing complications—and the added focus on nursing care will mean that nurses will have to be more accountable. Thus nurses will need to be more engaged in quality improvement efforts and documenting outcomes. The role of the nurse case manager will become even more important in this model, especially in monitoring the recovery of patients—especially high-risk patients—who are chronically ill. The goals are to prevent complications, prevent delays in discharge, and facilitate smooth transitions to the next level of care or a discharge to home care.

Health and Performance Improvements

Another recent trend in health care is termed health and performance improvements (HIP), and is focused on prevention. Outcomes in this model include (1) improved access to quality, preventive-oriented community services; (2) the patient's and family's knowledge, skills, and motivation for self-care; and (3) continuity of care, where there are few disruptions in services and transitions go smoothly, facilitated by a collaborative healthcare team. The team is patient and family centered in HIP programs, providing comprehensive preventive services to people residing in the community (Meyer, 2009, pp. 28–31).

OUTCOMES MEASUREMENT

Effectiveness cannot exist without quality; likewise, quality cannot exist without positive outcomes. Further research is needed to delineate the causal relationships between structure (i.e., the institutional culture, the leadership, and staff support), the process (i.e., the way patients are managed), the results of the interventions or outcomes, and the quality of care.

The following outcomes are commonly measured in healthcare settings:

- *Clinical Outcomes:* information about the results of patient diagnosis and treatment (e.g., mortality, LOS, rates of infections, recidivism rates, use of restraints, skin breakdown and pressure ulcers, blood glucose control, use of catheters and the length of their use, mechanical ventilation rates and the rates of pneumonias, and rates of nosocomial infections).
- *Economic Outcomes:* the use of health resources (direct costs) and the inability to use the same resources for other worthwhile purposes (opportunity costs, saved days, cost savings). Costs associated with adverse events.
- *Health Outcomes:* the outcomes that patients experience both physically and mentally (i.e., the quality of life, including death, functional

disability, appearance, pain, anxiety, and peace of mind); patient satisfaction. Outcomes may be immediate, such as inconvenience, discomfort, or acute adverse effects, or they may be delayed, such as subsequent changes in physiological or functional status that would not have occurred in the absence of the intervention.

▪ *Institutional Outcomes:* collaborative (interdisciplinary) practice; provision of high-quality care; effective use of resources; a positive and supportive environmental culture (i.e., a culture of caring), cost containment and effectiveness, decreased wait time in the emergency room, effective leadership and management (Huber, 2006; Kleinpell, 2007; Marshall, 2008).

CONSIDERATIONS WHEN ESTABLISHING OUTCOMES MANAGEMENT PROGRAMS

Numerous healthcare accrediting bodies, researchers, and governmental agencies are actively attempting to identify appropriate and valid outcomes measures, with their ultimate goal being to create national quality indicator databases. As yet, no comprehensive classification of nursing-sensitive patient outcomes or standardized measures exists, except the American Nurses Association (ANA) Report Card, nor does such a system exist for nursing case management. Contemporary research must be directed at assessing the content validity and nursing sensitivity of indicators and measurement outcomes for nursing practice. Outcomes and indicators should be field tested in a variety of settings for nursing practice and case management. Nurses and nurse case managers must measure, evaluate, and validate what they do and how their services affect the nation's health and healthcare systems. Clinical performance is quantifiable—hence the importance of outcomes research in nursing practice.

THE AMERICAN NURSES ASSOCIATION REPORT CARD

The development of the ANA Report Card for Acute Care Settings is one of the major accomplishments of the ANA, which has long sought to develop quality indicators for nursing practice (Huber, 2006). In 1995, the ANA's board of directors proposed the development of a report card for nursing in acute care settings, in response to the mandate from accrediting organizations for outcomes measurements. Outcomes measures can provide insight into structural components and care processes that may influence quality (Duffy & Korniewicz, 2002). The ANA developed specific indicators for the ANA Report Card (see

TABLE 13-5 Nursing Outcomes Indicators for Acute Care Settings

- Nosocomial infection rates
- Patient fall rates
- Patient satisfaction with nursing care
- Patient satisfaction with pain management
- Patient satisfaction with educational information
- Patient satisfaction in general with care
- Maintenance of skin integrity
- Nursing job and staff satisfaction

TABLE 13-6 Four Structural Indicators for Outcomes Management

- The staffing mix of nurses, licensed practical nurses, and unlicensed staff caring for patients in an acute care setting
- The ratio of registered nurses with direct patient care responsibilities to practical nurses and unlicensed workers (expressed as full-time employees [FTEs])
- The total number of hours worked by nursing staff with direct patient care responsibilities on acute care units per patient per day
- The impact of time available for nursing care related to the rate of nosocomial infections

Source: Duffy & Korniewicz, 2002.

Table 13-5), including the methods by which each indicator was to be calculated.

Table 13-6 lists four indicators that were identified by the ANA as structural or organizational indicators. They could also serve as environmental indicators, however.

Nurses and nurse case managers should use the ANA Report Card as a basis to continue to refine the outcomes indicators used for their profession. Given that the ANA Report Card documents the number of nurses per patient, the ANA is using the results as a way of communicating to decision makers that reducing the number of qualified and experienced nurses per patient (i.e., the nurse–patient ratio) may jeopardize the quality of care. The ANA has published several books addressing the studies related to staffing and the staff mix and the influence of these factors on patient care outcomes.

Several other agencies have developed "report cards" for outcomes. For example, the American Hospitals Association, in conjunction with the American Medical Colleges, developed the Hospital Quality Initiative for this purpose. Also, the National Committee for Quality Assurance (NCQA) developed "The State of Health Care Quality" tool to collect data on the quality of health care for accreditation purposes. Many other instruments are available as well (Data and Research Resource Center and Library, 2006).

THE ENVIRONMENTAL (ORGANIZATIONAL) CULTURE IN NURSING

There is growing concern about staffing ratios, which take into account both the number of patients assigned to a nurse and the patient's acuity (ANA, 2000/2008). In particular, the ANA has been studying nurses' views on workplace safety. Fifty-five percent of the nurse participants in an ANA study believed that the organizational climate affected the safety of both nurses and their patients. A majority of the participants who were surveyed claimed that nurses were feeling pressured to work harder and longer and that the workplace was becoming increasingly stressful, which they believe affected the quality of care, because they were often tempted to take shortcuts. The same pressures also increased the number of needle-stick injuries to nurses (*The American Nurse*, 2008).

Increasingly, nurse scientists have been focusing on the care environment —that is, the organizational culture. *Culture* is defined as the values, beliefs, norms, expectations, and assumptions that are shared by a group of people that link them to a group or an organizational system (Long & Byers, 2007). In one study, eight tools were developed and selected to measure the work environment. The researchers concluded that a positive work environment leads to the avoidance of medication errors, safety for the patient, and improves the quality of nursing care (Long & Byers, 2007).

A second study by Aiken, Clarke, Sloane, Lake, and Cheney (2008) examined the work environment in relation to nurses' job satisfaction, burnout, and the intention of leaving, along with the quality of care, mortality rates, and failure to rescue patients. These researchers found that improved staffing, emphasizing hiring of registered nurses and better educated and more skilled nurses, improved the care environment. They concluded that investing in staff development produced good relationships between physicians and nurses, and improved the quality of management and supervision, which in turn resulted in better patient outcomes. They claimed that these are the characteristics found in Magnet hospitals (i.e., hospitals that have been recognized by the American Nurses Association and the American Nurses Credentialing Center as providing superior nursing care), which allow these facilities to attract and retain quality employees.

Another study by Boltz, Capezuti, Bowar-Ferres, et al. (2008) examined nurses' perceptions of the geriatric nursing practice environment in the hospital. These researchers found that the quality of geriatric care was greatly influenced by the degree of organizational support that the nurses experienced. Three factors were identified as the most influential: (1) available resources; (2) institutional values regarding older adults; and (3) the degree of collaboration among the members of the healthcare team.

TABLE 13-7 Nursing Outcomes Indicators

---

1. Behavioral status
2. Functional status
3. Knowledge about the illness and treatment
4. Family functioning, family strain
5. Safety
6. Symptom control and interventions
7. Quality of life
8. Goal attainment
9. Client satisfaction
10. Costs and resource utilization

Source: Marek, cited in Huber, 2006.

TOOLS, INSTRUMENTS, AND INDICATORS FOR HOME HEALTH CARE

Nursing outcomes were developed by Marek (1989, 1997, cited in Huber, 2006), who identified the 10 indicators listed in Table 13-7.

Various organizations developed tools for accreditation during the 1990s. For example, the **Health Plan Employer Data Information Set (HEDIS)** was developed by the National Committee for Quality Assurance (NCQA). HEDIS is a data and information set used to rate managed care organizations that provide home health care; it is intended for use by employers, who examine the information when selecting health plans for their employees that include home health care. The HEDIS database contains multiple measures focusing on the following areas:

- The quality and effectiveness of care
- Access and availability of care
- Satisfaction with care
- Health plan stability
- Use of services and their costs
- Informed care choices and descriptive information about the health plan

The survey gathering this information is administered annually to the members of each managed care organization. Progress toward meeting the U.S. Public Health Service's *Healthy People 2010* goals is also examined. This information is made available to clients, employers, and insurers, enabling them to make comparisons among managed care organizations (Clevenger, 2008; Huber 2006).

The **Omaha System** has been used for more than 25 years to answer two basic questions: (1) What are the most frequently occurring clinical problems?

and (2) Which interventions are implemented for the most frequent problems? Four categories of activities are assessed in this system (Table 13-8), and a problem rating scale (a Likert-type scale) has been designed to measure the patient's progress related to the identified activities. A study of the Omaha System by Erci (2005) demonstrated that a case management program in home health has a significant influence on outcomes related to specific problems, especially in the areas of education, counseling, treatment, case management, and surveillance.

OUTCOMES MEASUREMENT IN ACUTE CARE SETTINGS

Table 13-9 identifies the instruments used to measure outcomes in acute care settings.

TABLE 13-8 Categories of Activities Assessed by the Omaha System

1. Health teaching, guidance, and counseling
2. Treatment and procedures
3. Case management (coordination, advocacy, and referral)
4. Surveillance (detection, critical analysis, and monitoring)

TABLE 13-9 Instruments for Outcomes Management

Protocols	Tools to predict the critical targets that a patient is to achieve within a specified period to time, along with the efficient use of resources.
NCM care plans	Plans that identify goals, outline nursing interventions, and provide for the evaluation of patient outcomes.
Practice guidelines	Clinical guidelines based on algorithms that are both evidence based and related to the diagnosis and management of the patient's clinical condition.
Critical pathways	Guidelines based on standards of practice for all disciplines involved in the patient's care. The guidelines are based on evidence-based standards of practice. The pathway serves as a roadmap that specifies the critical incidents and interventions that must occur along the patient's path to recovery. It maps the time and the sequence of interventions for a specific diagnosis.
Care map	A multidisciplinary comprehensive care plan that includes a current and retrospective analysis of variances from the patient's plan of care.

Sources: Huber, 2006; Whitehill, 2005.

Clinical/Critical Pathways

A **clinical pathway (CP)** is a multidisciplinary management tool that depicts important events that should take place sequentially on a day-to-day basis, while the patient is in the hospital (Schriefer & Botter, 2001). These tools were first introduced in 1985 by the New England Medical Center, which sought to incorporate expected outcomes within specific time frames (Cohen & Cesta, 2005; Rossi, 2003). They have also been defined as structured multidisciplinary patient care plans that document diagnostic and therapeutic interventions performed by nurses, physicians, and other team members for a particular diagnosis or procedure. CPs are time-specific blueprints for planning a patient's treatment during hospitalization to meet predetermined outcomes.

Clinical pathways evolved from protocols, algorithms, and standards of care, in response to the movement toward diagnosis-related groups (DRGs). These guidelines were developed to assist healthcare providers in determining the preferred pathway to obtain the best outcomes in the shortest period of time (Whitehill, 2005). Good outcomes are the result of consistent quality care.

Clinical pathways differ from nursing care plans in the following ways:

- CPs are targeted to a client's specific DRG. In other words, CPs are specific to a diagnosis and are not patient centered, but may be modified to individualize the plan according to the patient's needs.
- CPs are interdisciplinary (identifying who does what and when), and identify the collaborative partners on the team.
- CPs contain a timeline (hours, days, weeks, or phases).
- CPs identify and measure specific outcomes (clinical, functional, system process, financial, patient satisfaction).
- CPs monitor the patient's progress to identify any variances (e.g., patient/family, caregiver, internal system, external systems deviations) (Whitehill, 2005).

Because CPs are so diagnostically specific, they were found not to be applicable in psychiatric settings. For example, the symptoms experienced by one patient with schizophrenia may differ drastically from the symptoms experienced by another patient with the same diagnosis, who may also have a different course of the disease. Some organizations have now abandoned CPs; for example, most hospitals in the Triad area of North Carolina (Winston-Salem, Greensboro, and High Point) are no longer using them. Nevertheless, CPs can still be found in some hospital units, so the case manager should still be aware of this planning and evaluation tool.

Multidisciplinary Action Plans

The terms "clinical pathways," "multidisciplinary plans," and "multidisciplinary action plans" (MAPs) are frequently used interchangeably (Rossi, 2003). The MAP developed from CPs as case management grew into a more multidisciplinary collaborative practice. Care maps accomplish similar goals and outcomes as CPs. They increase the ease of evaluating cost-effectiveness and quality of care, focus on standards of care for specific types of diagnoses, identify variances in the delivery of care, and link CQI to collaborative practice and integrated resource allocation, patient care outcomes, and cost reimbursement systems. Care maps encompass a multidisciplinary plan of care for coordinating the interdisciplinary interventions and provide a central place for documenting each of the discipline's interventions (Cohen & Cesta, 2005). One of the best outcomes that has resulted from the widespread use of care maps has been improved communication among the disciplines.

Variances

Variances are deviations from expected outcomes or events. Four types of variances are distinguished:

- *Operational variances:* broken equipment; departmental delays; larger system delays; problems with insurance coverage; discharge delays because of lack of access to home care services or home equipment.
- *Healthcare provider variances:* deviations from the plan of care; physician practice variations; differing levels of expertise and experience among nurses, physicians, and other providers.
- *Patient variances:* refusal to comply; changes in physical and emotional status; changes in family status.
- *Unmet clinical indicators:* patient functioning; mental acuity; the ability to perform a return demonstration on home equipment prior to discharge (Mateo, Matzke, & Newton, 2002)

OTHER MEASUREMENT TOOLS FOR DETERMINING QUALITY

Benchmarking

With benchmarking, the data of one institution are compared to the data of another facility that has been identified as both a comparable institution and an excellent one. Benchmarking compares actual practice to best practice (Foster, 2003). It is a process of measuring what exists against what is identified as best (Pelletier & Albright, 2006). Benchmarking compares the data from one's own institution or one's own performance with the best practices or performance of another professional or healthcare organization using quality indicators across institutions (Hogan & Nickitas, 2009; Sullivan & Decker, 2009). The ability to benchmark or to compare data from one institution to another excellent institution contributes to developing standards of care (Goode, 2005).

Evidence-Based Practice

Evidence-based practice (EBP) has been defined as the use of the most current evidence when making patient care decisions based on valid research. It is the process of integrating clinical knowledge and expertise with the best available clinical evidence obtained from the results of systematic research (Mateo, 2001). It is the application of research findings to clinical practice to improve outcomes. According to Marshall (2008), this best practice also applies to nursing management, which implies that the nurse leader/manager uses the best evidence in making both clinical and organizational decisions.

The goals of EBP are to standardize interventions by healthcare professionals, thereby reducing the variations of medical practice across geographical areas. Ideally, cost savings will be the result of standardizing care, thus enhancing best practices and eliminating poor practices. EBP should guide decision making so that the decision maker is the right person, who has the right information, which is received at the right time (Cohen & Cesta, 2005).

The application of the latest research findings should guide the healthcare provider in decision making to evaluate the efficacy of alternative treatments. The individual clinician's expertise is integrated with the best available research evidence from systematic studies in making patient care decisions (Rossi, 2003). Table 13-10 lists the various sources from which to obtain the best evidence.

According to Quick, Nordstrom, and Johnson (2006), the implementation of evidence-based medicine is being driven by the demand for public reporting of outcomes data. Documenting and publicly reporting clinical outcomes; financial performance; patient, physician, and employee satisfaction; and good relationships with payers leads to financial success for hospitals.

Analysis of Cost–Benefit Ratios

Documenting savings is absolutely necessary for the survival of case management. Reports that illustrate financial savings for the institution versus the

TABLE 13-10 Sources of Best Evidence

1. Pathophysiology
2. Cost-effectiveness analysis
3. Benchmarking
4. Clinical expertise
5. Infection control
6. International, national, and local standards
7. Quality improvement and risk data
8. Retrospective or current chart reviews
9. Patient preference related to cultural and religious beliefs
10. Research
11. Internet sources
12. Websites
13. Literature
14. Colleagues
15. Professional standards of practice
16. Patient surveys and other measurement tools (may be designed for specific purposes by national organizations, or by healthcare institutions, or by a healthcare discipline to meet its current needs for documentation)

Source: Rossi, 2003.

costs of a case management program should be analyzed and reported in terms of the cost–benefit ratio—that is, dollars saved versus dollars spent (Mullahy, 2004). A cost–benefit analysis compares patient outcomes with the costs of equipment and technology, the overall costs of treatment (including the salaries of the health professionals), and program costs (Austin & Wetle, 2008). The report of this ratio should go to important stakeholders, such as the chief executive officer (CEO), the chief financial officer (CFO), and the director of nursing (DON). This kind of cost–benefit analysis should be ongoing; it should not only communicate the dollar savings, but also document the other benefits of case management to patients, staff, and the overall institution (Mullahy, 2004). The analysis should include the staff's experiences of having a nurse case manager available to them and to their patients and should document the patient care needs that were addressed by the nurse case manager.

Included in the cost–benefit analysis report are the savings that are directly related to the work of the nurse case manager, proving that this role reduced the cost of care and was worth the cost of the case management program (*hard savings*). A reduction of payer denials, reduced costs due to improved care coordination, and reduced duplication of services are also direct savings that may be attributable to the work of the nurse case manager (Daniels & Ramey, 2005). For example, in one hospital, the number of "frequent flyer" visits to the emergency department (ED) made by one patient declined after a nurse case manager and her social worker partner worked with the patient, along with the community primary care provider, to teach the patient about the appropriate use of the ED and alternative community agencies that are readily available. The smaller number of ED visits saved the hospital thousands of dollars (Bristow & Herrick, 2002).

Early case finding is another outcome that should be addressed in the cost–benefit analysis. Early case finding by identifying a pending acute problem may reduce costs in the long term (*soft savings*). For example, hospitalizing a diabetic patient before a diabetic crisis occurs reduces potential complications. The nurse case manager may then refer the patient to a dietician and diabetic classes to ensure better self-management in the future. Initially, the costs may be higher, but the eventual outcomes are improved and costs are saved.

Saving hospital days by timely discharges also results in cost containment. These kinds of soft savings (indirect savings) may or may not directly result from case management but still save money—for example, in the form of fewer postoperative complications, a reduction in readmission rates, fewer nosocomial infections, and improved transitions from one level of care to the next. Although indirect costs may be difficult to quantify, they should be included in the cost–benefit analysis report.

Case managers must document the value of what they do. After each case has been closed, a summary of the case manager's interventions and the outcomes for each patient, along with a financial analysis of the dollars spent versus dollars saved, should be included in the final cost–benefit report (Mullahy, 2004).

PROGRAM EVALUATION

Evaluation is the collection and analysis of information, using various methodological strategies, to determine the relevance, progress, efficiency, effectiveness, performance, and effects of a program on healthcare outcomes (Vann, 2006). It is an investigative process to determine whether the program outcomes match the expectations (Sullivan & Decker, 2009). Various strategies can be used to determine the efficiency, effectiveness, and impact of a case management program (Vann, 2006). Evaluation provides nurse case managers with the chance to conduct research, while collecting outcomes data to substantiate the worth of the case management program (Cohen & Cesta, 2005). Table 13-11 identifies the methods most frequently used in program evaluation.

TABLE 13-11 Strategies Used in Program Evaluation

- Data collection.

- Monitoring: tracking performance over time.

- Outcome measures: data that indicate the results of an action or intervention in meeting the goals of the program. Outcomes are often used to measure success, such as the state of the patient's health following an intervention.

- Process measures: the behaviors and activities of the healthcare providers—for example, teaching the patient self-care and having the patient correctly do a return demonstration.

- Trend analysis (time-series analysis): an examination of performance over time that determines whether changes in performance occur at a time when a new program or a new intervention is implemented.

Source: Vann, 2006.

The sources of data with which to evaluate case management services should have the following characteristics: relevancy, reliability, and validity. The sources of these data may be reports, online or hard-copy data, analysis of process and outcomes data, documentation systems, program descriptions, case studies, monitoring systems, surveys, and trend analysis.

Vann (2006) described a multimodel evaluation plan, applied to community settings, using different strategies that are applicable for evaluating case management programs in diverse settings. She developed an evaluation/planning tool that focused on pediatric patients whose care was covered by Medicaid. Vann found that designing an evaluation plan for community case management was a challenge because the community services vary so widely, the case managers come from different disciplines, and case management services often operate within complex health delivery systems with different organizational cultures. Thus it proved difficult to isolate the outcomes of case management from other services that were offered in the same setting.

Vann (2006) concluded from this study that, because of the continuing emphasis on cost containment, case management programs must routinely evaluate their strengths and weaknesses. Agencies should establish an evaluation plan to determine the quality of their programs, thereby enabling them to continually improve their programs and their clinical outcomes. Multimodel strategies are the best approach to evaluating community case management services. Nurse case managers and disease managers should be actively involved in conducting research on patient care outcomes.

■ SUMMARY

Data-based decision making in case management is required; thus it is essential for case managers to collect the right data to document their interventions, the patient's responses, and the outcomes. Data-driven decision making is a key part of the modern-day case manager's job (Barton & Skiba, 2005).

Outcomes are the endpoints to be used when evaluating patient care and program effectiveness. Evaluation should be conducted continuously within the healthcare organization. The challenge is to build a patient-centered multidisciplinary model to determine outcomes that includes clinical endpoints, functional status, patient and family well-being, patient and staff satisfaction, and cost–benefit ratios that demonstrate the delivery of cost-effective, quality care. Both nursing and case management programs need to constantly evaluate the effectiveness of their interventions to meet the desired outcomes (Huber, 2006).

The case management department must document its financial contributions to the organization and the improvements in the quality of care attributable to its work. Outcomes data must consistently be collected, analyzed, and disseminated to the appropriate stakeholders, so as to support the existence of the case management program (McGettigan & Marshall, 2003). Without good documentation of its effectiveness, case management will be past history, rather than an essential part of the future of nursing and health care. As data analysis becomes more sophisticated and public reporting more accessible to the consumer, program managers will also be expected to collect and analyze outcomes. The "mantra" of both case management and disease management must be "Begin with the outcomes in mind" (Howe, 2005, p. 4).

■ CASE STUDIES

You work for a home healthcare agency that serves a large at-risk pediatric population. Recently, a number of urinary infections have been diagnosed in those children with indwelling catheters. The data suggest a 25% increase in the infection rate over the past 6 months. The home care company has been notified that these data may influence its reimbursement rates in the future. Describe the plan of action you would implement to decrease the infection rate and improve patient outcomes.

■ DISCUSSION QUESTIONS

1. What is the difference between outcomes measurement and outcomes management?
2. Why is case management outcomes driven rather than process driven?
3. What have been the driving forces influencing outcomes?
4. What are clinical pathways?

■ CLASSROOM EXERCISES

Working with your classmates, answer the following questions:

1. Which outcomes measures are used to assess your unit's effectiveness? Where are those data stored?
2. Are the outcomes data shared with the staff?
3. How are the outcomes data used to improve care?
4. Identify and discuss the most frequently used outcomes indicators.
5. Discuss appropriate documentation of outcomes measures.

■ RECOMMENDED READINGS

Aiken, L. H., Clarke, S. P., Sloane, D. M., Lake, E. T., & Cheney, T. (2008). Effects of hospital care environment on patient mortality and nurse outcomes. *Journal of Nursing Administration, 38*(5), 223–229.

Aliotta, S. L. (2006). Key functions and direct outcomes of case management. In E. L. Cohen & T. G. Cesta (Eds.), *Nursing case management: From essentials to advanced practice applications* (4th ed., pp. 415–421). St. Louis, MO: Elsevier/ Mosby.

Marshall, D. R. (2008). Evidence-based management: The path to best outcomes. *Journal of Nursing Administration, 38*(5), 295–307.

Rosenthal, M. B. (2007). Nonpayment for performance? Medicare's new reimbursement rule. *New England Journal of Medicine, 357*(16), 1573–1575.

■ REFERENCES

Aiken, L. H., Clarke, S.P., Sloane, D. M., Lake, E. T., & Cheney, T. (2008). Effects of hospital care environment on patient mortality and nurse outcomes. *Journal of Nursing Administration, 38*(5), 223–229.

Aliotta, S. L. (2006). Key functions and direct outcomes of case management. In E. L. Cohen & T. G. Cesta (Eds.), *Nursing case management: From essentials to advanced practice applications* (4th ed., pp. 415–421). St. Louis, MO: Elsevier/ Mosby.

American Nurses Association (ANA). (2000/2008). *Executive summary: Nurse staffing and patient outcomes in the inpatient hospital setting.* Retrieved from http://www.nursingworld.org/FunctionalMenuCategories/MediaResources/ PressReleases/20

American Nurses Credentialing Center (ANCC). (2008). Modifying the Magnet model: The shape of things to come. *American Nurse Today, 3*(7), 22.

Austin, A., & Wetle, V. (2008). Health care providers: Nurses. In *The United States health care system: Combining business, health and delivery* (pp. 71–83). Upper Saddle River, NJ: Pearson/Prentice Hall.

Barton, A .J., & Skiba, D. J. (2005). The data-driven health care environment. In E. L. Cohen and T. G. Cesta (Eds.), *Nursing case management: From essentials to advanced practice applications* (4th ed., pp. 444–461). St. Louis, MO: Elsevier/ Mosby.

Boltz, M., Capezuti, E., Bowar-Ferres, S., Norman, R., Secic, M., Kim, H., et al. (2008). Hospital nurses' perceptions of the geriatric nurse practice environment. *Journal of Nursing Scholarship, 40*(3), 282–289.

Bristow, D. P., & Herrick, C. A. (2002). Emergency department case management. *Lippincott's Case Management, 7*(6), 243–254.

Centers for Medicare and Medicaid Services (CMS). (2005/2007). *Press release: Medicare "Pay for Performance P4P" initiatives.* Retrieved from http://www.cms. gov/apps/media/press/factsheet.asp?Counter=1343

Clevenger, K. (2008). Care of clients in the home setting. In M. J. Clark (Ed.), *Community nursing: Advocacy for population health* (5th ed., p. 577–602). Upper Saddle River, NJ: Prentice Hall.

Cohen, E. L., & Cesta, T. G. (2005). *Nursing case management: From essentials to advanced practice applications* (4th ed.). St. Louis, MO: Elsevier/Mosby.

Daniels, S., & Ramey, M. (2005). *The leader's guide to hospital case management.* Sudbury, MA: Jones and Bartlett.

Data and Research Resource Center and Library. (2006). *Key topic guide series: Quality measurement/outcomes. Report cards.* Retrieved from http://www. mahealthdata.org/data/library/10-outcomes.html

Duffy, J. F., & Korniewicz, D. M. (2002). *Quality indicators: Outcomes measurement using the ANA safety and quality indicators. ANA Continuing Education until December 31, 2002.* Retrieved from http://www.nursingworld.org/mods/archive/ mod72ceomfull.htm

Erci, B. (2005). Global case management: The impact of case management on client outcomes. *Lippincott's Case Management, 10*(1), 2–38.

Field trends: Coordination reduces Medicare spending. (2009, June/July). *Case in Point*, 16.

Foster, A. P. (2003). Quality management for case managers. In P. A. Rossi (Ed.), *Case management in health care* (2nd ed., pp. 734–749). Philadelphia: Saunders.

Goode, C. J. (2005). Outcomes effectiveness and evidence based practice. In E. L. Cohen & T. G. Cesta (Eds.), *Nursing case management: From essentials to advanced practice applications* (4th ed., pp. 572–579). St. Louis, MO: Elsevier/ Mosby.

Hogan, M. A., & Nickitas, D. M. (2009). *Nursing leadership and management: Reviews and rationales.* Upper Saddle River, NJ: Prentice Hall.

Howe, R. (2005). *The disease manager's handbook.* Sudbury, MA: Jones and Bartlett.

Huber, D. L. (Ed.). (2006). Measuring and managing outcomes. In *Leadership and nursing case management* (3rd ed., pp. 869–883; Glossary, pp. 885–892). Philadelphia: Saunders/Elsevier.

Kirchheimer, B. (2008), Wrestling with a new reality. *Nursing Spectrum, 4*(4), 30–31.

Kleinpell, R. M. (2007, May). APNs: Invisible champions. *Nursing Management, 38*(15), 18–22.

Long, T., & Byers, J. F. (2007). A review of organizational culture instruments for nurse executives. *Journal of Nursing Administration, 37*(1), 21–31.

Marshall, D. R. (2008). Evidence-based management: The path to best outcomes. *Journal of Nursing Administration, 38*(5), 295–307.

Mateo, M. A. (2001). Using evidence-based practice in providing care. *Lippincott's Nursing Case Management, 6*(1), 19–23.

Mateo, M. A., Matzke, K., & Newton, C. (2002). Designing measurements to assess case management outcomes. *Lippincott's Case Management, 7*(6), 261–266.

McGettigan, B. S., & Marshall, D. R. (2003). Effective reporting of case management outcomes. *Lippincott's Case Management, 8*(6), 237–240.

Meyer, L. C. (2009, June/July). Health and performance improvement (HPI). *Case in Point*, 28–30. Retrieved from http://www.guidedcare.org/pdf/CaseInPoint_ HPI_060109.pdf

Mullahy, C. M. (Ed.). (2004). Financial and quality assurance reporting: Cost–benefit analysis reports. In *The case manager's handbook* (3rd ed., pp. 297–404). Sudbury, MA: Jones and Bartlett.

Pelletier, L. R., & Albright, L. A. (2006). Quality improvement and health care safety. In D. L. Huber (Ed.), *Leadership and nursing care management* (3rd ed., pp. 827–867). Philadelphia: Saunders/Elsevier.

Quick, B., Nordstrom S., & Johnson, K. (2006). Using continuous quality improvement to implement evidence-based medicine. *Lippincott's Case Management, 11*(6), 305–315.

Rosenthal, M. B. (2007). Nonpayment for performance? Medicare's new reimbursement rule. *New England Journal of Medicine, 357*(16), 1573–1575. Retrieved from http://www. content.nejm.org/egi/content/full/357/16/1573

Rossi, P. A. (2003). Case *management in health care* (2nd ed.). Philadelphia: Saunders/Elsevier.

Roussel, L., & Swansburg, R. C. (2006). Performance appraisal. In L. Roussel, R. C. Swansburg, & R. J. Swansburg (Eds.), *Management and leadership for nursing administrators* (4th ed., pp. 437–468). Sudbury, MA: Jones and Bartlett.

Schriefer, J. A., & Botter, M. L. (2001). Clinical pathways and guidelines. *Outcomes Management in Nursing Practice, 5*(3), 95–98.

Sullivan, E. J., & Decker, P. J. (2009). *Effective leadership and management in Nursing* (6th ed.). Upper Saddle River NJ: Pearson/Prentice Hall.

The American Nurse. (2008, July/August). In brief: Workplace study, p. 5.

Vann, J. C. (2006). Measuring community-based case management performance. *Lippincott's Case Management, 11*(3), 147–157.

White, A.B. (2004). Case management and the national quality agenda: Partnering to improve the quality of care. *Lippincott's Case Management, 9*(3), 132–140.

Whitehill, C. (2005). A model of emergency department case management: Developing strategies and outcomes. In E .L. Cohen & T. G. Cesta (Eds.), *Nursing case management applications: From essentials to advanced practice* (4th ed., pp. 166–177). St. Louis, MO: Elsevier/Mosby.

Wright, B. B. (2006). Quality management. In L. Roussel, R. C. Swansburg, & R. J. Swansburg (Eds.), *Management and leadership for nurse administrators* (4th ed., pp. 407–427). Sudbury, MA: Jones and Bartlett.

Ethical Issues in Nursing Case Management

Laura J. Fero
Charlotte A. Herrick

14

■ Outline

■ OBJECTIVES

1. Discuss the reasons to study ethics.

2. Define the terms that are commonly used in ethical and philosophical discussions.

3. Identify the core values in the Nursing Code of Ethics.

4. Compare and contrast philosophical models that can be applied to solving an ethical dilemma.

5. Identify the ethical principles that should guide the actions of the nurse case manager.

6. Discuss the challenges that the nurse case manager faces when solving ethical dilemmas.

7. Describe the steps in ethical decision making and the competencies necessary to determine the answer to an ethical question.

8. Describe the objectives and functions of the interdisciplinary healthcare team while participating on an ethics committee.

9. Discuss the relationship between ethics and the law.

INTRODUCTION

Ethics is a branch of philosophy that attempts to deal with important questions involving human conduct. Because of the complexity of health care today and the advancement of technology, there is a need to attend

TABLE 14-1 Reasons for Studying Ethics

- To improve sensitivity to ethical issues
- To enhance awareness of making ethical decisions
- To improve the ability to foresee consequences
- To enhance self-awareness of one's own values, which may or may not conflict with others' values
- To improve the ability to systematically make ethical decisions based on logic and appropriate rationale rather than based on intuition
- To assist the nurse case manager to strive for ethical competence

to the values conflicts and ethical problems, which are often critical to decision making in health care. For these and other reasons (Table 14-1), the study of ethics has become important to nursing and nursing case management (NCM).

Myths Commonly Found in Healthcare Ethics

Ethical principles provide guidelines for practice, but they do not provide all of the answers and are not a "quick fix." Following are some myths about ethics that need to be addressed in the healthcare setting.

The healthcare professional can apply appropriate ethical principles and come up with the right answer.

The definition of a dilemma is that *there is no one right answer.*

Ethical principles make values and other principles irrelevant.

No set of values or principles is irrelevant, nor should any one set of values or principles have priority over others. The nurse case manager must choose which values or principles have priority and act accordingly.

There is only one right way to make an ethical decision and to do an ethical analysis.

There is no one right way to make a decision. The nurse case manager must consider the patient's beliefs, values, and rights as well as his or her own, including the nurse's Code of Ethics and the case manager's Standards of Practice. Ethical models can guide decision making for logic and consistency. When the nurse case manager makes a decision about an ethical issue, he or she should be able to clearly articulate the rationale for that decision and the steps followed in reaching that conclusion.

Definitions

Ethics is a branch of philosophy that attempts to answer questions about broad issues of morality, values, and human conduct, using universal principles to guide decision making. It guides individual and professional conduct by stating the ideal conduct. Ethical principles provide standards that may be at a higher level than the law. The law adheres to minimum standards of conduct and, if the law is breached, there are legal consequences (Nielsen, 2002).

Morals are the established rules of conduct to guide behavior, which determine right or wrong. Inherent in morals are judgmental implications.

Values are the intrinsic worth of objects, customs, norms, and behaviors, which may change over time. Values are standards of choice that provide a frame of reference as we integrate, appraise, and explain events and relationships.

Values clarification is a conscious process of identifying and ranking the importance of one's own values that guide personal and professional decisions. Values clarification enhances self-awareness and is important for nurses and case managers, so that they can achieve the following goals:

- Determine one's own values and beliefs
- Make decisions that are congruent with one's own values
- Identify priorities
- Enhance decision making, which motivates or determines action (Simon, Howe, & Kirschenbaur, 1972, cited in Hogan & Nickitas, 2009)

Personal values are standards that are chosen to guide one's personal behavior. To determine your own values, follow these steps:

1. Establish a hierarchy of values.
2. Prioritize your values and rank-order them from the most to the least important.
3. Choose freely what is important to you to guide your behavior.

Professional values are the core values of a profession—that is, the strongly held beliefs about good professional practice. Values are the fundamentals regarding nursing and case management strategies. Professional values set a standard of behavior higher than the legal standards (Hogan & Nickitas, 2009).

Most professions have developed an **ethical code of conduct** (code of ethics) that identifies the core values of the profession. Codes of ethics are guidelines for professional practice, including nursing practice and the practice of case management. The nurse case manager must—for both legal and ethical reasons—follow the codes of professional conduct developed by the American

Nurses Association (ANA) and the Case Management Society of America (*Standards of Practice for Case Management*) and the Commission for Case Management Certification (*Code of Professional Conduct for Case Managers with Disciplinary Rules, Procedures and Penalties*) (ANA, 2006; Moreo & Lamb, 2003; Mullahy, 2004, pp. 131–141).

Rights are just and valid claims. Rights give us dignity and protection and are derived from human needs. There are three types of rights:

- *Legal rights:* backed by laws
- *Probable rights:* likely to be backed by law if the case went to court
- *Human rights:* based on maintaining human dignity

CORE VALUES IN NURSING PRACTICE

Core values in nursing practice can be found in the ANA's Code of Ethics. Some of these values are highlighted here:

- A commitment to serve others—individuals, groups, and communities
- Respect for the rights of patients and others
- Caring
- Respect for the dignity and the uniqueness of each individual
- A commitment to lifelong learning and continuing competence
- Honesty and integrity
- A concern for the welfare of people and society
- Protection of the patient's rights to privacy and safety
- Responsibility and accountability to the patient, family, and profession (ANA, 2006)

The Patient's Bill of Rights

The Patient's Bill of Rights is posted in most all nursing care units in hospitals. See Table 14-2.

The Nurse's Bill of Rights

Table 14-3 summarizes the Nurse's Bill of Rights.

Duties are associated with rights; for every right there is a duty. There are three types of duties:

- *Legal duties:* obligations prescribed by law, which relate to role status or position (e.g., the Nurse Practice Act)
- *Protection of human rights*, including patient rights

TABLE 14-2 The Patient's Bill of Rights

Patients have the right to:
- Emergency treatment
- Informed consent
- All invasive medical procedures with written consent
- Confidentiality and privacy
- Palliative care
- Patient advocacy
- Research and human experimentation with written consent
- Protection from medical malpractice
- Organ donation and transplantation

TABLE 14-3 The Nurse's Bill of Rights

Nurses have the right to:
- Practice in a manner that fulfills their obligations to society and to those who receive nursing care.
- Practice in an environment that allows the nurse to act in accordance with professional standards and legally authorized scope of practice.
- Work in an environment that supports and facilitates ethical practice in accordance with the code of ethics for nurses and its interpretive statements.
- Freely and openly advocate for themselves and their patients without fear of retribution.
- Receive fair compensation for their work, consistent with their knowledge, experience, and professional responsibilities.
- Work in an environment that is safe for themselves and their patients.
- Negotiate the conditions of their employment, either as an individual or collectively, in all practice settings.

Source: Wiseman, 2001, p. 57.

- *Ethical duties:* responsibilities based on ethical principles or a professional code of ethics, such as the ANA Code of Ethics (Taylor, 2005, pp. 362, 363)

PHILOSOPHICAL MODELS FOR ETHICAL DECISION MAKING

Philosophical models for ethical decisions essentially evolved from two basic philosophical systems of thought: deontology and utilitarianism. Deontology, which emerged from Judeo-Christian theology, is based on ethical rules such as the Ten Commandments. Utilitarianism was advanced by the philosopher John Stuart Mill, who espoused the rule "The greatest good for the greatest number" (Beauchamp & Childress, 2001).

The Deontological Model

The roots of "deontology" are *deon*, meaning "deity," and *logos*, meaning "discourse." This school of thought grew out of the Judeo-Christian tradition, as espoused by writers such as Thomas Aquinas and Immanuel Kant. In this model, rules, values, morals, and ethics are determined from the word of God and, therefore, are unchangeable. Moral principles are laid by divine order; they are fixed and require adherence to universal principles. The nature of an act is inherently moral or immoral without regard for the consequences. The focus is on the act, *not* on the outcome. According to Kant, moral imperatives are absolutes and include autonomy, freedom, dignity, self-respect, and respect for individual rights. He subscribed to an ethical model in which there are no exceptions and the rules are absolutely binding. According to Aquinas, actions are appropriate, if they are in accord with the principles of nature. The Ten Commandments are the key principles handed down by God and, therefore, serve as the rules of nature. In simple terms, this philosophy can be summarized as "the end does not justify the means."

Steps in Decision Making Using the Deontological Model as a Guide

1. Identify the problem.
2. List the rules and principles according to the Ten Commandments.
3. List the alternative solutions according to the rules and principles.
4. Compare and contrast the solutions.
   - Is there one alternative that is consistent with the rules? If so, there is only one right action.
   - Are there several alternatives that are consistent with the rules? If there are several right actions, then prioritize them and select one as long as it abides by the Ten Commandments.
   - If there is no solution to the dilemma, appeal to a higher power or redefine the dilemma.

The Teleological/Utilitarian Model

The *teleological model*, which is also known as the utilitarian model, emerged from the works of the 19th-century philosopher John Stuart Mill. The more contemporary models are basically an outgrowth of the utilitarian model. In this model, rules, values, morals, and ethics are flexible so that they can best meet the needs of the greatest number of people. Consequences determine what is good. There are no hard-and-fast rules. Instead, the utilitarian philosophy is process oriented. According to Mill, the greatest good for the greatest number of people that causes the least harm should be the guiding principle. An act is right if it is at least as good as the consequences of an alternative act. The end justifies the means. Mill also believed in the Golden Rule: Do unto others as you would have them do unto you.

Steps in Decision Making Using the Utilitarian Model as a Guide

1. Perception of the problem: Frame an ethical statement.
   - List the conditions.
   - Identify the "who."
   - Define the "what."
2. List your personal values.
3. List the patient's and family's values.
4. List the alternatives, and list the consequences of each alternative.
5. Compare the consequences with the ethical principles and values.
6. Is the solution consistent with ethical values and principles? Examples of ethical principles include equality, justice, inflicting no harm, and promoting good.
7. What is the greatest good for the greatest number involved in the dilemma?
8. Make the decision based on how consistent is it with ethical principles and moral values.
9. Apply a short test: Would I be satisfied to have this action done to me? (Austin & Wetle, 2008; Beauchamp & Childress, 2001; Hogan & Nickitas, 2009).

The Herrick/Smith Model

The Herrick/Smith model was developed by Herrick and Smith (1990) for undergraduate students taking a course in nursing ethics, who had never had a course in philosophy. The instructors found that the ethical/philosophical models were confusing to undergraduate nursing students. At the same time, these students were very familiar with the nursing process. Consequently, the instructors designed a model that integrated concepts from the various philosophical models, the ANA Code of Ethics, and concepts from values clarification that were part of the nursing process. The Herrick/Smith model was later applied to geriatric nursing education and to the care of patients in an AIDS outpatient clinic. The purpose of the redesigned model was to teach undergraduate nursing students ethical decision making, using a framework that they already understood (Doolittle & Herrick, 1992; Herrick & Smith, 1990).

In this model, consequences are examined and predictions are made before a plan is implemented or actions are taken. Because decisions are made based on predictions of consequences, the model is based on a teleological system of thought. Table 14-4 summarizes the Herrick/Smith model.

ETHICAL PRINCIPLES

Three primary principles should guide ethical decision making: respect for persons, beneficence, and justice (Roussel, 2006). Principles to guide the nurse case manager's practice are listed and defined here:

Respect for persons and their autonomy: Personal liberty and freedom, where the individual determines the course of action, according to a plan chosen by him or her. It includes (1) the freedom to decide and (2) the freedom to act. To decide and act freely, one must (1) know the facts and (2) be free of coercion.

Fidelity: Loyalty, responsibility, accountability, duty to others. This principle includes professional ethical codes and advocacy, which may involve the protection of the patient against the preferences of society.

Beneficence/malfeasance: Do only good. Do no harm!

Justice: Equality; fair and equitable distribution of resources.

Paternalism: Protection of the weak, vulnerable, and disenfranchised.

Double effect (iatrogenicity): One may rightfully cause evil, if the following four conditions are present and verified:

1. The act itself for which the evil is caused is good or morally neutral.
2. The intent is to have a good effect; the evil is only secondary.
3. The good effect may not come about by means of an evil intent.
4. There must be a grave reason from permitting the evil to occur.

Veracity: The obligation to tell the truth.

Confidentiality: Respect for the confidences provided to you as a healthcare professional. The *patient's right to privacy.*

Generalizability: An act is right if there is the ability to generalize its maxim; it is wrong if it is not generalizable.

Egoism: The greatest benefit is to an individual to maximize personal benefits.

Altruism: Regard for the welfare of others. Do the greatest good for the greatest number of people.

Sources: Aiken, 2004; Beauchamp & Childress, 2001; Cooper, 2006; Guido, 2001; Hogan & Nickitas, 2009; Roussel, 2006.

TABLE 14-4 The Herrick/Smith Model

	Herrick/Smith Model	Nursing Process
Step 1	**Gather Data** **Subjective Data:** Thoughts, feelings, values, beliefs, cultural and religious backgrounds **Objective Data:** • Gather the facts • Ascertain the conditioning factors • Determine the moral and ethical issues • Identify the conflicts	**Assessment** **Subjective Data:** Patient's complaints **Objective Data:** • Signs and symptoms • Observable behaviors
Step 2	**Define the Problem** • Delineate the dilemma	**Problem Definition** Nursing diagnosis
Step 3	**Planning** • Examine the alternatives • List the ethical principles and rules • List the moral/legal rights and obligations • Apply the principles, rights, and obligations to the dilemma • Determine the patient's and family's expectations • List the alternatives and the consequences of each alternative • Determine who should make the decision	**Planning** Set goals Develop an intervention plan
Step 4	**Select a Plan** • One right plan • Several right plans—if all are equal, then choose by preference • If there is no "right plan," then appeal to a higher authority (Consult with an ethicist: pastoral care or an ethics committee.) • Reassess or select the best alternative	**Decision Making** Decide on priorities
Step 5	**Action** • Carry out the plan	**Implementation** Implement the plan
Step 6	**Evaluate** • Prize the decision • Advocate for what is the best possible solution	**Evaluation** Examine the outcomes and compare the results with the goals

ETHICAL CHALLENGES IN CASE MANAGEMENT

The challenges for the nurse case manager are numerous, yet the NCM role is a fulfilling one. Some of the challenges involve role expectations—for example, the drive to "be all things to all people" and the lack of training and education in NCM (many nursing schools do not teach case management, even though it is one of the fastest-growing roles for nurses today). Keeping up with the constant changes in legislation and changes in insurance policies is a challenge. One of the most frustrating experiences for the nurse case manager may result from a lack of administrative support, especially when budgets are tight. Frequently, nurse case managers find themselves at the center of ethical controversies and must have the skills to deal with them (Hendricks & Cesar, 2003). The focus of the discussion here is healthcare ethics from the nurse case manager's perspective.

Ethical Issues and Considerations

The primary role of the nurse case manager is to be an advocate. Case managers are under pressure from healthcare organizations, employers, and insurance companies to contain costs. They are the stewards of healthcare resources—yet they are also advocates for the patient. Frequently, the most difficult dilemma is deciding where the nurse case manager's allegiance belongs. Frequently, the nurse case manager is in the middle of a controversy. If the nurse case manager is handling worker's compensation cases, the challenge is that employers want the patient to return to work as soon as possible—sometimes before the injured worker has fully recovered. Common dilemmas faced by nurse case manager are the need to play an advocacy role on behalf of the patient, while containing costs, dealing with conflicting values, and experiencing a conflict of duties (Hendricks & Cesar, 2003).

Many decisions are made on a daily basis that require a balancing act between two ethical principles, or between conflicting duties, or between the rights of patients and their families' wishes, or between divided loyalties. The nurse case manager struggles with unique situations that may cause many nurse case managers to question themselves and their colleagues (McGonigle, Mastrian, & Pavlekovsky, 2007).

Often, the nurse case manager faces a clash between organizational ethics and professional ethics (Cooper, 2006). Balancing the interplay of various religious, social, cultural, political, and economic factors has become more important as the society has become more diverse (O'Donnell, 2007). As the demand for improvements in healthcare entities' financial performance continues to grow, nurse case managers, who have a more global picture of the patient's world, may find themselves at center stage in many of these ethical controversies. The balancing act between the health are institution's needs and the concerns of the nurse case manager to provide quality care for the patient is a primary concern.

Ethical Dilemmas Frequently Encountered by Nurse Case Managers

The following list includes some of the common examples of the ethical dilemmas that have been identified in the case management literature:

1. Balancing the benefits and the harmful side effects of a proposed medical treatment.
2. Disclosure, informed consent, and shared decision making.
3. Family issues (conflicts among family members).
4. Advocacy: Which priorities for which stakeholders? Quality care versus financial stewardship.
5. Divided loyalties: loyalty to the patient, the family, the employer, and the insurance company. Frequently the nurse case manager works for the insurance company.
6. Relationships between clinicians and patients.
7. Professional integrity and accountability.
8. Cost-effectiveness and the allocation of resources. Equality versus rationing resources. Expensive technologies and a patient's inability to pay for sophisticated medical treatments.
9. Balancing the rights of one patient versus the rights of other patients. Equal distribution of available resources.
10. Withdrawal of treatment, including discharges that occur too soon.
11. Issues of cultural and religious beliefs and healthcare beliefs.
12. Considerations of power and powerlessness. Often nurse case managers feel helpless to deal with physicians, the hospital, and the insurance companies, while still providing support and quality care to the patient (Taylor, 2005).
13. Respecting the client's choices and values, even though the healthcare team doesn't agree with them.
14. Advocating for vulnerable populations. If the patient is an undocumented alien, the dilemma translates into what is best for the patient versus what is best for the hospital, the insurance company, and society—a four-way dilemma.
15. Dealing with the clash between professional ethics and organizational or business ethics.
16. Denial of services.
17. Unclear advance directives and other end-of-life issues (Cooper, 2006; Hendricks, 2008; Hendricks & Cesar, 2003).

Quality of care will be examined following a closer examination of denial of services and end-of-life issues.

Denials by Third-Party Payers

Although nurse case managers cannot determine whether a service is medically appropriate, this role may require that the nurse case manager determine whether a request is covered under the patient's health plan or if the provider falls within the contracted provider network. If the patient must be denied services, the nurse case manager should help the patient secure another option, or inform the patient that he or she must pay for the service without the benefit of third-party coverage, or inform the patient that he or she may appeal the decision. In this case, the nurse case manager may be the bearer of bad news, and may be conflicted about the potential outcomes from the denial of services. In the case of denial for services, for a nurse case manager to be held legally liable for negligence, the following points must be proven:

- The nurse case manager breached his or her duty by making an inappropriate decision.
- The nurse case manager breached his or her duty in a manner that resulted in injury or damage.
- The withholding of payment was unreasonable in view of applicable standards of care.
- The breach of duty was the actual and the legal cause of the resulting injury or damage (Hendricks & Cesar, 2003, p. 57).

In no way is this discussion meant to be a comprehensive description of what the nurse case manager must deal with in making coverage decisions. Nevertheless, it does give the reader a brief introduction to healthcare issues that are related to ethical dilemmas and nursing case management. The discussion does not imply that the nurse case manager is the only healthcare professional facing these dilemmas. Patient care and health care have become extremely complex, and all parties are struggling to figure out how the country and its citizens will pay for health care.

End-of-Life Issues

Another dilemma for the nurse case manager may relate to his or her ability to influence the allocation of resources, particularly in regard to life-sustaining care (i.e., end-of-life care). Life-sustaining treatment may be extremely costly and beyond the family's financial reach. The case manager often has a better perspective of the patient's and family's desires and resources and can accomplish a lot on behalf of patients. The following list provides a guide as to what the nurse case manager can do in influencing end-of-life decision making:

1. The nurse case manager can facilitate decision making and can serve as negotiator when differences arise among the healthcare team and family members. Different perspectives are inevitable among family members, physicians, and other healthcare providers, as well as with the nurse case manager's own value system.
2. The nurse case manager may have a better understanding of the patient's, family's, and others' perspectives when conflicts arise.
3. The nurse case manager can explore options and compare their consequences, and then present them to the patient and family as well as the healthcare team.
4. The nurse case manager should examine the quality-of-life issues as well as the resources and costs attached to those issues.
5. The nurse case manager should not be the lone angel, but must be an integral part of a supportive healthcare team that makes decisions collaboratively.

Wisser (2006) provided some guidelines that are not necessarily ethical principles but are helpful in thinking about end-of-life decisions. They include the following ideas:

- Medicine excels at keeping people alive, but not necessarily living with quality of life.
- There is a big difference between what we *can do* and what we *should do*.
- By keeping the patient alive, are we prolonging the dying process?
- There is always room for hope and sometimes miracles do happen, but perhaps God has cast the final vote and we must come to acceptance.
- At some point an indecision becomes a decision.

Working with end-of-life issues is both rewarding and frustrating. The case manager is the patient's advocate—and the patient's *best interest* must be the primary focus of care. Even so, the nurse case manager must also be family centered, taking into consideration the welfare of the family members while honoring the patient's and family's values. Healthcare institutions must create a culture that integrates ethical principles with quality patient care.

Quality-of-Care Issues Identified by the Institute of Medicine

In its 2001 report *Crossing the Quality Chasm*, the Institute of Medicine (IOM) recommended some fundamental changes in the U.S. healthcare system to achieve better quality of care. Specifically, it included six goals for improvement:

- Safety
- Effectiveness
- Patient-centered care
- Care to be provided in a timely manner
- Efficiency
- Equitable care

It is the duty of the nurse case manager to assist the healthcare team to reach these goals (Finkelman & Kenner, 2007). These three issues are among the many ethical issues that nurse case managers and other healthcare professionals deal with on a daily basis.

MAKING ETHICAL DECISIONS

Levels of Ethical Thinking

Prior to making a decision, the nurse case manager should examine the philosophical/ethical models, identify the principles involved, examine the laws and other customary rules such as hospital protocols, and then make a decision that is based on a systematic process of decision making. Many different models have been developed for ethical decision making. For the nurse case manager, it is essential to learn one well and use it consistently. Most models are based on one of the philosophical systems of thought, combined with a problem-solving model.

Analyzing Ethical Dilemmas

Many problem-solving/decision-making models exist. The model described here is just one of many. The nurse case manager should select the model that is comfortable for him or her, so that the nurse case manager can systematically process the dilemma while under pressure during a crisis.

Ethical Dilemmas

Ethical dilemmas occur when situations have no clear-cut solutions. Dilemmas have the following characteristics:

- A conflict between two ethical principles—such that if one principle is honored, then another is violated

- Only two unsatisfactory solutions are possible, which require a choice between two unfavorable alternatives
- A conflict of rights and obligations
- A conflict of values between the nurse and the hospital, physician, patient or family, or another professional
- A pitting of professional ethics against personal religious values and morals (Cooper, 2006, pp. 742–754)

Steps to Analyzing an Ethical Dilemma and Finding Potential Solutions

1. Who are the actors?
2. Who has the ultimate decision-making power?
3. Who is ultimately responsible and accountable?
4. Who should carry out the decision?
5. What are the principles involved?
6. What are the conflicting variables?
7. What is the context of the dilemma?
8. What are the parameters that are fixed, such as the law? (*Remember:* Sometimes the law and ethics overlap, and both must be examined.)
9. What are the time factors and when must the decision be made?
10. Define the dilemma.

Identifying Potential Solutions

1. What are the alternatives?
2. What are the inherent features of each alternative?
3. What are the potential consequences for each alternative?
4. Which is the *best* alternative and which is the *worst?* (List all alternatives in the form of a hierarchy.)
5. Choose the best solution *or* gather more data.
6. Implement the solution.
7. Evaluate the outcomes.

CHARACTERISTICS OF ETHICAL COMPETENCE

Commitment to the Patient's Well-being

The nurse case manager is trusted to act in ways that advance the best interests of the patient, who is entrusted to his or her care.

Responsibility and Accountability

Nurse case managers hold themselves and their colleagues accountable for their practice.

The Ability to Act as an Effective Patient Advocate

The nurse case manager must ensure that the patient's needs are met, especially when the bottom line may be based on cost-effectiveness achieved at the expense of quality patient care. The nurse case manager must advocate for those who cannot advocate for themselves, such as emotionally and mentally impaired persons, children, the homeless, non-English-speaking immigrants, and the elderly.

The Ability to Mediate Ethical Conflicts

Ethical conflicts may arise among the patient, his or her significant others, the healthcare team, other professionals, and other interested parties (e.g., payers). The following forces are all contributing to ethical conflicts in health care today:

- Multiple therapeutic options are available, and there is a lack of consensus about their medical efficacy, benefits, and side effects.
- Demands for scarce resources may lead to rationing of those resources based on risk–benefit ratios or based on who is deemed worthy (or not worthy) of receiving a procedure.
- Moral pluralism and greater cultural diversity among populations may lead to conflicts about values and differing healthcare beliefs about what is appropriate care (Sheikh, 2000).

The Ability to Recognize and to Respond to the Ethical Dimensions in Clinical Practice

This capability includes recognition of the following sources of discord:

- Threats to human dignity
- Limited access to healthcare services
- Conflicts in interests and values of patients, professionals and the nurse case manager
- Technology versus humanity
- Costs versus quality
- Prioritizing scarce resources
- Role conflicts: gatekeeper versus advocate; advocate versus steward of scarce resources

The Ability to Critique New Healthcare Technologies

Changes in the way we define, administer, deliver, and finance health care in light of its potential to influence the health of humans' well-being was central to the 2008 presidential debate about health care (Hendricks, 2008). New technologies are changing the practice of case management. However, we will need to critique the newest technologies and their consequences, including the results or outcomes of these technologies, especially for beginning- and end-of-life care (Rossi, 2003; Taylor, 2005). We are increasingly applying electronic applications to support the case management process but, as Carneal and colleagues (2008) noted, that is no standardized application of new technologies. Are we sacrificing quality for efficiency?

Advocacy Competencies

Case managers must facilitate the relationships among clients, providers, healthcare agencies, and insurers, while primarily focusing on the patient. First they must advocate for the patient, second for the agency where they are employed, and third for the insurance company (Tahan, 2005). Lobbying federal and state legislatures about changing healthcare policies or lobbying hospital administrators for changes in policies and procedures or to acquire more patient care resources are other forms of advocacy.

Support for Patient Autonomy

The nurse case manager is duty-bound to help the patient act in his or her own best interests—for example, through the following actions:

- Protect the rights of patients with decision-making capacity so that self-determination is supported (autonomy)
- Facilitate communication among the patient and family, caregivers, and others
- Document patient preferences
- Prepare the patient for advance directives
- Identify morally and legally surrogate decision makers and support them
- Develop agency policies that identify the caregivers involved and procedures used to identify the appropriate decision makers

Identification of Patient Well-being

In assessing the patient's condition, the nurse case manager must identify ways to support the patient's well-being:

- Weigh the benefits and burdens of therapies
- Ensure that the patient's priorities are addressed
- Ensure continuity of care during service transitions or transfers
- Weigh the moral relevance of the third-party interests (family caregivers, the institution, the insurance company, and society) (Taylor, 2005)

Strategies That Can Be Employed by the Nurse Case Manager

Good Communication Skills and Good Interpersonal Relationships

Communicating with team members, family, and the patient can help the nurse case manager to advocate on the patient's behalf. Teaching the patient and family about the disease process and the options for treatment can ensure that they make wise decisions in their own best interest. Resolving disagreements that may arise between team members, the patient, and family further enhances the quality of care.

In addition, the nurse case manager can facilitate timely communication among individuals on the healthcare team so as to open a discussion around ethical dilemmas. Working together, they can identify and address system-related problems and factors that contribute to recurrent ethical dilemmas.

Acquiring Adequate Resources to Provide Quality Health Care

The nurse case manager fills a brokering role by identifying appropriate services and resources that are available to the client and family. The nurse case manager should appeal the denials by insurance companies, so that the resources needed by the patient are available.

ETHICS COMMITTEES

An ethics committee is an interdisciplinary institutional forum for addressing a wide range of subjects related to health care-oriented ethical dilemmas. The purpose of such a committee is to help the healthcare organization develop ethical guidelines for treating patients with complex conditions, where the treatment plan involves conflicting decisions. Ethics committees were created during the 1970s and have continued to be an integral part of healthcare organizations. Their emergence coincided with the advent of more advanced technology and the perceived need to better support healthcare professionals in their decision-making processes. Ethics committees support healthcare professionals while they wrestle with difficult ethical decisions.

Ethics committees also serve as patient advocates, educators and consultants, and advisors. Their members review ethical dilemmas and assist healthcare providers to develop a plan of care, using ethical principles and ethical decision-making models that address the values of the patient, the family, the healthcare team, and the hospital. The ethics committee is also involved in revising institutional policies to follow ethical principles and principles of family-centered care.

Members of the ethics committees come from many of the healthcare disciplines, but usually are people who are in charge of policies involving patient care. The goal of the committee is to come to a consensus, using an unbiased and systematic approach. Nurses and nurse case managers are frequently members of ethics committees.

Members' responsibilities include maintaining up-to-date knowledge of ethical and legal principles, medical conditions, and standards of care. They should have a working knowledge of current literature regarding evidence-based practice. The functions of an ethics committee are to identify problems, use ethical and legal principles to guide decisions, and then advise practitioners accordingly (Cooper, 2006; Hendricks & Cesar, 2003; Roussel, 2006; Sullivan & Decker, 2005; Taylor, 2005; Wiseman, 2001).

■ SUMMARY

Ethical factors are an inherent part of today's healthcare environment. The following factors contribute to ethical conflicts:

- The availability of multiple therapeutic options
- Distribution questions related to scarce resources and the growing need to contain costs
- An increasingly diverse society with differing cultural beliefs and values
- Technologies that sustain life, in cases where the same patients might have died in the past

Competing loyalties that require balancing the needs of the patient and other stakeholders, as well as the needs of the nurse case manager, may lead to an ethical dilemma. Respecting the unique needs of the individual is an essential part of the nurse case manager's advocacy role. Standardization of care through the development of critical pathways and other clinical measurements has ensured that standards for quality care now exist that can be used as guidelines for treatment. Even so, the nurse case manager should be aware that the focus on technology and outcomes may interfere with a focus on family- and patient-centered care. Role conflicts are common among nurse case managers, who often must balance their responsibilities as coordinator, facilitator, and advocate against their role as gatekeeper.

Providing care to a growing number of uninsured and underserved persons, including illegal immigrants, is not only stressing the U.S. health system, but also placing pressure on the nurse case manager in terms of advocacy. Tighter allocation of scarce resources is likely during times of economic downturns, testing the nurse case manager's ability to act as the "steward" of these resources (Cohen & Cesta, 2005; Tahan, 2005; Taylor, 2005; Wisser, 2006).

Ethical dilemmas involve conflicts of principles, conflicts of evidence, conflicts between unsatisfactory alternatives, conflicts between roles and obligations, and conflicts related to the values and beliefs held by patients, family members, and providers. In some cases, ethical principles may conflict with laws. In the healthcare realm, a conflict that seems universal is the conflict between costs and quality of care.

Ethics committees wrestle with these conflicts, along with challenges associated with the rapidly expanding technological healthcare system and an increasingly costly system of care. Unfortunately, the chief executives of managed care companies make salaries in the millions of dollars, while healthcare providers' salaries remain under intense scrutiny (Finkelman, 2006; Roussel, 2006; Sullivan & Decker, 2005).

Nurse case managers must be knowledgeable about the legal aspects of their practice and understand how ethical and legal issues may overlap (Table 14-5). Ethical and legal issues may intertwine in guiding professional actions. Contrary to public opinion, the law cannot totally be separated from ethics, as many rules of law are based on ethical values (Harris, 2007). The principles common to ethical issues that also guide legislation include autonomy, beneficence, nonmalfeasance, and justice—all of which form the basis of many of society's laws. Nevertheless, the law always has the last word when a dilemma arises. The law is also associated with punishment. For example, it may be ethical and humane to assist a terminally ill patient who is in a great deal of pain to commit suicide, but it is against the law! (And Dr. Jack Kevorkian eventually went to jail, if case you have forgotten.)

TABLE 14-5 The Overlap Between Laws and Ethical Principles

	Legal	Illegal
Ethical	**Informed consent** is both legal and ethical.	**Euthanasia** is ethical (according to many) but is illegal.
Unethical	**Abortion** is unethical (according to many) but is legal.	**Nonemergency medical treatment given without informed consent** is both unethical and illegal.

Whenever an overlap between legal and ethical issues occurs, the law reigns supreme. Of course, the law is the guideline for a *minimal* level of behavior, while ethical principles provide guidelines for the *highest* level of behavior. Thus ethical principles may require that the nurse case manager or other citizens do more than the law requires (Fattorusso & Quinn, 2007). The disparity between the law and ethics is greatest in regard to health care. Current laws require only access to health care in an emergency; the principle of beneficence is frequently ignored, which results in healthcare disparities and lack of access to health care for many Americans, who are ineligible for care other than emergency care (Harris, 2007). This situation may change in the future, but only if some type of healthcare reform becomes a reality. If the status quo remains, then the only care for the uninsured will be emergency care at the expense of the hospital, its patients, and the local citizens.

CASE STUDIES

Pick one of the following case studies to discuss.

1. A baby is born with multiple anomalies that are almost incompatible with life, yet the family wants everything done to save the baby. What should be the role of the case manager on the ethics committee?
2. A patient is borderline incompetent and refuses nursing home placement despite all indications of the need for a nursing home. Her refusal is delaying her discharge from the acute care hospital. The matter has come before the ethics committee. What should the role of the case manager be?
3. A battered spouse or elderly person elects to return to a known abusive situation. What should the role of the case manager be in the emergency room?
4. A family wants a loved one removed from life support but meets resistance from the medical team, because a clearly defined advance directive was not in place. The case is now before the ethics committee. What should the role of the case manager be?

DISCUSSION QUESTIONS

1. What is the purpose of an ethics committee?
2. Describe the historical background of ethics committees, and explain how they were originally formed.
3. Who should serve on an ethics committee?
4. What is the role of the case manager on an ethics committee?
5. Why do ethical conflicts occur?

■ CLASSROOM EXERCISES

1. Attend an ethics committee meeting in your facility or the one where you are having your clinical experience. Describe the meeting.
2. Describe an ethical dilemma and apply a philosophical model to guide the decision-making process.

■ RECOMMENDED READINGS

American Nurses Association (ANA). (2006). *The code of ethics for nurses: With interpretive statements*. Washington, DC: Author. Retrieved from http://www. nursingworld.org/ethics/code/ethicscode150.htm

McGonigle, D., Mastrian, K., & Pavlekovsky, K. (2007). Ethical realism revisited. *Professional Case Management, 12*(3), 184–187.

O'Donnell, L. T. (2007). Ethical dilemmas among nurses as they transition to hospital case management: Implications for organizational ethics. *Professional Case Management, 12*(3), 160–169.

■ REFERENCES

Aiken, T. D. (2004). *Legal, ethical and political issues in nursing* (2nd ed.). Philadelphia: F. A. Davis.

American Nurses Association (ANA). (2006). *The code of ethics for nurses: With interpretive statements*. Washington, DC: Author. Retrieved from http://www. nursingworld.org/ethics/code/ethicscode150.htm

Austin, A., & Wetle, V. (Eds.). (2008). Ethical issues in health care. In *The United States health care system: Combining business, health, and delivery* (pp. 12–13). Upper Saddle River, NJ: Pearson/Prentice Hall.

Beauchamp, T., & Childress, I. (2001). *Principles of biomedical ethics* (5th ed.). New York: Oxford University Press.

Carneal, G., Frater, J., Stricker, P., & Pock, R. (2008). Is technology changing the practice of case management? *Case in Point, 6*(5), 26–27.

Cohen, E. L., & Cesta, T. G. (2005). *Nursing case management: From essentials to advanced practice applications*. St. Louis, MO: Elsevier/Mosby.

Cooper, R. W. (2006). Legal and ethical issues. In D. L. Huber (Ed.), *Leadership and nursing care management* (3rd ed., pp. 733–754). Philadelphia: Saunders/Elsevier.

Doolittle, N., & Herrick, C. A. (1992). Ethics in aging: A family decision making paradigm. *Educational Gerontology, 18*(4), 395–408.

Fattorusso, D., & Quinn, C. E. (2007). *A case manager's study guide: Preparing for certification* (3rd ed., pp. 58–63). Sudbury, MA: Jones and Bartlett.

Finkelman, A. W. (2006) *Leadership and management in nursing.* Upper Saddle River, NJ: Pearson/Prentice Hall.

Finkelman, A. W., & Kenner, C. (2007). *Teaching IOM: Implications of the Institute of Medicine reports for nursing education.* Silver Spring, MD: American Nurses Association.

Guido, G. W. (2001). *Legal and ethical issues in nursing* (3rd ed.). Upper Saddle River, NJ: Prentice Hall.

Harris, D. M. (Ed.). (2007). The relationship between law and ethics. In *Contemporary issues in health care law and ethics* (pp. 7–10). Chicago: Health Administration Press.

Hendricks, A. G., & Cesar, J. (2003). How prepared are you? Ethical and legal challenges facing case managers today. *Case Manager, 14*(3), 56–61.

Hendricks, T. J. (2008). Practice matters: How the candidates want to change health care. *American Nurse Today, 3*(9), 36–38.

Herrick, C. A., & Smith, J. E. (1990). Ethical issues in the care of AIDS patients. *Nursing Forum, 24*(3&4), 35–46.

Hogan, M. A., & Nickitas, D. M. (2009). *Nursing leadership and management: Reviews and rationales.* Upper Saddle River, NJ: Pearson/Prentice Hall.

Institute of Medicine. (2001). *Crossing the quality chasm: A new health system for the 21st century.* Washington, DC: National Academy of Sciences.

McGonigle, D., Mastrian, K., & Pavlekovsky, K. (2007). Ethical realism revisited. *Professional Case Management, 12*(3), 184–187.

Moreo, K., & Lamb, G. (2003). NCMSA updates standards of practice for case management. *Case Manager, 14*(3), 52–54.

Mullahy, C. M. (Ed.). (2004). Ethical responsibilities of the case management profession. In *The case manager's handbook* (3rd ed., pp. 117–144; glossary, pp. 697–715). Sudbury, MA: Jones and Bartlett.

Nielsen, M. (2002). How ethical principles affect case management: A real-life example. *Case Manager, 13*(3), 68–71.

O'Donnell, L. T. (2007). Ethical dilemmas among nurses as they transition to hospital case management: Implications for organizational ethics. *Professional Case Management, 12*(3), 160–169.

Rossi, P. A. (Ed.). (2003). Introduction to complex care: Ethical issues. In *Case management in health care* (2nd ed., pp. 438–442). Philadelphia: Saunders.

Roussel, L. (2006). Ethical principles for the nurse administrator. In L. Roussel, R. C. Swansburg, & R. J. Swansburg (Eds.), *Management and leadership for nurse administrators* (4th ed., pp. 45–54) Sudbury, MA: Jones and Bartlett.

Sheikh, A. (2000). Universal ethics. Dealing with ethics in a multicultural world [Abstract]. *Cultural Diversity*. Retrieved from lltext.asp?resultSeId=R0000000&hit Num=8&BooleanTerm=culture5diversity&fuzzTy

Sullivan, E. J., & Decker, P. J. (2005). Legal and ethical issues. In *Effective leadership and management in nursing* (6th ed., pp. 70–87). Upper Saddle River, NJ: Pearson/Prentice Hall.

Tahan, H. A. (2005). Essentials of advocacy in case management. *Lippincott's Case Management, 10*(3), 136–144.

Taylor, S. C. (2005). Ethical issues in case management. In E. L. Cohen & T. G. Cesta (Ed.), *Nursing case management: From essentials to advanced practice applications* (4th ed., pp. 361–379). St. Louis, MO: Elsevier/Mosby.

Wiseman, R. (2001). The ANA develops bill of rights for registered nurses. *American Journal of Nursing, 101*(11), 55–57.

Wisser, S. (2006). To die or not to die. *Lippincott's Case Management, 11*(2), 107–110.

Legal Issues in Nursing Case Management

Laura J. Fero
Charlotte A. Herrick

15

■ OBJECTIVES

1. Define legal terms and concepts that apply to health care, including the different types of laws, torts, malpractice, libel, types of liability, and negligence.

2. Identify the nurse case manager's professional obligations and legal responsibilities.

3. Describe standards of practice, State Boards of Nursing and their duties to administer Nurse Practice Acts, licensure, and the potential benefits of multistate licensure.

4. Discuss the legal issues and concerns related to case management, including risk management, denial of services, compliance programs, and ethical issues such as informed consent, confidentiality, and the impact of the Health Insurance Portability and Accountability Act (HIPAA) on a patient's right to privacy.

5. List the recommendations and guidelines for a nurse case manager concerned about the legalities of practice.

INTRODUCTION

Professional obligations and responsibilities guide nursing practice and case management practice. Standards of practice, the policies and procedures of the institution where the nurse or case manager works, and codes of ethics also guide nursing and case management practice. If the nurse or nurse case manager fails to meet his or her responsibilities and obligations, fails to follow the agency's policies and procedures, or fails to abide by the American Nurses Association's (ANA's) Standards of Practice or the Standards of Practice published by the Case Management Society of America (CMSA), then he or she is potentially at risk for a malpractice suit.

Outcomes management is important to assess the quality of care and its cost-effectiveness and to identify areas of needed improvements. The nurse case manager must also examine recent clinical research to apply evidence-based practice to current nursing case management practice. It behooves the nurse case manager to know the law and to stay up to date, because the law changes over time as legislative policies change (Harris, 2003).

In some instances, ethical and legal issues may overlap (e.g., in regard to confidentiality and informed consent). The right to self-determination or autonomy and the right to privacy are now governed by two laws: the Client Self-Determination Act and the Health Insurance Portability and Accountability Act (HIPAA).

Many situations involving complex medical and nursing issues are not covered by the law; instead, ethical principles of professional conduct and standards of practice serve as guidelines in these areas. If the law does apply, however, it takes precedence over ethical principles. It is important for the nurse case manager to bridge the two realms—that is, ethical and legal issues—when planning and delivering care and/or planning transfers to another level of care or planning discharges.

In this chapter, legal terms and concepts are defined and legal issues that are important to the practice of nursing and nursing case management are examined. Thus the chapter offers a brief overview of various legal issues that pertain to a nurse case manager's practice.

DEFINITIONS

Laws are rules and regulations that govern people's behavior and their relationships with others, and that have been established by authority, society, or custom (Aiken, 2004). With laws, rules of conduct are established and enforced in a legal sense. Laws prohibit extremes in behavior so that people can live without fear for their safety or for their property (Sullivan & Decker, 2005). Five types of laws are defined here: administrative law, statutory law, common law, civil law, and tort law. The latter two are closely related.

Administrative law focuses on the laws created by a multitude of administrative agencies, as empowered by the executive branch of the government. Certain statutes grant authority to administrative agencies to establish standards, interpret statutes, and enact rules and regulations that will ensure that the specific intentions of the statute have been met. State Boards of Nursing are authorized by Nurse Practice Acts (statutory law) to write rules and regulations governing the practice of nursing. A State Board of Nursing is an example of an administrative agency (Hogan & Nickitas, 2009; Sullivan & Decker, 2005).

The legislative branch of the government enacts **statutory laws**, which empower the federal, state, and local authorities. Licensing laws for healthcare providers are examples of statutory laws that are designed to protect the public from harm, such as health care provided by an incompetent medical or nurse practitioner. Other statutory laws that affect nursing practice place limitations on the scope of practice and aim to ensure that any health care provided is both ethical and legal. In addition to the self-determination and confidentiality acts, health care-related legislation includes "living will" legislation and protective and reporting laws (Hogan & Nickitas, 2009; Sullivan & Decker, 2005).

The Nurse Practice Act is a statutory law that defines the scope of nursing practice within a specific state (Sullivan & Decker, 2005). Each state's statutes authorize individuals to perform designated skills and services. To practice nursing, a person must hold a valid state license, which means that the person may practice nursing within the limits of the legal standards of practice, as designated by the state's constitution (Cooper, 2006; Hogan & Nickitas, 2009).

Common laws are derived from earlier court decisions that set precedents (Cooper, 2006; Sullivan & Decker, 2005, p. 71)—that is, they are established by custom or tradition. A precedent means that a lower court will follow the decisions that were previously made by a higher court. Awareness of common law assists nurses to function within the boundaries of their role and to advocate for nursing practice.

Civil laws concern the rights and responsibilities of private individuals and protect their rights. Remedies usually involve some type of monetary compensation or a civil dispensation, such as court-ordered therapy or community service, rather than jail time. Civil law related to nursing is also considered to include tort law, involving negligence, personal injury, or malpractice. Nurses can also be involved in other legal procedures having to do with civil law, such as worker's compensation, breach of contract, divorce law, or custody hearings in a court of law (Cooper, 2006).

Tort law is a type of civil law, whereby a person does something wrong to another person or does something wrong to his or her property. A tort law addresses wrongful acts, whether unintentional or intentional. In an *intentional tort*, the action was intended to do harm. When liability under tort laws is established, the court usually requires the defendant to pay money for the damages to those who were mistreated. Nurses and nurse case managers should be familiar with this area of the law and knowledgeable about how it affects their practice (Cooper, 2006; Hogan & Nickitas; 2009; Sullivan & Decker, 2005).

TABLE 15-1 Definitions of Assault and Battery

Assault
• A threat or attempt to threaten
• A threat along with the ability to execute the threat
• The fear of harmful contact which is neither consented to nor privileged
Battery
• The intentional assault or the unlawful touching or striking another person
• Unlawful touching, resulting in bodily contact, if it is neither consented to nor privileged

Source: Roussel & Merrill, 2006.

Torts are civil wrongs against a person or property, whether intentional or unintentional, that can be redressed in a court proceeding. Legal terms that are intertwined with torts include malpractice and negligence (Cooper, 2006; Roussel & Merrill, 2006). If a patient is touched by a healthcare professional without informed consent, it may be interpreted as assault and battery (Table 15-1).

Constitutional law limits the power of governing bodies to what is written in the constitution (Aiken, 2004).

KEY LEGAL TERMS IN HEALTH CARE: MALPRACTICE, LIABILITY, AND NEGLIGENCE

Malpractice

Malpractice results from a failure of a health professional to act as another professional with the same knowledge and education would have acted, according to the recognized standards of practice and under similar circumstances (Cooper, 2006). Malpractice occurs when a professional's actions fall short of the standards defined in the state's Nurse Practice Act, defined by institutional policies of the healthcare agency, identified in federal guidelines and professional organizations, and set out in The Joint Commission's standards, and there is a breach of duty that causes an injury to the patient (Hogan & Nickitas, 2009). Malpractice suits may result from unethical conduct or a lack of skills; in other words, the healthcare professional's performance did not meet the standard of care (Hogan & Nickitas, 2009).

A healthcare professional could be accused of malpractice (and negligence, discussed later in this section) for a variety of reasons. For example, the nurse or the nurse case manager may have failed to observe a significant change in the patient's condition, did not document the change in the patient's condition, and failed to report the change to the appropriate responsible persons, such as a supervisor or physician, or the nurse or the nurse case manager did not document what the follow-up care entailed (Rossi, 2003).Other common causes of malpractice suits against nurses are (1) failure to closely monitor a patient in the recovery room, (2) using equipment incorrectly, (3) mistakes in medication administration, (4) failure to monitor the fetal heart rate during labor, and (5) not providing a safe environment. Other factors that have been identified as increasing the number of malpractice suits are (1) delegating without providing proper supervision, (2) early discharge without the appropriate follow-up, (3) improper assessment of the patient's condition, (4) lack of knowledge about new technologies, (5) a breach of confidentiality, and (6) not getting informed consent (Fattorusso & Quinn, 2007; Hogan & Nickitas, 2009).

The nursing shortage has also been blamed for nurses failing to provide care that is up to current standards. There have been claims that the patient-to-staff ratio is too high to practice safely and that often nurses are working overtime to staff the units. Fatigue can cause errors.

In summary, a malpractice suit can occur in the following circumstances:

- When a health professional failed to act according to the standards of practice
- When the health professional is unskilled or negligent

To win the suit, the plaintiff must prove the following points:

- A patient–healthcare professional relationship existed.
- There was a failure by the health professional to conform to the standard of practice.
- An actual injury resulted from the healthcare professional's intervention.
- There is a causal relationship between the professional's interventions and the patient's injury (Rossi, 2003; Roussel & Merrill, 2006; Swansburg, 2002).

Other causes of malpractice litigation may include uncalled-for behavior, poor interpersonal relationships, and failure to clearly communicate to the patient or the patient's family about the illness and its treatment (Fattorusso & Quinn, 2007). According to Fattorusso and Quinn (2007), most cases of malpractice occur not because of medical or nursing mismanagement, but rather because of poor patient–provider relationships or failure to fully inform patients and their families about the course of treatment. The case manager may be able to prevent unnecessary litigation by facilitating good interpersonal relationships between the patient and family and the healthcare team. However, to justify the suit, there must be a perceived injury to the patient due to substandard care (Fattorusso & Quinn, 2007).

Medical malpractice is primarily a matter of state law, thus tort reform proposals are at the state government level. However, lately, starting with the Clinton administration, Congress has considered proposals for malpractice reform at the federal level (Harris, 2003).

Liability

Liability may be defined as accountability, responsibility, obligation, or the state of being bound by law. It should not be confused with **libel** (or *slander*), which consists of malicious accusations about a professional's reputation that expose the professional to ridicule and disgrace; in libel (the written form) or slander (the spoken form), the accusations are false and are intended to harm the person's reputation (Roussel & Merrill, 2006).

Several types of liability are distinguished. *Legal liability* occurs when the law imposes a civil obligation on a person to compensate for an injury that was the consequence of poor judgment or an inappropriate act (Cooper, 2006).

Corporate liability arises because hospitals are responsible for the credentials of their medical and nursing staff and must monitor the care delivered in their facility. They are responsible for hiring qualified personnel, as well as supervising those employees' activities. Hospitals must actively intervene on behalf of the patient when the care is substandard. Organizations are responsible for the care that is provided to the patient and for any unprofessional conduct of their employees (Fattorusso & Quinn, 2007; Sullivan & Decker, 2005).

The legal concept of *respondeat superior* means that an employer is vicariously liable for the negligent acts or any omissions of care by an employee, including the negligent actions of doctors or nurses (Cooper, 2006; Fattorusso & Quinn, 2007; Finkelman, 2006; Sullivan & Decker, 2005).

Under *personal liability*, each person is held accountable and responsible for his or her individual actions, including acts of omission. Ignorance of the law is no excuse. Thus, when a law exists and the nurse violates it, the nurse is liable and is subject to criminal charges (Roussel & Merrill, 2006).

Professional liability is a legal concept describing the obligation of a professional person to pay a patient for damages caused by the professional's act of omission, commission, or negligence. Professional liability describes the monetary responsibility of defendants to their clients. This concept of liability lies at the heart of malpractice (Mullahy, 2004). *Liability limits* exist because there are limits to the amount of money the insurance company will pay to satisfy a claim against the insured professional; the defendant must pay the remainder of the claim that is owed to the client. It is important for the nurse case manager to be aware of and understand the risks of professional liability (Fattorusso & Quinn, 2007).

In *negligence liability*, a hospital or health maintenance organization may be held liable for an injury to a patient that was caused by a lack of proper care. If the physician is an employee of the hospital, then the hospital can be held liable vicariously for his or her negligence. If the physician is an independent contractor, however, then the hospital may or may not be vicariously liable for the physician's actions. However, the law is not totally clear about all possible relationships. For example, if the physician is an agent of a health maintenance organization (HMO), then the HMO may be liable under the doctrine of corporate negligence, because it is the responsibility of the HMO to screen and monitor the healthcare providers who participate in its network (Harris, 2003).

Negligence

Negligence involves wrongful acts that harm another person or their property. It can be either intentional or unintentional. *Intentional negligence* involves a voluntary and willful act that is intended to cause harm. *Unintentional negligence* is the failure of an individual to perform or not perform an act that a reasonable person would do or not do, under the same circumstances (Sullivan & Decker, 2005). For example, negligence may arise from the failure of the nurse or the nurse case manager to provide care required by the patient's condition (Cooper, 2006). Negligence is professional conduct that falls below the standard of care (Roussel & Merrill, 2006; Swansburg, 2002).

Table 15-2 identifies the four elements of negligence. To prove negligence against a nurse case manager, the court must make the following findings:

- The nurse case manager made a decision that resulted in injury or damage.
- The nurse case manager committed a breach of duty that was either the actual or the legal cause of the resulting injury.

TABLE 15-2 Four Elements of Negligence

- Duty is owed to the patient, which the professional is obligated to provide.
- There was a breach of duty.
- A breach of duty caused the patient's injury.
- The patient suffered harm or was injured because of negligence.

Source: Cooper, 2006.

TABLE 15-3 Professional Obligations of the Nurse Case Manager

- Identify potential risks so as to reduce them.
- Apply ethical/legal principles to manage risks.
- Assess the degree of adherence to the laws that govern health care.
- Interpret the meaning of the laws and convey the meaning to the healthcare team.
- Monitor the quality of services the patient receives and the outcomes.
- Assure compliance with regulatory guidelines, standards of practice, and evidence-based practice (Roussel & Merrill, 2006; Swansburg, 2002).
- Be accountable for his or her own specific acts and for the acts of those to whom he or she delegates a patient's care (Cooper, 2006).

TABLE 15-4 Major Legal Responsibilities of the Nurse Case Manager (Imposed by Civil Law)

- Maintain the standards of care.
- Respect the rights of patients and families.
- Assess the patient systematically.
- Create a plan of care based on the patient's condition.
- Supervise the implementation of the plan of care that is appropriate to meet the patient's needs.
- Follow the policies and procedures of the institution.
- Advocate for what is right for the patient using the appropriate chain of command of the organizational hierarchy.
- Ensure that medications are administered properly (i.e., giving the right drug, in the right dose, to the right patient, by the right route, and at the right time).
- Respond to the patient's and family's complaints, and monitor the patient's condition to ensure safety and to meet the patient's and family's needs.
- Educate the patient about the illness, treatment, risks, and benefits.
- Adequately supervise the patient's care by providers under the case manager's supervision.
- Monitor each patient's progress.

Source: Rossi, 2003.

Professional Obligations and Legal Responsibilities

Table 15-3 outlines the professional obligations of a nurse case manager. The nurse case manager is obliged to apply ethical and legal principles to provide satisfactory services and maintain the quality of care (Table 15-4). The nurse case manager or leader should constantly scan the environment for new ethical/legal issues and trends (Roussel & Merrill, 2006; Swansburg, 2002).

It is the *fundamental duty* of the nurse to observe and recognize when significant events have occurred that must be reported to the appropriate persons. The nurse or nurse case manager must follow up if the response from a higher authority is insufficient.

NURSES AND NURSE CASE MANAGERS: STANDARDS OF PRACTICE

Standards of Care

The CMSA has developed standards of practice for case management, which it updates periodically (Moreo & Lamb, 2003). The standards governing the primary case manager's role and functions were identified by Mullahy (2004) as "assessment, planning, facilitation, and advocacy" (p. 15).

The following documents should be referenced to ensure that the standard of care is being met:

- ANA standards
- Licensing statutes
- Nurse Practice Acts
- Policies and procedures manuals

Policies and Procedures

When a nurse is responsible for performing procedures that require skills or judgments beyond the usual scope of practice, a standardized procedure or protocol must be written to cover the procedure and authorized by the health-care agency. Policies and procedures serve as documents to standardize care, set standards, and guide practice (Sullivan & Decker, 2005). Policies are value statements that serve as guidelines for practice that define the "shoulds" and "oughts" for medical, nursing, and nurse case management practice (Jones, 2006).

Organizational Standards

Organizational standards are written to comply with established standards of care. The organization must provide adequate staffing with qualified personnel; otherwise, it may be held liable under the doctrines of respondeat superior and corporate liability if an injury occurs.

Licensure

Nurse Practice Acts

The first state to enact a Nurse Practice Act was North Carolina. Boards of Nursing govern Nurse Practice Acts. The Board of Nursing administers the statutory laws that define nursing, mandates a set of standards for licensure, mandates licensure examinations, regulates schools of nursing, sets standards for nursing curricula taught in schools of nursing, reviews and requires continuing education for license renewal, investigates reports of violations, disciplines violators of nurse practice laws, and regulates advanced practice nurses (Cooper, 2006; Hogan & Nickitas, 2009; Swansburg, 2002). In the United States, Boards of Nursing in all states administer similar nursing statutes (Hogan & Nickitas, 2009). The state authorizes those individuals who meet the state's designated qualifications to perform nursing skills and provide nursing services (Sullivan & Decker, 2005).

Licensure sets limits on the nurse's activities within the designated scope of practice (Cooper, 2006; Swansburg, 2002; Roussel & Merrill, 2006; Sullivan & Decker, 2005). The scope of practice is defined by each state within its Nurse Practice Act. The intention in regulating the scope of practice is to ensure the public's health and safety. State governments are mandated to provide oversight for the health, welfare, and safety of the public (Anthony, 2006).

Multistate Licensure

Multistate licensure is the process whereby two or more states mutually recognize licensure in the other state(s) (see Chapter 1) (Sullivan & Decker, 2005). A new initiative from the National Council of State Boards of Nursing is in the process of establishing interstate agreements that would mutually recognize the nurse's or nurse case manager's license, thereby allowing nurses and nurse case managers to practice in more than one state. Even if the nurse case manager is practicing in a different state from where the patient resides, he or she is still responsible for meeting the standards of the nurse case manager's home state as well as the state where the patient resides. Disciplinary action can be taken by both the nurse case manager's residential state and the patient's state if these licensure requirements are not met (Skiba, Sorenson, McCarthy, & Brownrigg, 2005; Sullivan & Decker, 2005).

As healthcare delivery has begun to cross more geographic boundaries via telehealth, the traditional standards of practice and licensure on a state-by-state basis are no longer working, according to Skiba et al. (2005). Questions of licensure have become increasingly complex. The National Council of State Boards of Nursing has proposed that an interstate licensing initiative be passed by states to govern nurse case managers who provide disease management and telehealth services across state boundaries (Table 15-5). The standards of practice must be agreed to and adhered to by the Compact states to ensure the quality of the care provided (Skiba et al., 2005). The CMSA has endorsed the

TABLE 15-5 Advantages and Disadvantages of the Interstate Nursing Compact

Advantages
- Need only one state license
- Decreased financial outlay
- Decreased personal malpractice liability
- Decreased administrative costs of maintaining multiple state licenses
- Easier verification of credentials for employers
- Mobility

Disadvantages
- Responsible to multiple State Boards of Nursing
- Cannot practice out of state if the nurse has a restricted license or is subject to disciplinary action by a state nursing board

Source: Fattorusso & Quinn, 2007, p. 83.

concept of multistate licensure, given that so many case managers and disease managers cross state lines daily.

LEGAL ISSUES AND CONCERNS

For case managers, it is essential to stay abreast of numerous legal issues and concerns:

- Risk management
- Denial of services
- Compliance programs
- Informed consent
- Confidentiality (HIPAA)
- Competence
- Brokering referrals, transfers, and discharges

Risk Management

Risk management is the identification of real and potential hazards so as to control the risk of financial loss due to legal liability. Assessment should be performed on an ongoing basis. As coordinators, facilitators, and managers of care, nurse case managers should pay close attention to outcomes to ensure that the outcomes meet the predetermined patient care goals. They should monitor the care that is delivered to ensure that it is in compliance with the requirements and standards of the healthcare organization and the standards of the regulatory and accreditation agencies (Tahan, 2005).

TABLE 15-6 Strategies to Reduce the Risk of Liability

1. Identify patterns and trends through internal audits and claims.
2. Report individual risk-related incidents, taking steps to reduce the liability.
3. Engage in product evaluation.
4. Develop appropriate informed consent protocols.
5. Evaluate patient care settings to determine risks and ensure safety.
6. Prevent occurrences likely to pose liability concerns for the organization, oneself, or one's teammates.
7. Use only reputable providers.
8. Develop written guidelines for decision making.
9. Document all patient contacts.
10. Record patient participation in decision making.
11. Establish quality assurance programs.
12. Assess the quality of the patient's care to comply with the standards of practice.
13. Implement grievance procedures.
14. Address all patient concerns.
15. Keep the patient's physician well informed.
16. Investigate all patient care problems and find solutions to them.
17. Work closely with the legal department and the risk management department.

Sources: Fattorusso & Quinn, 2007; Roussel & Merrill, 2006; Swansburg, 2002.

The Nurse Case Manager's Role as a Risk Manager

The risk manager should develop a complete description of the case management system, including the nurse case manager's role, and should document all plans to improve the quality of care. The goal for the nurse case manager/risk manager is to limit liability as much as possible. Table 15-6 outlines some recommendations to reduce the risk of a potential lawsuit.

Incident Reports

An *incident* is any deviation from a routine event. Incident reports document an untoward event and are considered an internal risk management tool. They are used to collect and analyze data for the purpose of determining risk-control strategies. After the analysis, such reports are used to identify the operational error(s) that contributed to the incident so that the error can be corrected immediately and a potential lawsuit averted. The reports of adverse events should be confidential, and copying the information is considered a breach of confidentiality (Hogan & Nickitas, 2009; Roussel & Merrill, 2006; Swansburg, 2002).

Denial of Services

The liability of case managers related to denial of service is both an ethical and legal issue. Case managers must be knowledgeable about denials and the appeals process. As case managers have become more influential in patient care planning, patients' attorneys have likewise begun naming case managers as defendants in lawsuits concerning negligence related to premature hospital discharge or negligent denial of payment for services. Case managers should *not* comply with any unreasonable demands by managed care organizations (MCOs) or payers without formally protesting or stating their position in writing and reporting it to the hospital administration, the director of case management, and the physician. The case manager's role as advocate should take priority over his or her role as gatekeeper (Hendricks, 2003).

The healthcare agency should have an appeal management process. The nurse case manager should document all denials and provide rationales for them during the appeal process (Hendricks, 2003). He or she should appeal the denial after thoroughly reviewing the criteria and should negotiate with the payer to determine an agreed-upon criteria for payment. The case manager should persist and not give up too easily (Bower, 2005). When at all possible, try to anticipate denials and work proactively to prevent them (Alliota, 2005).

Compliance Programs

A compliance program is a program within the healthcare organization that seeks to develop policies, gather information, and help the hospital to comply with federal, state, and local regulations that govern healthcare institutions. Compliance programs are developed to help an organization avoid legal problems. Cady (2005) recommends that case managers be thoroughly familiar with the employer's compliance plan, as such a plan protects the hospital and its personnel from being accused of fraud or abuse. The goal is to prevent criminal or civil wrongdoing, thereby reducing penalties.

For the nurse case manager, it is important to closely review all claims submitted to a third-party payer to reduce the possibility of being accused of fraud. Compliance programs are established with the intent to minimize the losses from false claims and to reduce an agency's exposure to civil and criminal damages (Cady, 2005). Good documentation is essential as a defense against charges of fraud and abuse.

Implied Consent and Informed Consent

Consent is another issue that overlaps ethics and the law. Consent may be oral, implied by law, or apparent, implied by the person's consent; alternatively, it can be informed consent. *Implied by law* consent may be assumed in case of an emergency, even if the patient is not able to explicitly provide the consent. It may also arise when the person is unable to give consent but there is no reason the person would deny consent if capable of providing it, and a reasonable person in the same or similar circumstances would likely give consent (Finkelman, 2006, p. 294).

With **informed consent**, the underlying premise is that the patient has a right to determine what happens to his or her body. To give this type of consent, the patient must agree in writing to treatments after being fully informed of the treatment, the rationale for the treatment, and the risks and the benefits of the treatment. Informed consent is the authorization by the patient or the patient's legal representative for medical treatment, assuming that the patient or his or her representative has the capacity to understand the procedure and that the consent is voluntary after there has been a full disclosure of the facts. Legal capacity is determined by age and competency (Fattorusso & Quinn, 2007; Sullivan & Decker, 2005).

Informed consent is more than a document; it is a process. The consent form documents this decision-making process. To ensure that the process is valid, there must be a written consent form describing the informed consent process, and this document must be witnessed by a third party (Fattorusso & Quinn, 2007; Sullivan & Decker, 2005). In the absence of that consent, the physician, nurse, or nurse case manager may be held liable and accused of assault and battery or professional negligence for treatments given. Informed consent protects the patient's ethical right to self-determination and protects the health professional against charges of assault and battery (Fattorusso & Quinn, 2007; Swansburg, 2002).

Confidentiality

Privileged communications cannot be used against an accused in a court of law. These communications include communication between an attorney and a client, a physician and a patient, a clergy member and a member of the congregation, members of a family or household, and prospective and former employers (Roussel & Merrill, 2006; Swansburg, 2002). Confidentiality is the crux of the patient's right to privacy, and the healthcare provider's obligation is to protect that right.

In 1996, Congress passed the Health Insurance Portability and Accountability Act (HIPAA), which established a comprehensive standard for medical privacy (Aiken, 2004). Privacy considerations are another example of the overlap between ethical and legal issues. The right to privacy has traditionally been an ethical principle but, with the passage of HIPAA, it is now also a legal right in the United States. The purpose of the legislation was to improve the efficiency and effectiveness of information systems and to establish a common set of standards and requirements for performing and securing electronic information exchange, while still ensuring that patients' rights are protected (Table 15-7).

TABLE 15-7 Patients' Rights Under the Health Insurance Portability and Accountability Act (HIPAA)

Patients have the right to:
- Be informed of their right to privacy.
- Be informed as to who will see their records and for what purpose.
- Inspect and have a copy of the medical record and make amendments to the record.
- Provide the healthcare provider(s) with valid authorization to release health information. The patient must sign the authorization.
- Limit the information given to insurance companies.
- Know the purpose of a research study in which they may be enrolled.
- Give permission to the researchers to use their health information but only if all identifiable information is removed from the records.
- Decline to participate in a study at any time.
- Refuse to provide personal information that may be used for the purpose of marketing—for example, for use by pharmaceutical companies.

Sources: Finkelman, 2006; Mullahy, 2004.

TABLE 15-8 Safeguards for Preserving Confidentiality by Healthcare Providers

- Speak quietly when discussing patients' cases with family members in the waiting room or other public areas.
- Avoid using patients' names in public hallways and elevators.
- Post signs to remind employees to protect confidentiality.
- Keep file cabinets and/or record rooms under lock and key.
- Provide additional security for electronically maintained personal information.

Source: Stuart Brock, personal communication, University of North Carolina–Greensboro School of Nursing, class lecture NUR 541, Fall 2004.

The *Privacy Rule* defines how patient information may be used or disclosed; the *Security Rule* sets a baseline for standards regarding confidentiality and the integrity of patient information (Cyphert, 2006; Skiba, et al., 2005). HIPAA protects employers from excluding employees from receiving healthcare benefits because of a preexisting condition, and it makes sure that healthcare benefits are "portable." The Act provides opportunities for medication and healthcare savings accounts. More important, it establishes heavy penalties for institutions and healthcare providers who violate a patient's right to privacy. These penalties apply if healthcare providers and institutions reveal confidential information without the patient's permission (Mullahy, 2004).

Table 15-8 offers some recommendations for safeguarding the confidentiality of patients. When disclosing medical information, it is wise to wait for a legitimate request with a signed consent of the patient to transfer medical information to another designated party (Aiken, 2004). However, there are some exceptions to the rule of confidentiality, in which federally mandated reporting is required. Specifically, confidentiality must be breached when there are reportable events, such as abuse of children, spouses, and the elderly; coroner's cases; cases involving communicable diseases; violent injuries or the threat of violence (duty to warn); or the patient is thought to be a potential terrorist.

Competence

The nurse case manager must know the rules that govern mandatory reporting of unsafe practices. Some states have established laws on mandatory reporting of unsafe practices; however, mandatory reporting is a complex process involving both legal and ethical parameters. Most disciplinary actions involve an impaired healthcare professional and are drug or alcohol related (Sullivan & Decker, 2005). All nurse case managers should know their own organizations' reporting policies.

Clinical competence includes the following elements:

- *Educational competence:* including training, license, certification, and education.
- *Knowledge:* understanding organizational policies and procedures. Being familiar with the job description and the organizational chart. Are expectations congruent with standards of practice, with ethical and legal standards, and with your own values?
- *Clinical expertise:* the possession of the knowledge, skills, and abilities necessary to perform a job (Henning & Cohen, 2008). There are different levels of expertise, depending on a person's education and experience, as described in Benner's model (1984), and ranging from novice to expert (Benner, 1984, Henning & Cohen, 2008, Kelly-Heidenthal, 2003; Nicol, Fox-Hiley, Bavin, & Sheng, 1996).

Brokering Referrals, Transfers, and Discharges

Referral

The role of the nurse case manager as a coordinator means that he or she initiates referrals and coordinates services to facilitate the progress of the patient's transition to the next level of care. The goal is to provide a smooth transition from one level of care to the next level and to ensure continuity of care (Daniels & Ramey, 2006). The nurse case manager can be held accountable for errors made during or after the transfer of services to another healthcare provider.

Negligent Referral

The nurse case manager has the obligation to act in the best interest of the patient. To fulfill this obligation, he or she must investigate the competency and qualifications of the facility to which a referral is being made and the credentials of its providers. The nurse case manager should use reasonable care in making the referral. For example, the case manager should examine the current licensure and accreditation of the facility. He or she should closely examine the outcomes of cases similar to the one under consideration for referral. The facility's billing practices, insurance coverage, and records of any previous litigation that the facility might have experienced should be assessed (Mullahy, 2004). The more choices the nurse case manager offers the patient, family, or physician, the less risk there will be of being held liable for the referral.

Change of Provider/Transfers

The following recommendations apply when care of a patient is being transferred to another provider:

- Be sure to have a physician's order and the client's agreement prior to transferring a patient or changing providers.
- Follow up on referrals to evaluate the quality of care.
- Keep the payer informed about referrals.

Also, the nurse case manager must follow up after a patient is referred to another healthcare provider. The nurse case manager may be accused of neglect if he or she fails to evaluate, observe, monitor, and communicate with the family and with the new provider to whom the patient was transferred to make sure that the patient is receiving the care that he or she needs from a qualified healthcare provider. Table 15-9 offers some recommendations to facilitate discharge planning.

LEGAL ISSUES AND NURSING CASE MANAGEMENT: A REVIEW

It behooves all nurses and case managers to know the legal constraints that guide their practice. Today's healthcare environment is filled with lawyers. As one risk manager said, "Nurses, physicians, and other healthcare professionals are targets for potential lawsuits" (personal communication, risk manager from Wake Forest University/Baptist Medical Center, class lecture, University of North Carolina–Greensboro School of Nursing, NUR 541, 2003). Ethical and legal issues frequently overlap but the law takes precedence over ethical principles. Know your local, state, and federal laws. "I don't know" is no excuse!

Tables 15-10 and 15-11 offer some guidelines for your practice. *Stay safe!*

TABLE 15-9 Recommendations for Discharge Planning

1. Begin early—shortly after the patient's admission.
2. Match the patient's condition to the family's or caregiver's knowledge and skills.
3. Plan for special considerations or equipment.
4. A comprehensive assessment must be done prior to discharge planning.
5. Discharge planning should be a team endeavor, and decision making should include the patient, the family, the physician, and the nurse case manager, as well as other members of the team, especially the social worker.
6. Develop contingency plans for unexpected adverse events.
7. Responsibility and accountability for the discharge plan rest with the nurse case manager and the physician.
8. Communication between all relevant agencies should be ongoing, so that the transfer of information is expedited.
9. The nurse case manager should follow up regarding the patient's progress and the outcomes of the transfer or discharge. A thorough follow-up is essential!
10. The case manager is responsible for the quality of the outcomes regarding referrals, transfers, and discharges.

Source: Tahan, 2007.

TABLE 15-10 Recommendations for Nurse Case Managers to Avoid Liability

1. Work within the guidelines that govern the nurse case manager's practice settings. Examine the laws that govern case management in your state.
2. Develop a risk-management mentality to protect yourself, your company, and your patient.
3. Act according to your best judgment, and keep apprised of changes in the profession and in the healthcare industry.
4. Document all case management activities and decisions. Be sure you have a documented referral that allows you to supervise the care of the patient during the transfer.
5. Get legal advice as necessary. Have a lawyer review all contracts.
6. Purchase professional liability insurance.
7. Apply and obtain certification.

Source: Mullahy, 2004.

■ SUMMARY

In today's society, it behooves the nurse case manager to have a working knowledge of the law; the healthcare agency's policies and procedures; federal and state legislation that governs health care, including old, new, and pending legislation; and the standards of practice for nursing and case management. Nurse case managers are often confronted with difficult choices in clinical, professional, and organizational situations. They are held accountable and

TABLE 15-11 Ten Rules for the Nurse Case Manager

1. Know the law.
2. Document everything.
3. Do not make negative statements about a patient.
4. Question authority.
5. Stay educated.
6. Manage risks.
7. Do not hurry through a discharge—be careful!
8. Be discreet.
9. Use restraints wisely.
10. Be kind: Good rapport between the patient, the family, and the nurse case manager goes a long way toward preventing malpractice suits.

Source: Roussel & Merrill, 2006.

responsible for their actions, both legally and ethically. When nurses become defendants in lawsuits, other nurses will serve as expert witnesses in court; the latter nurses will weigh the nurse case manager's decisions and actions in terms of having made the right decision at the right time according to the standards of care, organizational standards, the law, and ethical principles. Thus nurse case managers must have knowledge of the legal issues that guide practice as well as be familiar with the best available evidence to guide current practice.

■ CASE STUDIES

Have you ever been involved in a legal action or threat of one in health care? How was the situation handled? What was the outcome? Discuss your experience with your peers.

■ DISCUSSION QUESTIONS

1. Why do case managers need to understand how legal liability relates to both clinical practice activities and their responsibilities for delegation and supervision?
2. What are the grounds on which case managers can be found legally liable for injuries to patients?
3. Which actions can the case manager take to protect against malpractice suits?

■ CLASSROOM EXERCISES

Interview a risk manager at a local healthcare organization, a legal nurse consultant, or someone who has served as an expert witness. What is their specific skill set?

■ RECOMMENDED READINGS

Alliota, S. L. (2005). Key functions and direct outcomes of case management. In E. L. Cohen & T. G. Cesta (Eds.), *Nursing case management: From essentials to advanced practice application* (4th ed., pp. 415–422). St. Louis, MO: Elsevier/ Mosby.

Bower, K. A. (2005). Case management: Life at the intersection of margin and mission. In E. L. Cohen & T. G. Cesta (Eds.), *Nursing case management: From essentials to advanced practice application* (4th ed., pp. 423–432). St. Louis, MO: Elsevier/Mosby.

Cady, R. F. (2005). Compliance and regulation. In E. L. Cohen & T. G. Cesta (Eds.), *Nursing case management: From essentials to advanced practice applications* (4th ed., pp. 397–411). St. Louis, MO: Elsevier/Mosby.

Moreo, K., & Lamb, G. (2003). CMSA updates standards of practice for case management. *Case Manager, 14*(3), 52–54.

Mullahy, C. M. (Ed.). (2004). The case manager as catalyst, problem solver and educator (pp. 1–25); Legal responsibilities of the case management profession (pp. 77–116); HIPAA (pp. 145–147); glossary (pp. 695–718). In *The case manager's handbook* (3rd ed.). Sudbury MA: Jones and Bartlett.

Skiba, D. J., Sorenson, L., McCarthy, M. B., & Brownrigg, V. J. (2005). Telehealth application to case management. In E. L. Cohen & T. G. Cesta (Eds.), *Nursing case management: From essentials to advanced practice application* (4th ed., pp. 384–396). St. Louis, MO: Elsevier/Mosby.

Tahan, H. A. (2005). The role of the nurse case manager. In E. L. Cohen & T. G. Cesta (Eds.), *Nursing case management: From essentials to advanced practice application* (4th ed., pp. 277–295). St. Louis, MO: Elsevier/Mosby.

Tahan, H. A. (2007). One patient, numerous healthcare providers and multiple care settings: Addressing the concerns of care transitions through case management. *Professional Case Manager, 12*(1), 37–46.

■ REFERENCES

Aiken, T. D. (Ed.). (2004), Nursing and the law. In *Legal, ethical and political issues in nursing* (2nd ed., pp. 35–81). Philadelphia: F. A. Davis.

Alliota, S. L. (2005). Key functions and direct outcomes of case management. In E. L. Cohen & T. G. Cesta (Eds.), *Nursing case management: From essentials to advanced practice application* (4th ed., pp. 415–422). St. Louis, MO: Elsevier/Mosby.

Anthony, M. K (2006). Professional practice and career development. In D. L. Huber (Ed.), *Leadership and nursing care management* (3rd ed., pp. 61–78). Philadelphia: Saunders/Elsevier.

Benner, P. (1984). *From novice to expert: Excellence and power in clinical nursing practice.* Menlo Park, CA: Addison-Wesley.

Bower, K. A. (2005). Case management: Life at the intersection of margin and mission. In E. L. Cohen & T. G. Cesta (Eds.), *Nursing case management: From essentials to advanced practice application* (4th ed., pp. 423–432). St. Louis, MO: Elsevier/Mosby.

Cady, R. F. (2005). Compliance and regulation. In E. L. Cohen & T. G. Cesta (Eds.), *Nursing case management: From essentials to advanced practice applications* (4th ed., pp. 397–411). St. Louis, MO: Elsevier/Mosby.

Cooper, R. W. (2006). Legal and ethical issues. In D. L. Huber (Ed.), *Leadership and nursing care management* (3rd ed., pp. 733–754). Philadelphia: Saunders/Elsevier.

Cyphert, S. T. (2006). The health care system. In D. L. Huber (Ed.), *Leadership and nursing care management* (3rd ed., pp. 198–199). Philadelphia: Saunders/Elsevier.

Daniels, S., & Ramey, M. (2006). Clinical management initiatives [Crossing the continuum]. In S. Daniels & M. Ramey (Eds.), *The leader's guide to hospital case management* (pp. 195–205). Sudbury, MA: Jones and Bartlett.

Fattorusso, D., & Quinn, C. E. (2007). *A case manager's study guide: Preparing for certification* (3rd ed.). Sudbury, MA: Jones and Bartlett.

Finkelman, A. W. (2006). Health care policy, legal issues and ethics in health care delivery. In A. W. Finkelman, *Leadership and management in nursing care: A nursing perspective* (pp. 276–313). Upper Saddle River, NJ: Prentice Hall.

Harris, D. M. (2003). *Contemporary issues in health care, law and ethics.* Chicago: American College of Healthcare Executives, Health Administration Press.

Hendricks, A. G. (2003). How prepared are you? Ethical and legal challenges facing case managers today. *Case Manager, 14*(3), 56–61.

Henning S. E., & Cohen, E. L. (2008). The competency continuum: Expanding the case manager's skill sets and capabilities. *Professional Case Management, 13*(3), 127–148.

Hogan, M. A., & Nickitas, D. M. (Eds.). (2009). Safety first: Legal rights and responsibilities. In *Nursing leadership and management.* Upper Saddle River, NJ: Pearson/Prentice Hall.

Jones, K. R. (2006). Health policy, health and nursing. In D. L. Huber (Ed.), *Leadership and nursing care management* (3rd ed., pp. 109–130). Philadelphia: Saunders/Elsevier.

Kelly-Heidenthal, P. (2003). First-line patient case management. *Nursing leadership and management*. Retrieved from http://www.delmarlearning.com/companions/content/0766825086/ppt/Chapter%2014.ppt

Moreo, K., & Lamb, G. (2003). CMSA updates standards of practice for case management. *Case Manager, 14*(3), 52–54.

Mullahy, C. M. (Ed.). (2004). The case manager as catalyst, problem solver and educator (pp. 1–25); Legal responsibilities of the case management profession (pp. 77–116); HIPAA (pp. 145–147); glossary (pp. 695–718). In *The case manager's handbook* (3rd ed.). Sudbury, MA: Jones and Bartlett.

Nicol, M. J., Fox-Hiley, A., Bavin, C. J., & Sheng, R. (1996). Assessment of clinical and communication skills: Operationalizing Benner's model. *Nurse Education Today, 16*(3), 175–179.

Rossi, P. A. (Ed.). (2003). Protecting oneself from malpractice. In *Case management in health care* (2nd ed., pp. 291–319). Philadelphia: Saunders.

Roussel, L., & Merrill, M. E. (2006). Health policy, legal and regulatory issues. In L. Roussel, R. C. Swansburg, & R. J. Swansburg (Eds.), *Management and leadership for nurse administrators* (4th ed., pp. 366–379). Sudbury, MA: Jones and Bartlett.

Skiba, D. J., Sorenson, L., McCarthy, M. B., & Brownrigg, V. (2005). Telehealth application to case management. In E. L. Cohen & T. G. Cesta (Eds.), *Nursing case management: From essentials to advanced practice application* (4th ed., pp. 384–496). St. Louis, MO: Elsevier/Mosby.

Sullivan, E. J., & Decker, P. J. (Eds.). (2005). Understanding legal and ethical issues. In *Effective leadership and management in nursing* (6th ed., pp. 67–83). Upper Saddle River, NJ: Prentice Hall.

Swansburg, R. C. (2002). Legal principles of nursing. In R. C. Swansburg & R. J. Swansburg (Eds.), *Introduction to management and leadership for nurse managers* (3rd ed., pp. 581–591). Sudbury, MA: Jones and Bartlett.

Tahan, H. A. (2005). The role of the nurse case manager. In E. L. Cohen & T. G. Cesta (Eds.), *Nursing case management: From essentials to advanced practice application* (4th ed., pp. 277–295). St. Louis, MO: Elsevier/Mosby.

Tahan, H. A. (2007). One patient, numerous healthcare providers and multiple care settings: Addressing the concerns of care transitions through case management. *Professional Case Manager, 12*(1), 37–46.

Index